CUTANEOUS

LYMPHOMAS

BASIC AND CLINICAL DERMATOLOGY

Series Editors

ALAN R. SHALITA, M.D.
Distinguished Teaching Professor and Chairman
Department of Dermatology
State University of New York
Health Science Center at Brooklyn
Brooklyn, New York

DAVID A. NORRIS, M.D.
Director of Research
Professor of Dermatology
The University of Colorado
Health Sciences Center
Denver, Colorado

CUTANEOUS LYMPHOMAS

edited by

Günther Burg
University Hospital of Zürich, Switzerland

Werner Kempf
University Hospital of Zürich, Switzerland

Associate Editors

Dmitry V. Kazakov
Medical Faculty Hospital, Pilsen, Czech Republic

Marshall E. Kadin
Beth Israel Deaconess Medical Center,
Harvard Medical School, Massachusetts, U.S.A.

Reinhard Dummer
University Hospital, Zürich, Switzerland

informa
healthcare

New York   London

Simultaneously published in the USA by Informa Healthcare, 52 Vanderbilt Avenue, 7th Floor, New York, NY 10017, USA.

Informa Healthcare is a trading division of Informa UK Ltd. Registered Office: 37–41 Mortimer Street, London W1T 3JH, UK. Registered in England and Wales number 1072954.

©2005 Informa Healthcare, except as otherwise indicated; Reissued in 2010

A CIP record for this book is available from the British Library.

Library of Congress Cataloging-in-Publication Data available on application

ISBN-13: 9780824729974

Orders may be sent to: Informa Healthcare, Sheepen Place, Colchester, Essex CO3 3LP, UK
Telephone: +44 (0)20 7017 5540
Email: CSDhealthcarebooks@informa.com
Website: http://informahealthcarebooks.com/

For corporate sales please contact: CorporateBooksIHC@informa.com
For foreign rights please contact: RightsIHC@informa.com
For reprint permissions please contact: PermissionsIHC@informa.com

Contents

Preface

This book covers the broad spectrum of cutaneous lymphomas, concentrating on definite nosologic entities and presenting new concepts. Various lymphoproliferative disorders with primary or secondary cutaneous involvement are described on the basis of our experience over three decades. Since the classical work found in Alibert's "Description des maladies de la peau, observées à l'hopital Saint Louis et exposition des meilleurs méthodes suivies pour leur traitement" there have been only a few monographs specifically dealing with the topic of cutaneous lymphomas. The goals of this volume are a description of cutaneous lymphomas using widely accepted terminolgy and the new WHO/EORTC classification, and presentation of the unique features of cutaneous lymphomas including their epidemiology, etiological and pathogenetic factors, diagnostic procedures, therapy, and prognosis. This book is addressed to dermatologists, oncologists, pathologists, hematologists, and others in disciplines dealing with hematopoietic disorders.

This book is the result of the cooperation of many people with special expertise in the field of lymphoproliferative disorders of the skin. We thank our associate editors and all the authors. This book is based heavily on our experience with patients followed at the Department of Dermatology of the University Hospital of Zürich. We are grateful to all colleagues who have been involved in the care of these patients. Their contributions range from clinical care to laboratory evaluations to scientific research. The following persons deserve special mention: Mrs. Beatrix Müller, Chief Dermatopathology Technician; Mrs. Margrit Johnson and Mr. Markus Bär, Clinical Photographers. Walter Burgdorf, M.D., was helpful with the language editing. Several funding organizations including the Swiss National Foundation provided substantial financial support for various scientific programs on cutaneous lymphomas and related disorders.

Finally, one of us (GB) wants to express his deep appreciation to his former mentor and teacher, Prof. Dr hc mult Otto Braun-Falco. Almost 20 years ago we wrote a book entitled *Cutaneous Lymphomas, Pseudolymphomas and Related Disorders* (Springer 1983). At that time, immunophenotyping and genotyping were just starting to become important tools in the study of cutaneous lymphomas. The current book highlights the progress in the understanding of cutaneous lymphomas since this classic work was written.

Günter Burg / Werner Kempf

Contributors

Stanislaw Buechner   Department of Dermatology, University of Basel, Basel, Switzerland

Günter Burg   Department of Dermatology, University Hospital, Zürich, Switzerland

Walter Burgdorf   Tutzing, Germany

Antonio Cozzio   Department of Dermatology, University Hospital, Zürich, Switzerland

Udo Döebbeling   Department of Dermatology, University Hospital, Zürich, Switzerland

Reinhard Dummer   Department of Dermatology, University Hospital, Zürich, Switzerland

Michael J. Flaig   Department of Dermatology, LMU, Munich, Germany

Michael Geiges   Department of Dermatology, University Hospital, Zürich, Switzerland

Philippa Golling   Department of Dermatology, University Hospital, Zürich, Switzerland

Monika Hess Schmid   Department of Dermatology, University Hospital, Zürich, Switzerland

Marshall E. Kadin   Beth Israel Deaconess Medical Center, Harvard Medical School, Boston, Massachusetts, U.S.A.

Dmitry V. Kazakov   Department of Dermatology, University Hospital, Zürich, Switzerland

Werner Kempf   Department of Dermatology, University Hospital, Zürich, Switzerland

Sonja Michaelis   Department of Dermatology, University Hospital, Zürich, Switzerland

Beatrix Müller   Department of Dermatology, University Hospital, Zürich, Switzerland

Frank O. Nestle   Department of Dermatology, University Hospital, Zürich, Switzerland

Christian A. Sander   Department of Dermatology, St. Georg Hospital, Hamburg, Germany

Roman Specker   Rehetobelstrasse, St. Gallen, Switzerland

Daniel W.P. Su   Department of Dermatology, Mayo Clinic, Rochester, Minnesota, U.S.A.

Abbreviations

CBCL	Cutaneous B-cell lymphoma
CL	Cutaneous lymphoma
CTCL	Cutaneous T-cell lymphoma
DLBCL	Diffuse large B-cell lymphoma
EORTC	European Organization for Research and Treatment of Cancer
FCC	Follicle center cell
FCL	Follicle center lymphoma
MF	Mycosis fungoides
NK	Natural killer cells
SS	Sézary syndrome
TCR	T-cell receptor
WHO	World Health Organization

1

Cutaneous Lymphomas—Historical Aspects

Michael Geiges, Werner Kempf, and Günter Burg
Department of Dermatology, University Hospital, Zürich, Switzerland

Roman Specker
Rehetobelstrasse, St. Gallen, Switzerland

The first detailed medical descriptions of skin diseases can be found in the medical literature at the end of the 18th century, when scientists started to use the concept of the skin as an organ. Before that time, it made no sense to describe details of skin changes as we do today, since they were thought to be only signs of an uneven distribution of internal body fluids. These disturbances could much better be diagnosed by examination of urine.

Giovanni Battista Morgagni (1682–1771) postulated the importance of tissue and organs. One of the first books of skin diseases regarding the skin as an organ was written by Anne Charles Lorry (1726–1783) in 1776. He also described tumors ["Fleischgewächse (Sarcome)"] that develop in the skin, grow, multiply, and fester. It is not possible to make a clear retrospective diagnosis of these lesions.

In 1806, Alibert (1768–1837) presented an extraordinary skin disease which he described in detail under the name of "Pian fungoides" in 1814 and as "Mycosis fungoides" in 1832 in his second volume of "Monographie des Dermatoses." He called this "a strange disorder of the skin with mushroom-like tumors" (1,2). The case he observed was a patient named Lucas. The disease began with a desquamating rash ("éruption furfuracée"). Lucas died 5 years later of illness with numerous tumors on his face and body.

With the clinical symptoms Alibert described and looking at the figure published in 1832 (Fig. 1), we would still diagnose the disease as mycosis fungoides.

In the atlas mentioned above, there is also the famous illustration of the "Arbre des Dermatoses" showing the classification of skin diseases Alibert created (Fig. 2). In this tree, we can find mycosis fungoides in the branch of the venerous diseases, as in the opinion of Alibert, it was a European form of the tropical disease "smallpox of Amboyna" or "pian ruboide" or yaws (Fig. 3).

The tropical disease "smallpox of Amboyna" had been described by Bontius (1592–1631) (3) (Fig. 4). Bontius identified the difference between this disease and

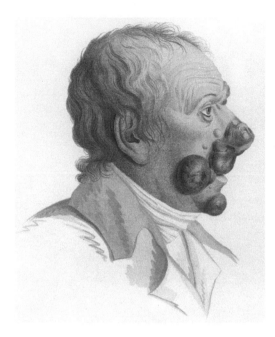

Figure 1   Patient "Lucas" (Monographie des Dermatoses, Alibert, 1832).

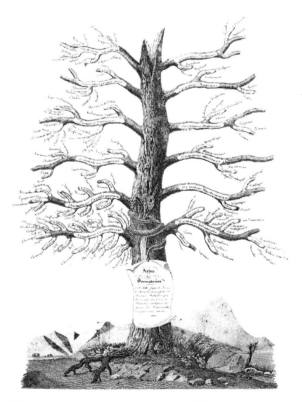

Figure 2   Arbre des dermatoses (Alibert, 1832).

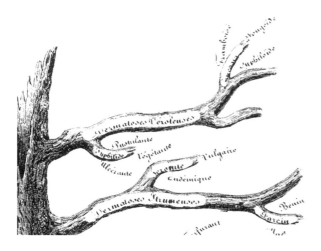

Figure 3 Details of Fig. 2 (branch of the veneral diseases).

syphilis (e.g., that it is not transmitted by sexual intercourse). After the death of Bontius, his notes had been published in 1658 by Gulielmo Piso in six books of his work "de Indiae utriusque re naturali et medica" (Fig. 5). It is worth noting that Alibert in 1832 copied part of the text from Bontius word by word.

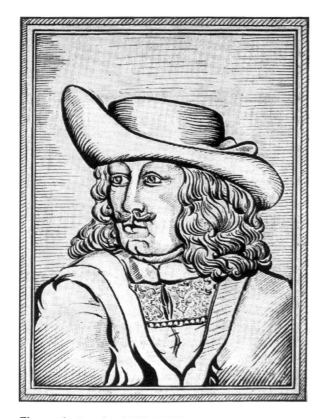

Figure 4 Bontius (1592–1631).

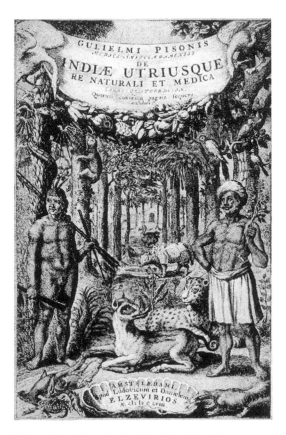

Figure 5 After the death of Bontius, his notes were published in 1658 by Gulielmo Piso in six books entitled "de Indiae utriusque re naturali et medica."

Although he gave the disease the name, it would be a mistake to say that Alibert was the first to describe a lymphoma of the skin, for at this time the etiology of the disease was completely unclear, neither were the characteristics of cancer defined nor was there a theory of cells as components of the body structure. White blood cells had not yet been discovered. Still believing that the atmosphere played an important role in the genesis of most diseases, Alibert was astonished that his patient in Paris got the disease in a climate that was much milder than that of Indonesia.

In the following decades, Alibert's description of mycosis fungoides has been discussed by many different authors and has often been compared with or used as a synonym for "Molluscum of Bateman," a disease Thomas Bateman (1778–1821) published which we can today diagnose as neurofibromatosis.

Another step towards the establishment of lymphomas of the skin was taken when it was recognized that the tumors represented an alteration of lymphocytes. The development of new staining techniques with some highly specialized stains made it possible to categorize the lymphomas. During the second half of the 19th century, the main emphasis was on observing skin biopsies and interpreting skin changes with the knowledge gained from histological changes.

In 1864, Heinrich Köbner (1838–1904) published the first histological description of a lymphoma of the skin and called it "beerenschwammähnliches Papillargeschwulst der Haut" (sponge-like papillary tumor of the skin). Along with many contemporaries, he assigned them to the "Granulationsgeschwülste" which develop as a response to some unknown agent. In 1845, Rudolf Virchow (1821–1902), one of the most famous advocates of the cell theory, created the term "lymphoma" for a group of tumors with structures similar to the lymphatic tissue, such as the intestinal follicles. Lymphoma was used to describe a tumor of lymphatic cells without differentiating between malignant proliferations and inflammatory hyperplasia. In his lectures, Virchow mentions the work of Köbner but still felt that mycosis fungoides was not a lymphoid disease but rather similar to yaws.

The first connections of mycosis fungoides with the lymphoid system were made in 1869. The microscopic studies of Xavier Gillot and Louis Antoine Ranvier (1835–1922) in Paris indicated that mycosis fungoides was caused by regeneration of lymphoid tissue in the skin. They considered mycosis fungoides as a cutaneous manifestation of lymphoma—called lymphadénie cutanée (4). It was Gillot who in his thesis was the first to describe different clinical stages of mycosis fungoides. He assigned the symptoms to four stages:

> Taches congestives (erythematous stage: itching and red colored patches)
> Plaques lichénoides (lichenoid stage: itching and different plaques with small papules)
> Tumeurs fongoïdes (fungal stage: mushroom-like tumors of different size)
> Ulcérations et cicatrices (the tumors are breaking up)

Ernest Bazin (1807–1878) published his three different stages one year later than Gillot. Nevertheless, he is today regarded as the original describer of the clinical stages of mycosis fungoides (5):

> Période érythémateuse (erythematous stage: red colored patches)
> Période lichénoide (the lichenoid stage: itching and different plaques with small papules)
> Période fongoïdique, mycositique (fungal stage: mushroom-like tumors of different size)

A second type of mycosis fungoides was found in 1885 by Emile Vidal (1825–1893) and Jean-Louis Brocq (1856–1928). They published a review of six cases as "Etude sur le mycosis fungoides." Their cases III, V, and VI corresponded to the stages of Bazin. But cases I, II, and VI were missing the typical initial stages. The disease started directly with tumors and its course was rapid and fatal. This type was called mycosis fungoides d'emblée.

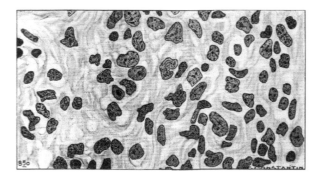

Figure 6 Histological drawing of atypical lymphocytes (Sézary, 1949).

In 1892, Frangois Hensi Hallopeau (1842–1919) and Ernest Besnier (1831–1909) wrote about a third variant of mycosis fungoides: the erythroderma type (6). All of the six cases they had observed began with a reddish rash over the entire body. They denied a connection to leukemia. It was Albert Franz Sézary (1880–1956) who at a meeting of the French Society of Dermatology and Syphiligraphy in February 1938 presented a patient with an erythroderma "avec présence de cellules monstrueuses dans le derme et le sang circulant" (with monstrous cells in the skin and circulating blood) as a leukemic variant of a reticulosis (cancer of lymphatic cells) of the skin—this disease nowadays still bears his name as an eponym (7) (Fig. 6).

The development of electron microscopy finally made it possible for Lutzner to describe the cells in Sézary syndrome with their cerebriform nuclei in detail. They are known today as "Lutzner cells" (8). In the following years, many research groups used electron microscopy, cytophotometry, and cytogenetics to search for connections of the different clinical aspects and diseases such as Sézary syndrome and mycosis fungoides. In 1975, Lutzner and others confirmed that they could be classified as entities in the spectrum of cutaneous T-cell lymphomas (9).

REFERENCES

1. Alibert JL. Description des Maladies de la Peau Observées à l'Hôpital St. Louis, Paris, Barrois, 1806.
2. Alibert JL. "Description des maladies de la peau" tome second, Paris, 1814.
3. Bontius J. De medicina Indorum libri IV, Piso, 1642.
4. Gillot X. "Thèse pour le doctorat en médecine: étude sur une affection de la peau décrite sous le nom de Mycosis fongoïde", Paris, 1869.
5. Bazin E. Leçons sur le traitement des maladies chroniques en général affections de la peau, Paris, 1870.
6. Besnier E, Hallopeau F. Sur les érythrodermies du mycosis fungoide. Ann Dermatol Syphiligr (Paris) 1892; III:987.
7. Sézary A, Bouvrain Y. Erythrodermie avec presence de cellules monstreuses dans derme et dans sang circulant. Bull soc Fr Dermatol Syphiligr 1938; 45:254–260.
8. Lutzner MA, Jordan HW. Ultrastructure of an abnormal cell in Sézary's syndrome. Blood 1968; 31:719–726.
9. Lutzner MA. NIH Conference: cutaneous T-cell lymphomas: the Sézary syndrome, 4mycosis fungoides, and related disorders. Ann Intern Med 1975; 83:534–552.

2

Unique Features of Cutaneous Lymphomas

Günter Burg and Werner Kempf
Department of Dermatology, University Hospital, Zürich, Switzerland

The skin as one of the body's largest organs has many unique clinical, histological, and immunologic features which are reflected in CL. The most frequent type of cutaneous lymphoma is mycosis fungoides (MF), the first detailed description of which was given by Alibert in his atlas published almost 200 years ago. The Italian Bontius had already mentioned almost 200 years earlier, a disfiguring disease in natives of the Malaccan islands (now part of Indonesia). This probably was the first report on what we designate today as MF. Sézary described in 1938 a leukemic and erythrodermic variant of MF, which had already been mentioned by von Zumbusch in 1915.Cutaneous T-cell lymphomas progresses through different stages usually designated as patches, plaques, and tumors. Therefore CTCL serves as a prototype disease to study lymphomagenesis from the very early stages to highly malignant diseases.

B-cell lymphomas also may arise in the skin, but are less frequent than their nodal counterparts. They were previously referred to as "reticuloses" or "reticulo-sarcomas" of the (1,2) before clearly being identified as having a B-cell lineage by the use of immunophenotyping in the 1980s (3). Their clinical, histological, and biological peculiarities provide enough evidence that they in fact represent nosologically distinct group of lymphomas.

Cutaneous lymphomas differ from nodal lymphomas and from other extranodal lymphomas in many respects. There are many physiologic and anatomic factors which help to explain various features of CL: just as in lymph nodes, the skin provides regions to which T cells or B cells, respectively, home preferentially, a variety of functionally different compartments and microenvironments.

Morphologically different patterns of CL can be distinguished. The epidermis, the subepidermal papillary dermis, the periadnexal areas, and the subcutaneous tissue are typical microenvironments for T-cell infiltrates. These areas contain antigen-presenting cells and postcapillary high endothelial venules and correspond to the perifollicular and interfollicular regions in lymph nodes. In contrast, the mid and deep dermis and their perivascular spaces are compartments to which B-lymphocytes home preferentially. In most forms of CL, there is a substantial dendritic cell/macrophage component in close association with the lymphoid component

(4), for example highlighted by networks of CD21-positive follicular dendritic cells in cutaneous B-cell lymphomas.

Phenotypically T-lymphocytes homing into the skin express distinct homing markers, e.g., E-selectin-binding epitopes (5). The cells express the cutaneous lymphocyte antigen (CLA), a tissue-selective homing receptor involved in directing T-cell traffic to inflamed skin which is recognized by mAb HECA-452 (6). They are memory/helper T cells (CD4+, CD45RO+). The skin is nourished by two interconnected vascular systems, the superficial vascular plexus coursing just beneath the epidermis and the deep vascular plexus located above the subcutaneous tissue. There is some evidence that expression of a specific homing receptor is able to direct lymphocyte traffic, not only to a distinct organ but also to a distinct vascular bed within one organ (7). As an example, the deficiency or absence of the adhesion molecule CDIIa/CD18 may contribute to the inability of the tumor cells to extravasate in intravascular malignant lymphoma (8).

Biologically CL differ from their nodal equivalents in several ways: (i) T-cell lymphomas are more common in the skin than B-cell lymphomas. (ii) Even histo- and cytomorphologically similar nodal and cutaneous lymphomas may have markedly different prognoses. Primary cutaneous CD30+ large cell lymphomas have a better prognosis than their nodal counterparts and than other cutaneous large cell lymphomas (9–11). Similarly, follicle center cell derived B-cell lymphomas of the skin or MALT-type lymphomas of the skin also have a much better prognosis than their nodal counterparts (12). (iii) Because of the likelihood of earlier diagnosis and often better prognosis, different *therapeutic strategies* are employed for the treatment of cutaneous lymphomas than for nodal and extranodal lymphomas (13–16). Both topical and systemic approaches are employed; a careful choice must be made depending on clinical stage and the distinct pathologic subtype of CL.

REFERENCES

1. Degos R, Ossipowski B, Cevatte J, Touraine R. Réticuloses cutanées (réticuloses histio-monocytaires). Ann Dermatol Syphiligr 1957; 84:125–152.
2. Gottron HA. Retikulosen der Haut. Stuttgart: Thieme, 1960; 501–590.
3. Burg G, Braun-Falco O. Cutaneous Lymphomas, Pseudolymphomas, and Related Disorders. Berlin: Springer, 1983.
4. Berger CL, Hanlon D, Kanada D, Dhodapkar M, Lombillo V, Wang N, Christensen I, Howe G, Crouch J, El-Fishawy P, Edelson R. The growth of cutaneous T-cell lymphoma is stimulated by immature dendritic cells. Blood 2002; 99:2929–2939.
5. Priest R, Bird MI, Malhotra R. Characterization of E-selectin-binding epitopes expressed by skin-homing T cells. Immunology 1998; 94:523–528.
6. Heald PW, Yan SL, Edelson RL, Tigelaar R, Picker LJ. Skin-selective lymphocyte homing mechanisms in the pathogenesis of leukemic cutaneous T-cell lymphoma. J Invest Dermatol 1993; 101:222–226.
7. Kunstfeld R, Lechleitner S, Groger M, Wolff K, Petzelbauer P. HECA-452+ T cells migrate through superficial vascular plexus but not through deep vascular plexus endothelium. J Invest Dermatol 1997; 108:343–348.
8. Jalkanen S, Aho R, Kallajoki M, Ekfors T, Nortamo P, Gahmberg C, Duijvestijn A, Kalimo H. Lymphocyte homing receptors and adhesion molecules in intravascular malignant lymphomatosis. Int J Cancer 1989; 44:777–782.
9. Kaudewitz P, Stein H, Dallenbach F, Eckert F, Bieber K, Burg G, Braun FO. Primary and secondary cutaneous Ki-1+ (CD30+) anaplastic large cell lymphomas. Morphologic, immunohistologic, and clinical-characteristics. Am J Pathol 1989; 135:359–367.

10. Beljaards RC, Kaudewitz P, Berti E, Gianotti R, Neumann C, Rosso R, Paulli M, Meijer CJ, Willemze R. Primary cutaneous CD30-positive large cell lymphoma: definition of a new type of cutaneous lymphoma with a favorable prognosis. A European Multicenter Study of 47 patients. Cancer 1993; 71:2097–2104.

11. Kaudewitz P, Kind P, Sander CA. CD30+ anaplastic large cell lymphomas. Semin Dermatol 1994; 13:180–186.

12. Pimpinelli N, Santucci M, Bosi A, Moretti S, Vallecchi C, Messori A, Giannotti B. Primary cutaneous follicular centre-cell lymphoma—a lymphoproliferative disease with favourable prognosis. Clin Exp Dermatol 1989; 14:12–19.

13. Nestle FO, Haffner AC, Schmid MH, Dummer R, Burg G. [Current therapy concepts in cutaneous T-cell lymphomas]. Schweiz Med Wochenschr 1997; 127:311–320.

14. Zackheim HS. Treatment of cutaneous T-cell lymphoma. Semin Dermatol 1994; 13: 207–215.

15. Piccinno R, Caccialanza M, Berti E, Baldini L. Radiotherapy of cutaneous B cell lymphomas: our experience in 31 cases. Int J Radiat Oncol Biol Phys 1993; 27:385–389.

16. Demierre MF, Foss FM, Koh HK. Proceedings of the International Consensus Conference on Cutaneous T-cell Lymphoma (CTCL) Treatment Recommendations, Boston, MA, Oct 1–2, 1994. J Am Acad Dermatol 1997; 36:460–466.

3

Cutaneous Lymphoma: A Prototype Neoplasia for Cancer Research

Günter Burg and Werner Kempf
Department of Dermatology, University Hospital, Zürich, Switzerland

Nodal lymphomas may go through a preneoplastic phase, but the initial subtle findings are clinically hidden, whereas in cutaneous lymphomas (CL), the tiniest changes can be seen and monitored clinically or with sequential biopsies during all stages of disease progression. Especially in cutaneous T cell lymphomas, there may be a long preneoplastic phase, which precedes the transition to overt malignant lymphoma. The life expectancy of patients suffering from these preneoplastic conditions is unaffected (1). These preneoplastic conditions are most interesting with respect to questions of the pathogenesis and of the early molecular changes as a normal lymphocyte transforms into a neoplastic cell.

Thus, CL reflect the whole spectrum of pathogenetic events in cancerogenesis. In our concept, the preneoplastic processes depend on a persistent antigenic stimulation and on a specific homing microenvironment. During disease progression and transformation into overt lymphoma, the tumor cells become less dependent on those stromal, cellular, or soluble microenvironmental factors.

REFERENCE

1. Zackheim HS, Amin S, Kashani-Sabet M, McMillan A. Prognosis in cutaneous T-cell lymphoma by skin stage: long-term survival in 489 patients. J Am Acad Dermatol 1999; 40:418–425.

4
Epidemiology

Günter Burg and Werner Kempf
Department of Dermatology, University Hospital, Zürich, Switzerland

The incidence and mortality rate of non-Hodgkin lymphoma (NHL) have increased substantially in many countries over recent decades (1,2). One possible explanation may be the increasing number of immunosuppressed patients who are at higher risk for cancer. Non-Hodgkin lymphoma is a common malignancy in those with HIV infection, in organ transplant recipients, and in primary immune deficiencies. Comparing the patterns of malignancy and immune parameters among these patients and the general population may elucidate the role of host response in controlling oncogenic factors, particularly viral infections (3). The percentage of extranodal NHL is between 25% and 35% in most countries, with the skin and the gastrointestinal tract being the most common extra-nodal sites (4).

CUTANEOUS LYMPHOMAS

The overall frequency of cutaneous lymphomas (CL) is about 0.3/100,000 inhabitants per year (5,6). Sixty-five percent of CL are T-cell types, 25% B-cell types, and the rest comprises rare or undefined types of lymphoproliferative skin infiltrates (7,8). Incidence rates of CL in different geographic regions at different periods as reported in the literature are given in Table 1. Differences in both classification and diagnostic criteria over time make comparison difficult (9).

CUTANEOUS T-CELL LYMPHOMAS

The most common cutaneous T-cell lymphomas (CTCL) is mycosis fungoides (MF). Most studies on epidemiology of CL refer to MF and most have been hampered by methodological issues (37). The increase in frequency of this subtype of CL is probably due to overdiagnosing MF by including non-MF CTCL and other conditions such as parapsoriasis into this group. Weinstock and others have reviewed the epidemiology of MF (17,37,38). The *incidence* from 1973 through 1992 in the United States was 0.36/100,000 persons per year. The age-adjusted incidence rate ratio of blacks to whites was 1.7 and that of Asians to whites was 0.6. There was no evidence of increasing incidence rates during the period 1983 through 1992 and stabilizing

Table 1 Summary of the Literature About the Incidence of Cutaneous Lymphomas

Author group (Ref.)	Geographic region	Classification used	Time span	Incidence per 100,000 per year	Clinical epidemio-logic	Population-based
Brennan and Coates (10)	New South Wales, Australia	ICD-9	72–95			×
Weinstock and Gardstein (11)	USA	ICD-9	73–92	MF-incidence: 1973–1974 = 0.18 1991–1992 = 0.45 1973–1984: All races = 0.29 Male = 0.41 Female = 0.19		×
Sukpanichnant and Sonakul (12)	Thailand	Working formulation/Rye	57–71		×	
Weinstock and Reynes (13)	USA	ICD-9	73–94			×
Dobson and Hancock (14)	UK	BNLI	70–95		×	
Ortega and Verastegui (15)	Mexico	Working formulation	90–92		×	
Iscovich et al. (16)	Israel	Working formulation	85–93	All cutaneous lymphomas Male = 1.18 Female = 0.63 MF: Male = 0.77 Female = 0.35		×
Newton et al. (4)	USA/Asia/Europe	ICD-9/ICD-0	?	All cutaneous lymphomas Puerto Rico (1978–1987) = 0.10		×

Reference	Location	Classification	Period	Notes		
Koh et al. (17)	USA	?	73–84	Thailand (1988–1989) = 0.02; Spain (1986–1987) = 0.01; England (1983–1987) = 0.18	×	×
Maksymiuk and Bratvold (18)	Saskatchewan	IWF	66–75		×	×
Devesa and Fears (19)	USA	ICD	69–88	SEER-data, see also (20)	×	
Bunker et al. (21)	Colorado	?	74–91		×	×
Hjelle et al. (22)	New Mexico	?	88–89		×	×
Weinstock (23)	USA	ICD-9/10	73–86		×	
Chuang et al. (24)	USA	?	70–84		×	×
Campbell et al. (25)	Nigeria	?	68–89		×	×
Liang et al. (26)	Hong Kong	IWF	75–89			×
Whittemore et al. (27)	USA	?	81–86		×	×
Linet et al. (28)	Sweden	?	61–79			×
Cartwright et al. (29)	Yorkshire	BNLI	79–84		×	
Alberts and Lanier (30)	Alaska	IWF	69–83		×	
Maeda and Jubashi (31)	Nagasaki	IWF	73–77		×	
Biggar and Horm (32)	USA and Puerto Rico	ICD-0	73–81	SEER-data, see also (20)	×	
McFadden and Nyfors (33)	Norway	?	60–80		×	
Dougan and Matthews (34)	Western Australia	ICD-9	60–69	MF-Incidence: 1960–1969 Male = 0.3 Female = 0.1	×	
Greene and Dalager (35)	USA	IWF	50–75		×	×
Tulinius (36)	Various	ICD-9			×	×

?, Classification scheme not indicated in the cited article.

thereafter. The age-adjusted incidence rates per 100,000 in a study from Israel were 1.18 and 0.63 for Jewish men and women, respectively (16). In a study from Switzerland looking at a total number of 426 lymphoproliferative skin infiltrates (9), CTCL were fond at a frequency of 1.0/100,000 per year (55% male and 45% female). This is much higher than the figures reported for the United States.

Among 650 North American cases followed with known dates of diagnosis and no history of prior malignancy, the median *survival time* was 7.8 years. Advanced age, black race, prior malignancy, and Sézary syndrome present at the time of diagnosis were each independently associated with poor prognosis (6). Mortality rates declined steadily from 1979 to 1991 (11). The Surveillance, Epidemiology, and End Results Program (SEER) of the National Cancer Institute includes nine population-based cancer registries, covering approximately 10% of the US population. Data were drawn from this base on the survival of all MF patients who were registered during the years 1973–1992. There was a total of over 10,000 person-years of follow-up for the 1633 patients studied. Relative survival changed little after 11 years, at which point it was 66% (20).

Genetic factors do not appear to be crucial in the early stages of CTCL. The rate of chromosomal aberrations, especially of chromosomes 1, 6, and 11, increase with the activity of the disease and has prognostic significance in patients with CTCL. Aberrations of chromosomes 8 and 17 are especially associated with active or progressive disease (39). Familial MF rarely has been reported (40,41).

EPIDEMIOLOGIC FACTORS INFLUENCING INCIDENCE AND MORTALITY RATES

Sex

Several surveys have revealed a predominance among males (38,42).

Age

Advanced age seems to be an adverse prognostic factor.

Race and Geographic Factors

Black race is associated with poorer survival (42). The prognosis of Asian and Hispanic patients were slightly but not significantly worse than those of whites, and there were no significant geographic differences related to prognosis. A survey on the incidence rate of CL (including MF and non-MF) in Israel showed that rates of CL were significantly lower in non-Jews (16). There is also a substantial geographic variation, showing high numbers of retrovirus-induced adult T-cell lymphoma/leukemia (ATL) in Japan and Caribbean (43).

Ultraviolet Radiation

The incidence of NHL is known to increase markedly following immune suppression. Exposure to ultraviolet radiation (UVR) may cause systemic immune suppression. Part of the recent increase in NHL incidence may be due to increased UVR exposure (1). The concept that sunlight exposure has contributed to the rising rates of NHL is not unequivocally supported (44). Moreover, this explanation is hard to accept for CTCL, since UVR is an efficient mode of treatment (45–47). Furthermore, there are clear indications of a considerable decrease in the death rate in MF following PUVA treatment (46).

Occupational Exposure

The influence of occupational exposures was suggested by the excessive MF mortality rates in countries where petroleum, rubber, primary and fabricated metal, machinery, and printing industries were located (42,48). In a more recent study, employment in a manufacturing occupation (especially petrochemical, textile, metal, and machinery industries) was shown to be a risk factor (38). Workers employed in the petroleum industry have limited evidence for excess leukemia and other lymphatic and hematopoietic neoplasms, and skin cancer (particularly malignant melanoma) (49). Furthermore, studies on exposure to benzene in a multinational cohort of more than 308,000 petroleum workers followed from 1937 to 1996 indicated that these workers were not at an increased risk of NHL (50).

Epidemiological studies assessing an association between hair dyes and the risk of cutaneous NHL in humans did not reveal a direct relationship (51).

Malignant lymphoma and multiple myeloma in New Zealand have been found to be linked with agricultural occupations (2). In a study performed in Sweden from 1961 to 1979, the risks of one or more types of lymphoproliferative malignancies (including MF) were significantly increased among women working in the agriculture and textile industries, housekeepers, and post office employees. Limitations of these linked-registry data include lack of detailed information on specific exposures and duration of employment, and the relatively small sizes of specific occupational cohorts (28).

In summary, so far no definite association between specific antigen exposures and MF has been established.

Other Risk Factors

An analysis of cases from US mortality statistics indicated that the cases of cutaneous T-cell lymphoma seemed to have a high frequency of antecedent allergies, fungal and viral skin infections, sun sensitivity, familial aggregation of lymphoma, and leukemia (38). An increased incidence of NHL was found in patients with a history of antecedent skin diseases (29). Patients with lymphomatoid papulosis have a significantly increased frequency of prior or coexisting lymphoproliferative disorders, an increased frequency of non-lymphoid malignant lesions, and exposure to radiation therapy (52).

CUTANEOUS B-CELL LYMPHOMAS (CBCL)

There are almost no data on the incidence of CBCL. In the same Swiss study (9), CBCL had an incidence of 0.35/100,000 per year (59% male and 41% female). The average ages were 50 and 62 years in male and female patients, respectively. CBCL seem to be more frequent in Europe than in other parts of the world.

REFERENCES

1. McMichael AJ, Giles GG. Have increases in solar ultraviolet exposure contributed to the rise in incidence of non-Hodgkin's lymphoma? Br J Cancer 1996; 73:945–950.

2. Pearce N, Porta M. Association of non-Hodgkin's lymphoma with rheumatoid arthritis [letter]. Am J Med 1986; 81:747–748.
3. Mueller N. Overview of the epidemiology of malignancy in immune deficiency. J Acquir Immune Defic Syndr 1999; 21(suppl 1):S5–S10.
4. Newton R, Ferlay J, Beral V, Devesa SS. The epidemiology of non-Hodgkin's lymphoma: comparison of nodal and extra-nodal sites. Int J Cancer 1997; 72:923–930.
5. Weinstock MA, Horm JW. Mycosis fungoides in the United States: increasing incidence and descriptive epidemiology. JAMA 1988; 260:42–46.
6. Weinstock MA, Horm JW. Population-based estimate of survival and determinants of prognosis in patients with mycosis fungoides. Cancer 1988; 62:1658–1661.
7. Burg G, Kerl H, Przybilla B, Braun-Falco O. Some statistical data, diagnosis, and staging of cutaneous B-cell lymphomas. J Dermatol Surg Oncol 1984; 10:256–262.
8. Burg G, Dummer R, Kerl H. Classification of cutaneous lymphomas. Derm Clinics 1994; 12:213–217.
9. Roth G. Kutane lymphome-eine klinisch epidemiologische analyse anhand des patient-engutes der dermatologischen klinik des USZ in den Jahren 1982–1999. Doctoral thesis, University Zürich, 2001.
10. Brennan P, Coates M. Second primary neoplasms following non-Hodgkin's lymphoma in New South Wales, Australia. Br J Cancer 2000; 82:1344–1347.
11. Weinstock MA, Gardstein B. Twenty-year trends in the reported incidence of mycosis fungoides and associated mortality. Am J Public Health 1999; 89:1240–1244.
12. Sukpanichnant S, Sonakul D. Malignant lymphoma in Thailand: changes in the frequency of malignant lymphoma determined from a histopathologic and immuno-phenotypic analysis of 425 cases at Siriraj Hospital. Cancer 1998; 83:1197–1204.
13. Weinstock MA, Reynes JF. Validation of cause-of-death certification for outpatient cancers: the contrasting cases of melanoma and mycosis fungoides. Am J Epidemiol 1998; 148:1184–1186.
14. Dobson LS, Hancock H. Localised non-Hodgkin's lymphoma: the Sheffield Lymphoma Group experience (1970–1995). Int J Oncol 1998; 13:1313–1318.
15. Ortega V, Verastegui E. Non-Hodgkin's lymphomas in Mexico. A clinicopathological and molecular analysis. Leuk Lymphoma 1998; 31:575–582.
16. Iscovich J, Paltiel O, Azizi E, Kuten A, Gat A, Lifzchitz-Mercer B, Zlotogorski A, Polliack A. Cutaneous lymphoma in Israel, 1985–1993: a population-based incidence study. Br J Cancer 1998; 77:170–173.
17. Koh HK, Charif M, Weinstock MA. Epidemiology and clinical manifestations of cutaneous T-cell lymphoma. Hematol Oncol Clin North Am 1995; 9:943–960.
18. Maksymiuk AW, Bratvold JS. Non-Hodgkin's lymphoma in Saskatchewan. A review of 10 years' experience. Cancer 1994; 73:711–719.
19. Devesa SS, Fears T. Non-Hodgkin's lymphoma time trends. Cancer Res 1992; 52: 5432s–5440s.
20. Weinstock MA, Reynes JF. The changing survival of patients with mycosis fungoides: a population-based assessment of trends in the United States. Cancer 1999; 85:208–212.
21. Bunker JD, Freeman JH, Jester JD, Golitz LE. Cutaneous T-cell lymphoma in Colorado 1974–1991. J Dermatol 1991; 18:369–376.
22. Hjelle B, Mills R, Swenson S, Mertz G, Key C, Allen S. Incidence of hairy cell leukemia, mycosis fungoides, and chronic lymphocytic leukemia in first known HTLV-II-endemic population. J Infect Dis 1991; 163:435–440.
23. Weinstock MA. A registry-based case-control study of mycosis fungoides. Ann Epidemiol 1991; 1:533–539.
24. Chuang TY, Su WP, Muller SA. Incidence of cutaneous T cell lymphoma and other rare skin cancers in a defined population. J Am Acad Dermatol 1990; 23:254–256.
25. Campbell OB, George AO, Shokunbi WA, Akang EE, Aghadiuno PU. Problems in the management of mycosis fungoides in Nigeria. Trop Geogr Med 1991; 43:317–322.

26. Liang R, Chiu E, Loke SL, Chan TK, Todd D, Ho F. Primary and secondary cutaneous lymphomas in Hong Kong Chinese. Hematol Oncol 1990; 8:333–338.

27. Whittemore AS, Holly EA, Lee IM, Abel EA, Adams RM, Nickoloff BJ, Bley L, Peters JM, Gibney C. Mycosis fungoides in relation to environmental exposures and immune response: a case-control study. J Natl Cancer Inst 1989; 81:1560–1567.

28. Linet MS, McLaughlin JK, Malker HS, Chow WH, Weiner JA, Stone BJ, Ericsson JL, Fraumeni JJ. Occupation and hematopoietic and lymphoproliferative malignancies among women: a linked registry study. J Occup Med 1994; 36:1187–1198.

29. Cartwright RA, McKinney PA, O'Brien C, Richards ID, Roberts B, Lauder I, Darwin CM, Bernard SM, Bird CC. Non-Hodgkin's lymphoma: case control epidemiological study in Yorkshire. Leuk Res 1988; 12:81–88.

30. Alberts SR, Lanier AP. Leukemia, lymphoma, and multiple myeloma in Alaskan natives. J Natl Cancer Inst 1987; 78:831–837.

31. Maeda H, Jubashi T. Epidemiological studies on malignant lymphoma in Nagasaki City, especially in relation to atomic bomb exposure. Gan No Rinsho 1987; 33:807–814.

32. Biggar RJ, Horm J. Incidence of Kaposi's sarcoma and mycosis fungoides in the United States including Puerto Rico, 1973–81. J Natl Cancer Inst 1984; 73:89–94.

33. McFadden N, Nyfors A. Mycosis fungoides in Norway 1960–80. A retrospective study. Acta Derm Venereol Suppl (Stockh) 1983; 109:1–13.

34. Dougan LE, Matthews ML. The effect of diagnostic review on the estimated incidence of lymphatic and hematopoietic neoplasms in Western Australia. Cancer 1981; 48:866–872.

35. Greene MH, Dalager NA. Mycosis fungoides: epidemiologic observations. Cancer Treat Rep 1979; 63:597–606.

36. Tulinius H. Epidemiology of non-Hodgkin's lymphoma. Strahlentheapie 1977; 153: 209–217.

37. Weinstock MA. Epidemiology of mycosis fungoides. Semin Dermatol 1994; 13:154–159.

38. Morales Suarez-Varela MM, Llopis Gonzalez A, Marquina Vila A, Bell J. Mycosis fungoides: review of epidemiological observations. Dermatology 2000; 201:21–28.

39. Karenko L, Sarna S, Kahkonen M, Ranki A. Chromosomal abnormalities in relation to clinical disease in patients with cutaneous T-cell lymphoma: a 5-year follow-up study. Br J Dermatol 2003; 148:55–64.

40. Shelley WB. Familial mycosis fungoides revisited. Arch Dermatol 1980; 116:1177–1178.

41. Baykal C, Buyukbabani N, Kaymaz R. Familial mycosis fungoides. Br J Dermatol 2002; 146:1108–1110.

42. Greene MH, Dalager NA, Lamberg SI, Argyropoulos CE, Fraumeni JF. Mycosis fungoides: epidemiologic observations. Cancer Treat Rep 1979; 63:597–606.

43. Takenaka T, Nakamine H, Oshiro I, Maeda J, Kobori M, Hayashi T, Komoda H, Hinuma Y, Hanaoka M. Serologic and epidemiologic studies on adult T-cell leukemia (ATL): special reference to a comparison between patients with and without antibody to ATL-associated antigen. Jpn J Clin Oncol 1983; 13:257–267.

44. Freedman DM, Zahm SH, Dosemeci M. Residential and occupational exposure to sunlight and mortality from non-Hodgkin's lymphoma: composite (threefold) case-control study [see comments]. Br Med J 1997; 314:1451–1455.

45. Herrmann JJ, Roenigk HJ, Hurria A, Kuzel TM, Samuelson E, Rademaker AW, Rosen ST. Treatment of mycosis fungoides with photochemotherapy (PUVA): long-term follow-up. J Am Acad Dermatol 1995; 33:234–242.

46. Swanbeck G, Roupe G, Sandstrom MH. Indications of a considerable decrease in the death rate in mycosis fungoides by PUVA treatment. Acta Derm Venereol 1994; 74:465–466.

47. Dimitrov B. Malignant melanoma of the skin and non-Hodgkin's lymphoma in USA: a comparative epidemiological study. Folia Med 1999; 41:121–125.

48. Greene MH, Pinto HA. Lymphomas and leukemias in the relatives of patients with mycosis fungoides. Cancer 1982; 49:737–741.

49. Ward EM, Burnett CA, Ruder A, Davis-King K. Industries and cancer. Cancer Causes Control 1997; 8:356–370.
50. Wong O, Raabe GK. A critical review of cancer epidemiology in the petroleum industry, with a meta-analysis of a combined database of more than 350,000 workers. Regul Toxicol Pharmacol 2000; 32:78–98.
51. La Vecchia C, Tavani A. Epidemiological evidence on hair dyes and the risk of cancer in humans. Eur J Cancer Prev 1995; 4:31–43.
52. Wang HH, Lach L, Kadin ME. Epidemiology of lymphomatoid papulosis [see comments]. Cancer 1992; 70:2951–2957.

5

The Lymphoid System

Marshall E. Kadin

Beth Israel Deaconess Medical Center, Harvard Medical School, Boston, Massachusetts, U.S.A.

The lymphoid system is comprised of B and T lymphocytes and dendritic antigen presenting cells. These cells have their origin in the bone marrow and undergo morphologic and functional maturation in peripheral lymphoid organs, including the thymus, lymph nodes, and spleen. Here circulating lymphocytes come into contact with antigen presenting cells which prime them for functional activity.

B lymphocytes originate in the bone marrow and mature within follicles located in the cortical region of the lymph nodes and spleen. Within the follicles, B lymphocytes come into intimate contact with antigen presenting follicular dendritic cells (CD21+) and helper T lymphocytes (CD3+ and CD4+). Plasma cells are mature antibody producing B cells which are concentrated in the medullary cords of the lymph node.

The thymus is the principal organ responsible for maturation of T lymphocytes. Immature T lymphocytes are concentrated in the cortical thymus and migrate into the medullary portion where they come into contact with thymic epithelial and dendritic cells. Immature thymocytes express terminal deoxynucleotidyl transferase (TdT), CD1a, CD5, and CD7, and coexpress CD4 and CD8. During maturation, they lose TdT, acquire CD3, and develop restricted expression of CD4 (helper) or CD8 (cytotoxic-suppressor) profiles. Mature T lymphocytes migrate to interfollicular T-zones of peripheral lymph nodes where they come into contact with specialized antigen presenting cells, known as interdigitating reticulum cells (IDC) and with Langerhans cells (LC) migrated from the skin.

Lymph nodes have an elaborate sinus system draining lymphatics and lined by specialized cells belonging to the mononuclear phagocyte system. These are mainly macrophage/histiocytes capable of particulate phagocytosis and give rise to sinus histiocytosis when stimulated by neighboring tissues and particulate matter. These cells are strongly positive for alpha-naphthyl butyrate esterase and express histiocyte lysosome/macrophage marker CD68. Langerhans cells which migrate to lymph nodes from the skin become concentrated in lymph node sinuses and paracortical T-zones in pathologic conditions, e.g., dermatopathic lymphadenitis and LC histiocytosis.

Normal skin has no lymphoid tissue. It does contain LC in the epidermis and dermal dendritic cells both of which originate from monocytes in the bone marrow. Bone marrow monocytes express specialized receptors for the Fc fragment of immunoglobulin. They can be recognized by diffuse cytoplasmic staining for nonspecific esterase (NSE) and alpha-naphthyl butyrate esterase. In contrast, LC have only focal perinuclear NSE and express CD1a and S100 antigens. Dermal dendritic cells express fascin, an actin bundling filament.

The lymphoid system is comprised of primary and secondary lymphoid organs. The primary lymphoid organs are the source of lymphoid precursors. Lymphoid progenitor cells are derived from pluripotent stem cells in blood islands of the yolk sac and later in the fetal liver and spleen. Later stages of development occur in the bone marrow. Naïve lymphocytes generated in the bone marrow circulate in the bloodstream to localize in peripheral lymph nodes and spleen where they come into contact with specialized antigen presenting cells. The secondary lymphoid organs are the lymph nodes, spleen, and mucosa-associated lymphoid tissues (MALT). Lymphoid tissues in the skin are sometimes referred to as skin-associated lymphoid tissues (SALT).

Pluripotent stem cells undergo lineage commitment and differentiation to B cells within the bone marrow microenvironment through the synergistic effects of interleukin-7 and stromal cell derived factor-1 (SDF-1) (1–3). T lymphocytes mature in the thymus. At about the 7th week of human fetal development, prothymocytes from the yolk sac and liver migrate to the thymus, and later from the bone marrow. Within the thymus, prothymocytes interact with thymic epithelial cells, macrophages, medullary dendritic cells, and LC which regulate T-cell development and negative selection under the influence of cytokines. Highly expressed CD30 enhances negative selection in the thymus and mediates programmed cell death via a bcl-2 sensitive pathway (4). Only about 2% of prothymocytes escape thymic negative selection and ultimately reach secondary lymphoid organs where they participate in adoptive immunity (5,6).

REFERENCES

1. Rosenberg N, Kincade PW. B-lineage differentiation in normal and transformed cells and the microenvironment that supports it. Curr Opin Immunol 1994; 6:203–211.
2. Namikawa R, Muench MO, de Vries JE, Roncarolo MF. The FLK2/FLT3 ligand synergizes with interleukin-7 in promoting stromal-cell-independent expansion and differeniation of human fetal pro-B cells in vitro. Blood 1996; 87:1881–1890.
3. Le Bien TW. B-cell lymphopoiesis in mouse and man. Curr Opin Immunol 1998; 10: 188–195.
4. Chiarle R, Podda A, Prolla G, Podack ER, Thorbecke GJ, Inghirami G. CD30 overexpression enhances negative selection in the thymus and mediates programmed cell death via a bcl-2 sensitive pathway. J Immunol 1999; 163:194–205.
5. Haynes BF, Heinly CS. Early human T cell development: analysis of the human thymus at the time of initial entry of hematopoietic stem cells into the fetal thymic microenvironment. J Exp Med 1995; 181:1445–1458.
6. Res P, Spits H. Developmental stages in the human thymus. Semin Immunol 1999; 11: 39–46.

6

Structure and Function of Secondary Lymphoid Tissues

Marshall E. Kadin

Beth Israel Deaconess Medical Center, Harvard Medical School, Boston, Massachusetts, U.S.A.

Lymph nodes have a well-defined architecture including sinuses, cortical, paracortical, and medullary regions (Fig. 1). Sinuses are potential spaces lined by sinus histiocytes which are professional macrophages (Fig. 2). Cortical areas of the lymph node contain lymphoid follicles which bring developing B lymphocytes into contact with antigen expressing follicular dendritic cells (Fig. 3). Naïve B cells are concentrated in the dark staining mantle zone surrounding the germinal center (GC) (Fig. 3). These mantle zone lymphocytes are small to medium sized, have dense chromatin, and express surface immunoglobulin M (IgM) and immunoglobulin D (IgD).

During the immune response to antigens, mantle zone lymphocytes migrate into the follicle GC where they proliferate and mature in response to antigen which is corecognized by helper T lymphocytes (CD3+ and CD4+). Following antigen stimulation, B lymphocytes are transformed into centroblasts which undergo immunoglobulin gene hypermutation. Centroblasts are large cells with vesicular nuclei with areas of chromatin clearing and one to several prominent nucleoli adjacent the nuclear membrane. Centroblasts undergo affinity maturation or apoptosis giving rise to the dark zone of the follicle (Fig. 4). Surviving centroblasts give rise to centrocytes which occupy the light or apical zone of the GC (Fig. 4). Centrocytes have elongated angular nuclei with diffuse chromatin and inconspicuous nucleoli.

The final step in B lymphocyte maturation is the development of plasma cells which are concentrated in the medullary cords of the lymph node. Plasma cells have an eccentric nucleus with coarsely clumped "cartwheel" chromatin, and lack prominent nucleoli. Plasma cells can accumulate large amounts of cytoplasmic immunoglobulin which appears as pink globules known as Russell bodies. If the accumulated immunoglobulin indents the nucleus, it may appear as an intranuclear inclusion known as a Dutcher body (Fig. 5). Because of their high content of carbohydrates, both Dutcher and Russell bodies stain with the periodic acid Schiff (PAS) stain which is inhibited by diastase. This is especially prominent with IgM which has the highest carbohydrate concentration of Ig heavy chains. Plasma cells can accumulate in the medullary cords and can also exit the lymph node through efferent lymphatics, returning to the circulation through the thoracic duct (1,2).

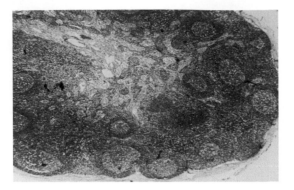

Figure 1 Architecture of normal lymph node—round secondary follicles of containing developing B lymphocytes occupy the outer portion (cortex) and are separated by and external to paracortical T-zone. The central portion includes the medullary cords containing mature plasma cells and sinuses lined by specialized macrophages.

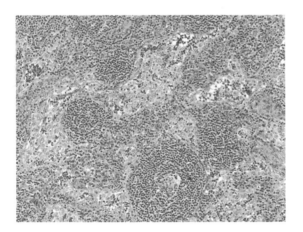

Figure 2 Lymph node with expanded sinuses containing pale-staining histiocyte/macrophages.

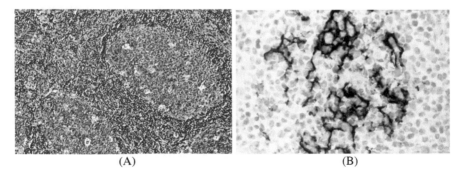

(A)   (B)

Figure 3 (A) Reactive follicle outlined by mantle zone of dark staining lymphocytes surrounding germinal center with lighter staining centroblasts and centrocytes, and starry sky macrophages. (B) Silver stain outlining arborizing fibers of follicular dendritic cells.

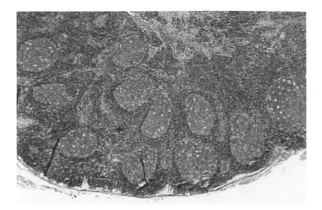

Figure 4 Lymph node with follicles polarized by outer dark zones containing centroblasts and apoptotic bodies and paler staining apical portions containing predominance of centrocytes.

Immunoblasts are also antigen-stimulated B or T lymphocytes which are found mainly in the interfollicular zone but may also occur in the GC. B immunoblasts are distinguished by abundant basophilic cytoplasm and large eccentric nuclei with a single prominent central nucleolus (Fig. 6). B immunoblasts may be immediate precursors to plasma cells.

T cells are concentrated in the interfollicular zone. The interfollicular zones have a diffuse dark-staining mottled appearance due to the presence of numerous small T lymphocytes and scattered pale-staining antigen presenting cells. The antigen presenting cells of the T zone include resident interdigitating reticulum cells (IDC), also known as T-zone histiocytes, and Langerhans cells (LC) which have migrated from the skin. Both IDC and LC have elongated finely grooved nuclei with pale chromatin, inconspicuous nucleoli, and a small rim of pale cytoplasm (Fig. 7). They cannot be distinguished at the light microscopic level. When examined with electron microscopy, only LC contain cytoplasmic Birbeck granules which are thought to arise from infoldings of the cell membrane (Fig. 7). Birbeck granules often have a "tennis racket" appearance. Both LC and IDC stain for CD1a and for S100 antigens which are not expressed by professional macrophages. They are only capable of

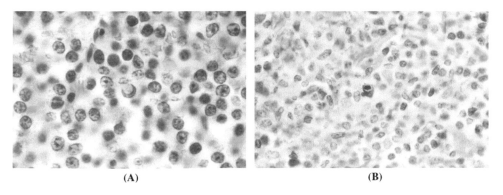

(A)　　　　　　　　　　　　　　　(B)

Figure 5 (A) Plasma cell with intranuclear inclusion (Dutcher body). (B) Periodic acid Schiff stain of Dutcher body.

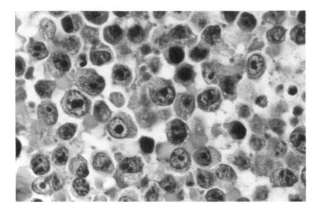

Figure 6 Immunoblasts with basophilic cytoplasm, eccentric nuclei, and prominent central nucleoli.

microphagocytosis or pinocytosis and do not contain cellular elements. They are potent antigen presenting cells.

The T zones contain a mixture of naïve and memory T cells. Naïve T cells, not been previously exposed to antigen, circulate continuously between lymph nodes and blood. They express high levels of L-selectin, permitting their attachment and rolling on the surface of high endothelial venules in lymph nodes. The rolling T cells are activated by a secondary lymphocyte chemokine, 6-C-kine (SLC) expressed on the luminal surface of high endothelial venules (3). The T cells are then activated by chemokine receptor CCR7 which allows them to bind tightly through lymphocyte functional antigen 1 (LFA-1) to intercellular adhesion molecule 1 (ICAM-1) expressed on venules. The resultant flattening of T lymphocytes on the endothelial cell surface allows them to exit the venule and accumulate in T-cell-rich areas of the lymph node where they are exposed to resident IDC. They are also exposed to antigen presenting LC and dermal dendritic cells which migrate to lymph nodes through afferent lymphatics. If a naïve T cell encounters antigen for which it has specificity in a skin draining lymph node, it becomes activated and acquires the characteristics of a memory T cell, expressing cutaneous lymphocyte antigen (CLA). Memory T cells

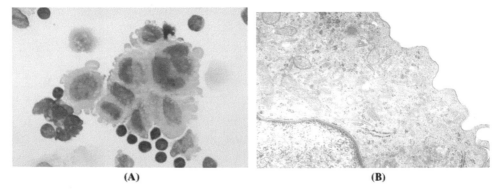

(A)   **(B)**

Figure 7 (A) Langerhans cells with elongated nuclei and abundant pale-staining cytoplasm with adjacent smaller lymphocytes. (B) Langerhans cell with Birbeck granule identified by electron microscopy.

have the capacity to migrate to the skin site where the antigen was first encountered, but also may retain the capacity to exit high endothelial venules in lymph nodes (reviewed in Ref. 4).

SPLEEN

In contrast to lymph node GCs where antigen is delivered through the lymphatic system, antigen enters GCs of the spleen through the blood stream. B lymphocytes are concentrated within GCs and surrounding mantle and marginal zones in the splenic white pulp. T lymphocytes are concentrated in the periarteriolar lymphoid sheaths (PALS). The spleen also contains a red pulp comprised of cords and sinuses lined by specialized cells of the mononuclear phagocyte system. These macrophages clear micro-organisms coated with antibody and complement from the bloodstream. The spleen is required for early adaptive response to circulating pathogens, such as occurs in bacterial sepsis.

MUCOSA-ASSOCIATED LYMPHOID TISSUES

Specialized lymphoid compartments underlie mucosal surfaces of the gut and bronchial epithelium. Lymphoid follicles which occur just beneath the epithelium throughout the small intestine and are known as Peyer patches. A subset of intestinal epithelial cells known as M cells are specialized for transport of bacteria and other antigens from the intestinal lumen to the Peyer patches where antigen-dependent B cell differentiation occurs (5).

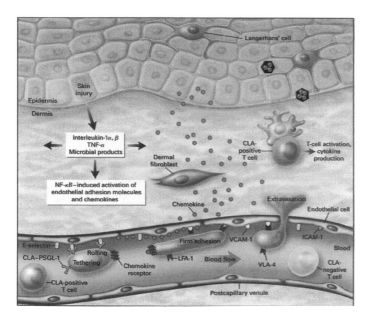

Figure 8 The binding of CLA on memory T cells to E-selectin and P-selectin on the luminal surface of cutaneous postcapillary venules initiates the process known as *tethering*. Tethering slows the movement of T lymphocytes which then upregulate expression of integrins $\alpha_1\beta_2$ (LFA-1) and $\alpha_4\beta_1$ (VLA-4) which bind to VCAM-1 and ICAM-1, respectively on the luminal surface of endothelial cells (8,9). Following tethering, the T lymphocytes become flattened on the endothelial cell surface in preparation for extravasation though the endothelial layer. (Reproduced from Fig. 2 of Ref. 4, Copyright 1999, Massachusetts Medical Society, all rights reserved.)

SKIN

Memory T cells are generated in lymph nodes draining the skin and recirculate back to the skin during inflammation or certain pathologic conditions, e.g., cutaneous T-cell lymphoma. The process of homing to the skin requires the binding of memory T cells to specialized receptors on endothelial cells (Fig. 8). The process of skin homing is mediated by CLA, a specialized form of P-selectin glycoprotein ligand expressed on the tips of microvilli of skin-homing T cells (6). Expression of CLA is critically dependent upon signals from the microenvironment, being upregulated by transforming growth factor-beta and to a lesser degree by interleukin-6 (7). Upon reaching the extravascular space, T cells are subject to chemotactic stimuli from sites of injury or infection. When exposed to antigen, they become activated and release inflammatory cytokines (chemokines) which amplify the inflammatory infiltrate. Chemokines are small (8–10 kDa) chemotactic cytokines, that act through G-protein-coupled receptors and are classified by the spacing of the cysteine residues near the amino terminus (10). The differential expression of chemokines and their receptors most likely contributes to the characteristic histopathology, anatomic sites of origin, and spread of lymphoproliferative disorders (11).

REFERENCES

1. Kroese FG, Timens W, Nieuwenhuis P. Germinal center reaction and B-lymphocytes: morphology and function. Curr Top Pathol 1990; 84:103–148.
2. MacLennan IC. Germinal centers. Annu Rev Immunol 1994; 12:117–139.
3. Campbell JJ, Bowman EP, Murphy K, Youngman KR, Siani MA, Thompson DA, Wu L, Zlotnik A, Butcher EC. 6-C-kine (SLC), a lymphocyte adhesion-triggering chemokine expressed by high endothelium, is an agonist for MIP-3beta CCR7. J Cell Biol 1998; 141:1053–1059.
4. Robert C, Kupper TS. Inflammatory skin diseases, T cells and immune surveillance. N Engl J Med 1999; 341:1817–1828.
5. Kerneis S, Bogdanova A, Kraehenbuhl JP, Pringault E. Conversion by Peyer's patch lymphocytes of human enterocytes into M cells that transport bacteria. Science 1997; 277:949–952.
6. Fulbrigge RC, Kieffer JD, Amerding D, Kupper TS. Cutaneous lymphocyte antigen is a specialized from of PSGL-1 expressed on skin-homing T cells. Nature 1997; 389:978–981.
7. Picker LJ, Treer JR, Ferguson-Darnell B, Collins PA, Bergstresser PR, Terstappen LWMM. Control of lymphocyte recirculation in man. II Differential regulation of the cutaneous lymphocyte associated antigen, a selective tissue-homing receptor for skin-homing T-cells. J Immunol 1993; 150:1122–1136.
8. Picker LJ, Kishimoto TK, Smith CW, Warnock RA, Butcher EC. ELAM-1 is an adhesion molecule for skin-homing T-cells. Nature 1991; 349:796–799.
9. Campbell JJ, Haraldsen G, Pan J, Rottman J, Qin S, Ponath P, Andrew DP, Warnke R, Ruffing N, Kassam N, Wu L, Butcher EC. The chemokine receptor CCR4 in vascular recognition by cutaneous but not intestinal memory T cells. Nature 1999; 400:776–780.
10. Mackay CR. Chemokines: what chemokine is that? Curr Biol 1997; 7:R384–R386.
11. Vermeer MH, Dukers DF, ten Berge RL, Bloemena E, Wu L, Vos W, de Vries E, de Tensen CP, Meiejer CJLM, Willemze R. Differential expression of thymus and activation regulated chemokine and its receptor CCR4 in nodal and cutaneous anaplastic large-cell lymphomas and Hodgkin's disease. Mod Pathol 2002; 15:838–844.

7

Ontogeny of Lymphoid Cells

Marshall E. Kadin

Beth Israel Deaconess Medical Center, Harvard Medical School, Boston, Massachusetts, U.S.A.

B-CELL ONTOGENY

Pre-B cells are the earliest committed B cell precursors and can be identified by the presence of B-cell receptor accessory chains CD79a and CD79b. The developing B cell undergoes immunoglobulin gene rearrangements mediated by a V(D) J recombinase complex, including recombination activation gene products RAG-1 and RAG-2, DNA-dependent protein kinase, and a DNA ligase (1). RAG-1 and RAG-2 are expressed at high levels during the early pro-B cell stage when IgH gene rearrangements occur and again at the pre-B cell stage when Ig light chain rearrangements are taking place. These enzymes flank the coding sequences of individual V, D, and J segments and mediate DNA recombination. Terminal deoxynucleotidyl transferase (TdT) adds N-nucleotides at the heavy chain joining regions leading to increased diversity of the antigen receptor genes (2). Pre-B cells express the product of an intact, fully rearranged heavy chain gene called μ. The pre-B cell receptor which is essential for B-cell development and maturation consists of two μ chains, two surrogate light chains, CD79a and CD79b (3).

RAG-1 and RAG-2 are expressed again at the next stage of B-cell development during which rearrangement of the Ig light chains κ and λ loci occurs. VκJκ gene rearrangements precede VλJλ genes. Approximately one-third of κ rearrangements are nonproductive in which case the recombination complex is activated at the λ locus. Immature B cells express IgM at the surface and are then able to interact with antigen for which they have specificity. From this stage on, B cell growth and differentiation are antigen dependent.

In the peripheral circulation, most immature IgM+ B cells become naïve mature IgM+, IgD+ B cells that can enter the spleen, lymph nodes, and MALT tissues where they are located primarily in the mantle zone. Upon recognition of antigen in the context of T-cell derived costimulatory signals, naïve mature B cells enter the primary follicles and initiate germinal center formation. Undifferentiated germinal center B cells called centroblasts proliferate in the dark zone where they undergo somatic mutation and Ig gene recombination. There is a high rate of apoptosis among centroblasts. B cells that bind antigen and receive cognate T cell help can survive the affinity maturation process and differentiate into centrocytes, which occupy the light zone of the germinal center. Differentiated centrocytes exit the lymph node as plasma cells or memory B cells.

CD19 and CD21, the receptor for C3d or complement receptor-2, colocalize with immunoglobulin to form the B-cell coreceptor complex. CD21 serves as receptor for Epstein–Barr virus. CD20 is a nonglycosylated protein that contains four transmembrane spanning domains and appears to function as a calcium channel (3,4). Cross-linking of CD20 causes activation of cytoplasmic kinases, phosphorylation of phospholipase-C, and mobilization of intracellular calcium stores (5). CD19, CD20, and CD21 are useful surface markers to detect B-cell lineage. They are accompanied by CD45 (leukocyte common antigen) tyrosine phosphatase, a large glycosylated membrane receptor that occurs in various isoforms generated by alternative splicing and by glycosylation of specific residues of the formed protein. Together, these functional markers can be used for diagnosis of B-cell lymphoproliferative disorders.

B-1 cells are a distinct subset of B cells committed to the production of natural antibodies. B-1 cells appear early in ontogeny and are distinguished from conventional B-2 cells by their expression of CD5, a cysteine-rich transmembrane protein (6). CD5 appears to modulate the response to antigen receptor engagement and, in autoreactive B cells, may limit cellular activation and proliferation in the context of antigen binding.

T-CELL ONTOGENY

Pluripotent cells from the bone marrow arrive in the thymus where they differentiate into CD2+ committed T cells, after which they undergo an orderly sequence of T-cell receptor (TCR) gene rearrangements, first involving the β chain gene, followed by γ and δ segments, and, if the $\gamma\delta$ gene product is nonfunctional, the α chain segment. Each stage of T-cell maturation is marked by a particular pattern of surface antigens. Triple-negative thymocytes lack CD3; double-negative thymocytes lack CD4 and CD8; and double-positive thymocytes express CD4 and CD8. Mature $\alpha\beta$ (type 2) thymocytes express CD4 or CD8. Thymic maturation occurs in the double-positive stage during which time the cells are selected for their ability to bind MHC and their lack of autoreactivity (7). Positive selection requires the interaction of thymocytes with thymic cortical epithelial cells expressing the MHC complexed with autologous peptides (8). Most thymocytes are rejected for export to the periphery based on their failure to recognize autologous MHC and thereby undergo apoptosis in the thymic medulla. Double-positive thymocytes that interact successfully with MHC-I develop into CD8+ cells and those that interact with MHC-II become CD4+ T-cells (9). Simultaneously, in a process referred to as negative selection, thymocytes that bind peptides derived from autologous structures with high affinity are eliminated (10).

γ/δ T CELLS

γ/δ T cells represent only a small number of peripheral blood lymphocytes but they are numerous in the skin and intestinal tract where they mediate an early response to pathogens (11). They can mediate cytotoxicity in the absence of antigen-specific priming. Their growth is stimulated by IL-7 and SCF secreted by epithelial cells

(12). The TCR is restricted and oligoclonal populations are present in the skin and gut. The TCRs are skewed for binding of common pathogenetic microbes and may be selected by environmental factors and infections in the host (13). Hepatosplenic and subcutaneous panniculitis-like γ/δ T-cell lymphomas are derived from different Vδ subsets of γ/δ T lymphocytes which correspond to the predominant γ/δ T-cell subsets normally found in the spleen and skin respectively(14).

NATURAL KILLER CELLS

Natural killer (NK) cells comprise about 10–15% of peripheral blood lymphocytes in adults (15). They are also numerous in the spleen but not in peripheral lymph nodes. Small numbers of NK cells are present in the liver, lung, and intestinal mucosa. Natural killer cells are cytotoxic cells which have the morphology of medium- to large-sized granular lymphocytes. The cytoplasmic granules contain phospholipids, proteoglycans, and cytotoxic proteins such as granzyme B and perforin (16). Natural killer cells do not rearrange any of the genes encoding the T-cell receptor chains nor express on their surface the CD3 antigen complex. Instead they express the FcγRIIA (CD16) and N-CAM (CD56) antigens (17). Cytotoxicity mediated by NK cells is non-MHC-restricted (18). Natural killer cells are capable of killing a variety of cell types, including tumor cells, virus-infected cells, and, in some instances, normal cells in the absence of previous deliberate or known sensitization. Natural killer cells interact with nonclassic MHC-I related molecules through inhibitory and activation receptors to identify targets for autologous killing (19). In this capacity, NK cells play a central role in the immune response to certain tumors. Natural killer cells are potent producers of interferon-gamma (IFN-γ) and granulocyte macrophage colony stimulating factor (GM-CSF), and are capable of producing other cytokines, including tumor necrosis factor-alpha (TNF-α) (32). Natural killer cells stimulated by micro-organisms or by cytokines, such as IL-12 and TNF, produce large amounts of IFN-γ and other cytokines that facilitate helper T-cell development.

Natural killer cells originate in the bone marrow from a common lymphoid precursor that gives rise to T, B, and NK cells (20). The cytokine IL-15 is particularly important in the differentiation and expansion of NK cells (21). Natural killer cell development is independent of the thymus.

MYELOID CELLS

Monocytes and myeloid cells are derived from common precursors in the bone marrow. Myeloid cells are distinguished by their content of primary and secondary specific granules which define them morphologically and functionally as neutrophils, eosinophils, basophils, and mast cells. Neutrophils are the most frequent myeloid cells and are among the principal effectors of the innate response to bacteria and fungi. Neutrophils can directly bind and engulf bacteria, which are cleared in the absence of humoral activity (22). Neutrophils and monocyte/macrophages express membrane-bound CD14, a glycosyl phosphatidlyinositol (GPI)-anchored scavenger receptor that binds bacterial lipopolysaccharide (LPS). CD14 is a conserved lipid transport protein that forms complexes in the plasma with LPS-binding protein (23). Upon engagement of surface CD14 by LPS, a cascade of inflammatory events is initiated including transcription of cytokines IL-1, IFN-γ, and adhesion molecules.

Some bacteria have evolved a mechanism to escape recognition by CD14 and can be engulfed only after opsonization by complement or antibody. After phagocytosis, bacteria enter neutrophil granules where they are subjected to a low pH and potent antimicrobial factors including cathepsins, lysozyme, elastase, and defensins as well as oxygen metabolites (24,25).

Circulating neutrophils express highly specialized surface receptors to facilitate chemotaxis and locomotion to sites of inflammation. The first phase of neutrophil interaction with endothelial cells is the rolling phase of leukocyte trafficking which is mediated by adhesion molecules known as leukocyte selectins (CD62L) on endothelial cells. Bacterial LPS and TNF-α upregulate endothelial cell expression of E-selectin (CD62E). The second or tethering phase of leukocyte migration is mediated by integrins and intercellular adhesion molecules (ICAMs). There are three leukocyte integrins each of which express a common β chain (β_2, CD18) and a distinct alpha chain (26). The ICAMs are immunoglobulin-related molecules that mediate intercellular adhesion and leukocyte activation and serve as endothelial cell surface counter-receptors for leukocyte β_2 integrins. When inflammation occurs, IL-8 and other factors augment neutrophil expression of β_2 integrins, causing neutrophils to adhere to the vascular endothelium and facilitating diapedesis of neutrophils from the blood vessel lumen into tissues (27).

Upon neutrophil activation, a respiratory burst occurs in which toxic oxygen metabolites including hydrogen peroxide are generated. The resulting chemical interactions generate hypochlorous acid, the neutrophil component responsible for the green color and odor that occurs where large numbers of neutrophils are present and also causes the green color of chloromas (granulocytic tumors) (24).

EOSINOPHILS

Eosinophils play a major role in the defense against parasites (28,29). They have bilobed nuclei and contain coarse granules, which contain arginine-rich basic proteins. These bind acidic eosin dye that accounts for their red appearance. Eosinophil granules contain eosinophil peroxidase, collagenase, cationic protein, and platelet activating factor (30). Eosinophils can cause tissue damage by the release of granule contents, which is regulated in part by a receptor for eotaxin expressed selectively on eosinophils (31).

The growth and maturation of eosinophils in the bone marrow is stimulated by GM-CSF, IL-3, and IL-5 (32). Eosinophils produce and secrete IL-5 which is overexpressed in diseases characterized by eosinophilia (32,33). Eosinophils recognize IgE bound to the surface of parasites through expression of low affinity IgE receptor CD23 (34) and the high affinity IgE receptor FcϵRI, which is expressed only upon activation (35). They then discharge their granules which damage the parasites.

BASOPHILS AND MAST CELLS

Basophils represent less than 1% of circulating granulocytes. They contain large granules comprising heparin and other sulfated or carboxylated acidic proteins, which appear blue with Wright–Giemsa stain. Basophils are closely related to mast cells and appear to play a role in the innate response to some infectious agents (36). Both basophils and mast cells express the high affinity IgE receptor FcϵRI (35). Mast cells are principal mediators of local and systemic hypersensitivity reactions such as anaphylaxis. They modulate vascular permeability through discharge of their granules which contain histamine, heparin, leukotrienes, proteases, and TNF-α (36). Degranulation of mast cells causes local vasodilatation and an increase in circulating neutrophils and monocytes. Lymphatic flow is also augmented, resulting in increased antigen from the tissue to regional lymph nodes. IgE crosslinking by antigen is required for mast cell activation and degranulation. The wheel and flare reaction characteristic of ectopic response to subcutaneous injection is mediated by mast cells in the dermis (37).

MONOCYTES AND MACROPHAGES

Monocytes mature from myelomonocytic precursors in the bone marrow during a process that is stimulated by growth factors including IL-3 and GM-CSF. After leaving the bone marrow, monocytes circulate for 1–3 days in the bloodstream. After leaving the blood stream, they mature in tissues as macrophages, Langerhans cells or dendritic cells specialized for phagocytosis and/or antigen presentation. Monocytes express Fc receptors for IgG (FcγRI and FcγRIIa; CD64 and CD32), respectively, and for IgA (FcαRI, CD89).

In the tissues, differentiated monocytes include Kuppfer sinus lining cells in the liver, microglial cells in the brain, and multinucleated cells comprising granulomas (38,39). Macrophage activation is largely dependent on interaction with type 1 helper T lymphocytes (Th1) cells which stimulate macrophages by secretion of IFN-γ. Peptides derived from digested microbes are presented by macrophages in the context of MHC-class II molecules, thereby driving the initial steps of adaptive immunity. Activated macrophages express high levels of CD40 and CD80, two molecules that are important for costimulation of T lymphocytes. Activated macrophages generate nitric oxide which has potent activity against diverse micro-organisms (40). Macrophages clear cellular and infectious debris at sites of cell death and infection through their ability to bind and ingest apoptotic material.

REFERENCES

1. Ramsden DA, van Gent DC, Gellert M. Specificity in V(D)J recombination: new lessons from biochemistry and genetics. Curr Opin Immunol 1997; 9:114–120.
2. Kamori T, Okada A, Stewart V, Alt FW. Lack of N regions in antigen receptor variable region genes of TdT-deficient lymphocytes. Science 1993; 261:1171–1175.
3. Torres RM, Faswinkel H, Reth M, Rajewsky K. Aberrant B cell development and immune response in mice with a compromised BCR complex. Science 1996; 272: 1804–1808.
4. Tedder TF, Engel P. CD20: a regulator of cell-cycle progression of B lymphocytes. Immunol Today 1994; 15:450–454.
5. Deans JP, Schieven GL, Suh GL, Valentine MA, Gilliland LA, Aruffo A, Clark EA, Ledbetter JA. Association of tyrosine and serine kinases with the B cell surface antigen CD20. Induction via CD20 of tyrosine phosphorylation and activation of phospholipase C-gamma and PLC phospholipase C-gamma 2. J Immunol 1993; 151:4494–4504.
6. Resnick D, Person A, Krieger M. The SRCR superfamily: a family reminiscent of the Ig superfamily. Trends Biochem Sci 1994; 19:5–8.

7. Sebzda E, Mariathasan S, Ohteki T, Jones R, Bachmann MF, Ohashi PS. Selection of the T cell repertoire. Annu Rev Immunol 1999; 17:829–879.
8. Von Boehmer H. Positive selection of lymphocytes. Cell 1994; 76:219–228.
9. Zuniga-Pflucker JC, Hones LA, Chin LT, Kruisbeek AM. CD4 and CD8 act as co-receptors during thymic selection of the T cell repertoire. Semin Immunol 1991; 3: 167–175.
10. Nossal GJ. Negative selection of lymphocytes. Cell 1994; 76:229–239.
11. Boismenu R, Havran WL. An innate view of gamma delta T cells. Curr Opin Immunol 1997; 9:57–63.
12. Laky K, Lefrancois L, von Freeden-Jeffry U, Murray R, Puddington L. The role of IL-7 in thymic and extrathymic development of TCR gamma delta cells. J Immunol 1998; 161:707–713.
13. Chowers Y, Holtmeier W, Harwood J, Morzycka-Wroblewska E, Kagnoff MF. The v delta 1 T cell receptor repertoire in human small intestine and colon. J Exp Med 1994; 180: 183–190.
14. Przybylski GK, Wu H, Macon WR, Finan J, Leonard DGB, Felgar RE, DeGiuseepe JA, Nowell PC, Swerdlow S, Kadin ME, Wasik MA, Salhany KE. Hepatosplenic and subcutaneous panniculitis-like $\gamma\delta$ T cell lymphomas are derived from different Vδ subsets of γ/δ T lymphocytes. J Mol Diag 2000; 2:11–19.
15. Trinchieri G. Biology of natural killer cells. Adv Immunol 1989; 47:189.
16. Moretta A. Molecular mechanisms in cell-mediated cytotoxicity. Cell 1997; 90:13–18.
17. Robertson MJ. Natural killer cell clinical studies: surface antigens of human natural killer cells. In: Kishimoto T, Kikutani H, von dem Borne AEGK, et al, eds. Killer Cells in Health and Disease. New York: Garland Publishing, 1998:317–329.
18. Takasugi M, Mickey MR, Terasaki PI. Reactivity of lymphocytes from normal persons on cultured tumor cells. Cancer Res 1973; 33:2898.
19. Lanier LL. NK cell receptors. Annu Rev Immunol 1998; 16:359–393.
20. Miller SC. Reduction and renewal of murine killer cells in the spleen and bone marrow. J Immunol 1982; 129:2282.
21. Williams NS, Klem J, Puzanov IJ, Sivakumar PV, Schatzle JD, Bennett M, Kumar V. Natural killer cell differentiation: insights from knockout and transgenic mouse models and in vitro systems. Immunol Rev 1998; 165:47.
22. Hampton MB, Kettle AJ, Winterbourn CC. Inside the neutrophil phagosome: oxidants, myeloperoxidase and bacterial killing. Blood 1998; 92:2007–3117.
23. Wright SD. CD14 and innate recognition of bacteria. J Immunol 1995; 155:6–8.
24. Matzner Y. Neutrophil pathophysiology. Semin Hematol 1997; 34:265–266.
25. Rorregaard N. Current concepts about neutrophil granule physiology. Curr Opin Hematol 1996; 3:11–18.
26. Gahmberg CG. Leukocyte adhesion: CD11/CD18 integrins and intercellular adhesion molecules. Curr Opin Cell Biol 1997; 9:643–650.
27. Brown EI. Neutrophil adhesion and therapy of inflammation. Semin Hematol 1997; 34:319–326.
28. Walsh GM. Human eosinophils: their accumulation, activation and fate. Br J Haematol 1997; 97:701–709.
29. Weller PF. Eosinophils. J Allergy Clin Immunol 1997; 100:283–287.
30. Weller PF. Eosinophils: structure and function. Curr Opin Immunol 1994; 6:85–90.
31. Ponath PD, Qin S, Post TW, Wang J, Wu L, Gerard NP, Newman W, Gerard C, Mackay CR. Molecular cloning and characterization of a human eotaxin receptor which is expressed selectively on eosinophils. J Exp Med 1996; 183:2437–2448.
32. Rothenberg ME. Eosinophilia. N Engl J Med 1998; 338:1592–1600.
33. Dubucquoi S, Desreumaux P, Janin A, Klein O, Goldman M, Tavernier J, Capron A, Capron M. Interleukin 5 synthesis by eosinophils: association with granules and immunoglobulin-dependent secretion. J Exp Med 1994; 179:703–708.
34. Sutton BJ, Gould HJ. The human IgE network. Nature 1996; 366:421–428.

35. Garman SC, Kinet JP, Jardetzky TS. Crystal structure of the human high-affinity IgE receptor. Cell 1998; 95:951–961.

36. Abraham SN, Arock M. Mast cells and basophils in innate immunity. Semin Immunol 1998; 10:373–381.

37. Marshall JS, Bienenstock J. The role of mast cells in inflammatory reactions of the airways, skin and intestine. Curr Opin Immunol 1994; 6:853–859.

38. Johnston RB Jr. Current concepts: immunology. Monocytes and macrophages. N Engl J Med 1988; 318:747–752.

39. Ziegler-Heitbrock HW. Heterogeneity of human blood monocytes: the CD14+ CD16+ subpopulation. Immunol Today 1996; 17:424–428.

40. MacMicking J, Xie QW, Nathan C. Nitric oxide and macrophage function. Annu Rev Immunol 1997; 15:323–350.

8

Histo- and Cytomorphology

Marshall E. Kadin

Beth Israel Deaconess Medical Center, Harvard Medical School, Boston, Massachusetts, U.S.A.

Inflammatory reactions in the skin usually contain a polymorphous infiltrate of T cells, B cells, plasma cells, tissue macrophages, Langerhans cells, dermal dendritic cells, and variable numbers of myeloid cells. The composition of the inflammatory cell infiltrate depends on the nature of skin injury or infection. In some conditions, such as Borrelia burgdorferi infections, secondary follicles with germinal centers are often seen. Reactive germinal centers in inflammatory conditions appear polarized with dark and light zones, have a starry sky appearance due to macrophages with ingested nuclear material from apoptotic cells, a high mitotic rate, and a distinct mantle zone of small round lymphocytes. In contrast, follicular lymphomas have a loss of polarity, few or absent starry sky macrophages, a low mitotic rate and an indistinct to absent mantle zone. In marginal zone lymphomas, the germinal centers may be partially replaced by centrocyte-like cells which are elongated B lymphocytes with small nuclei. Numerous plasma cells, with light chain restriction by immunohistochemistry, often in the superficial portion of the infiltrate, are characteristic of cutaneous marginal zone lymphomas, in contrast to the polyclonal plasma cells randomly dispersed and concentrated in perivascular sites in inflammatory conditions. Some degree of tissue eosinophilia and or neutrophilia is a common feature of hypersensitivity and arthropod bite reactions.

In nearly all inflammatory conditions, a mixture of cell types is seen. In contrast, lymphomas and leukemias show a clear predominance of one cell type or lineage. Usually the cells comprising the infiltrate represent a particular stage of cellular differentiation. Tumors derived from immature cells or blasts are revealed by a uniform population of medium to large cells with round to oval nuclei, fine evenly dispersed chromatin, and one to several small distinct nucleoli. The mitotic rate is high. In myeloid leukemias, some number of cytoplasmic granules can be detected in cells showing maturation. This is often most apparent in eosinophilic myelocytes. Chloracetate esterase or Leder stains for primary granules are helpful in establishing a diagnosis of myeloid leukemia.

Primary cutaneous T-cell lymphomas usually show some degree of epidermotropism in which malignant T cells with highly convoluted or cerebriform nuclei, often surrounded by halos, are found in the basal layer of the epidermis and sometimes concentrated in the upper layers of the epidermis comprising Pautrier microabscesses. The cerebriform cells are often found in juxtaposition with Langer-hans cells and one must be careful to distinguish benign collections of Langerhans cells with pale elongated and convoluted nuclei and pale cytoplasm, in inflammatory conditions, from collections of malignant T cells with dark round to oval highly convoluted nuclei, best appreciated by focusing up and down with 60–100 X oil objective lenses or electron microscopy.

9

Growth Patterns of Lympho- and Myeloproliferative Infiltrates of the Skin

Günter Burg and Werner Kempf
Department of Dermatology, University Hospital, Zürich, Switzerland

Marshall E. Kadin
Beth Israel Deaconess Medical Center, Harvard Medical School, Boston, Massachusetts, U.S.A.

Morphology always has a macrodimension seen at low power magnification as a silhouette or pattern and a microdimension which provides additional information on the cytological structure under high power magnification. Apart from histopathology and cytomorphology, special morphologic features may provide important information for categorizing lymphoproliferative skin infiltrates.

PRINCIPAL GROWTH PATTERN

In nodal lymphomas, the distinction between nodular or diffuse growth pattern has long been used as a major criteria for the discrimination of lymphoma subtypes (1). These terms are still very helpful in describing growth pattern of lymph node involvement.

   With respect to the skin, the terms "nodular" or "diffuse" reflect growth patterns which best can be compared with a ball or a disk, respectively, and which are quite different from their nodal counterparts.

   A *diffuse* (*disk-like*) cutaneous infiltrate spreads two-dimensionally within the subepidermal dermis over a large area (Figs. 1 and 2). It is preferentially composed of T lymphocytes and clinically presents as patches, flat plaques, or covers the total body in case of erythroderma. The typical growth pattern is horizontal, except for vertical extension along adnexal structures. It is typical for early stages of CTCL.

   A *nodular* cutaneous infiltrate usually is primarily located within the dermis and grows centrifugally three-dimensionally in all directions (Fig. 3). This pattern is mostly found in cutaneous B-cell lymphomas (CBCL) or in high-grade malignant large-cell lymphomas of both lineages, either primary or secondary, e.g. in cases of mycosis fungoides transforming into a high-grade malignant large-cell lymphoma. Nodular growth patterns in the skin may be small as in lymphomatoid papulosis

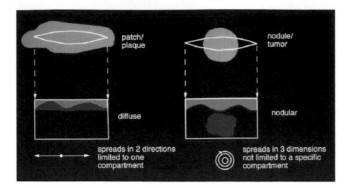

Figure 1 Schematic infiltration patterns in cutaneous lymphomas: diffuse (disk-like) vs. nodular infiltrates.

or large without restriction to preferential T- and B-cell compartments, sometimes reaching beyond biopsy borders.

There may be combinations of both growth patterns, if for example tumors develop within patches or within erythroderma.

GROWTH PATTERN IN CUTANEOUS LYMPHOMAS

There are five major patterns seen in cutaneous lymphoproliferative infiltrates, which on low power microscopic magnification give some information on the type of infiltrate and which first have been described and used as a conceptual basis for pattern diagnosis and classification of hematopoietic skin infiltrates in 1983 (2).

T-Cell Pattern

This pattern is characterized by a band-like loosely packed subepidermal infiltrate, showing epidermotropism of single cells and of clusters of cells into the epidermis

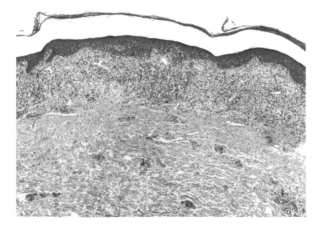

Figure 2 Superficial (disk-like) skin infiltrate in the upper and mid dermis with epidermotropism of lymphocytes.

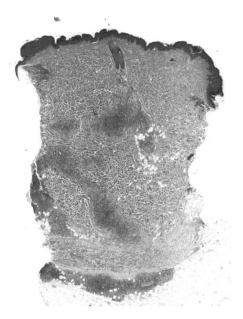

Figure 3 Nodular skin infiltrate in all dermal layers and separated from the overlying epidermis.

(Fig. 2). There also is marked subepidermal edema. The infiltrate usually contains eosinophils and plasma cells, in addition to small lymphocytes. The prototypical diseases which reflect this pattern are mycosis fungoides and other low-grade malignant CTCL.

B-Cell Pattern

This is a well-demarcated nodular infiltrate with convex margins, composed of densely packed small lymphocytes in the dermis, without significant interstitial infiltration but obliterating local tissue structures (Fig. 3). The subepidermal papillary compartment of the dermis usually is free of infiltrate, unless a concomitant diffuse subepidermal T-cell component is present. This type of pattern is prototypically found in low-grade malignant B-cell lymphomas such as MALT-type marginal zone lymphoma or follicle center lymphoma of the skin.

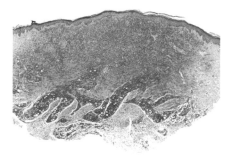

Figure 4 Diffuse growth pattern with an infiltrate in all dermal layers. This growth pattern is found for example in diffuse large B-cell lymphoma.

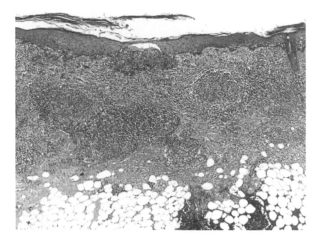

Figure 5 Pseudolymphomatous growth pattern with a superficial and a deeper nodular infiltrate.

Diffuse Growth Pattern

There is diffuse infiltration of the whole dermis with or without epidermotropism. Both the band-like feature of T-cell pattern and the nodular feature of B-cell pattern are lacking, even though the macroscopic correlates are usually large nodules or tumors. The cells are usually medium to large size. This pattern is typically seen in highly proliferative large B- or T-cell lymphomas or in non-lymphoid proliferations such as histiocytic tumors (Fig. 4).

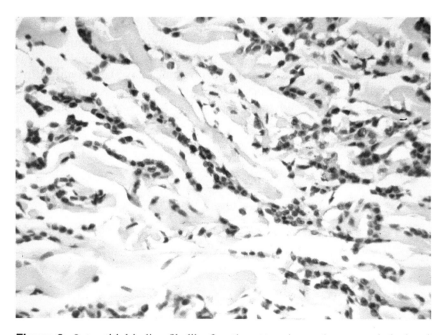

Figure 6 Interstitial indian file-like frouth pattern in myelomonocytic leukemia.

Pseudolymphomatous Growth Pattern

The mixture of a (disk)-like T-cell pattern and a nodular B-cell pattern with a rather concave boundary and with interstitial spread is indicative for a reactive pseudolymphomatous process as seen in scabies or insect bites (Fig. 5).

Interstitial Growth Pattern

Indian file-like spread of infiltrating cells (Fig. 6) is typically seen in myeloproliferative skin infiltrates. Diagnosis can be suggested on the basis of this typical growth pattern and the cell morphology, but has to be confirmed by appropriate phenotyping.

GROWTH PATTERNS OF MYELOPROLIFERATIVE INFILTRATES IN THE SKIN

Chronic leukemias of lymphoid or myeloid origin tend to present with perivascular accumulations of leukemic cells. In contrast, acute leukemias or blast crisis of chronic myelogenous leukemia typically demonstrate interstitial dermal as well as perivascular patterns of infiltration.

REFERENCES

1. Rappaport H. Tumors of the Hematopoietic System. Washington: Armed Forces Institute of Pathology, 1966.
2. Burg G, Braun-Falco O. Cutaneous Lymphomas, Pseudolymphomas and Related Disorders. Berlin, Heidelberg, NewYork, Tokyo: Springer-Verlag, 1983.

10

Stepwise Approach to the Diagnosis of Lymphoproliferative Skin Infiltrates and Related Disorders

Monika Hess Schmid, Günter Burg, and Werner Kempf
Department of Dermatology, University Hospital, Zürich, Switzerland

A stepwise approach is required for establishing diagnosis in CL, combining data of history, clinical features, morphologic and immunophenotypic data as well as the results of molecular studies (Fig. 1).

HISTORY

Patients with cutaneous T-cell lymphoma (CTCL) will recall a preceding chronic dermatitis for many years that may have been considered as therapeutically resistant chronic contact dermatitis, atopic dermatitis, eczema, or psoriasis. Because of histologic unspecific morphology of the prelymphomatous patch stage and the difficulty in distinguishing those changes from inflammatory skin diseases in early stages, it may take an average of 2–10 years until a definite diagnosis can be established (1,2).

Despite detailed investigations of pre-existing allergies or biologic (e.g. viral), physical or chemical exposures no evidence of the hypothesized association was found (3–5). However, patients with CTCL are at increased risk of some other malignancies, presumably because of the immunosuppressive effects of the disease and the exposure to potentially carcinogenic therapies (6,7).

In contrast to CTCL, which evolve usually over a period of years and decades from erythematous patches, plaques into tumoral lesions, CBCL have a relatively brief history of a few weeks or months without a prelymphomatous stage.

CLINICAL FEATURES

The wide spectrum of CL includes disorders with similar clinical and histological features, but highly variable biologic behavior. Even within one subgroup of CL such as CTCL, there are many different clinical entities such as mycosis fungoides (MF), Sézary syndrome, pagetoid reticulosis, or granulomatous slack skin.

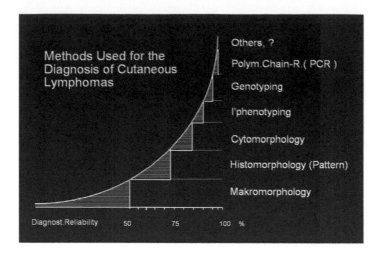

Figure 1 Stepwise approach of diagnosis in cutaneous lymphomas.

The prototype of CTCL is MF (8–10) which represents 70% of all CTCL. Mycosis fungoides is usually characterized by the sequential appearance of patches (flat, erythematous macules, or minimally elevated lesions with fine scale) in a pre-lymphomatous stage developing into thin (well demarcated, infiltrated, elevated erythematous lesions) and thick (thickness over 1 mm) plaques and finally into tumors (red-brown nodules) which tend to ulcerate. Even though this is a stepwise progression with biological breakpoints, these three phases may overlap or occur simultaneously (11). In 10–20% of CTCL patients, the disease may spread to extra-cutaneous sites such as lymph nodes, peripheral blood, and occasionally other organs (lungs, spleen, liver, and gastrointestinal tract) (2,9,11–13).

Besides this classical presentation, MF can present in many different ways which may produce diagnostic difficulties. For example, bullous (14), follicular (15,16), subcutaneous (17,18), granulomatous (19), hyperkeratotic (12,20) hyper-(21) or hypopigmented (22) forms of MF have been reported.

Sézary syndrome is a leukemic variant of CTCL characterized by erythroderma with scaling, edematous swelling of the skin ("anasarca"), alopecia, onychodystro-phy, palmoplantar hyperkeratosis excessive itching (10), and even pain (11,23,24). There is prominent lymphadenopathy. The diagnostic criteria recently have been redefined by the International Society of Cutaneous Lymphomas (25).

CBCL present from the beginning with infiltrated plaques, nodules, or tumors without scaling or ulceration and are usually confined to one body area. The head and neck area seems to be preferentially involved (8).

REFERENCES

1. Jorg B, Kerl H, Thiers BH, Brocker EB, Burg G. Therapeutic approaches in cutaneous lymphoma. Dermatol Clin 1994; 12:433–441.
2. Duvic M. Current treatment of cutaneous T-cell lymphoma. Dermatol Online J 2001; 7:3.
3. Tuyp E, Burgoyne A, Aitchison T, MacKie R. A case–control study of possible causative factors in mycosis fungoides. Arch Dermatol 1987; 123:196–200.

4. Whittemore AS, Holly EA, Lee IM, Abel EA, Adams RM, Nickoloff BJ, Bley L, Peters JM, Gibney C. Mycosis fungoides in relation to environmental exposures and immune response: a case–control study. J Natl Cancer Inst 1989; 81:1560–1567.

5. Wood GS, Salvekar A, Schaffer J, Crooks CF, Henghold W, Fivenson DP, Kim YH, Smoller BR. Evidence against a role for human T-cell lymphotrophic virus type I (HTLV-I) in the pathogenesis of American cutaneous T-cell lymphoma. J Invest Dermatol 1996; 107:301–307.

6. Olsen EA, Delzell E, Jegasothy BV. Second malignancies in cutaneous T cell lymphoma. J Am Acad Dermatol 1984.

7. Kantor AF, Curtis RE, Vonderheid EC, van Scott EJ, Fraumeni JJ. Risk of second malignancy after cutaneous T-cell lymphoma. Cancer 1989; 63:1612–1615.

8. Burg G, Kempf W, Heaeffner AC, Nestle FO, Hess Schmid M, Doebbeling U, Mueller B, Dummer R. Cutaneous lymphomas. Curr Problems Dermatol 1997; 9:137–204.

9. van Doorn R, Van Haselen CW, van Voorst Vader PC, Geerts ML, Heule F, de Rie M, Steijlen PM, Dekker SK, van Vloten WA, Willemze R. Mycosis fungoides: disease evolution and prognosis of 309 Dutch patients. Arch Dermatol 2000; 136:504–510.

10. Scarisbrick JJ, Whittaker S, Evans AV, Fraser-Andrews EA, Child FJ, Dean A, Russell-Jones R. Prognostic significance of tumor burden in the blood of patients with erythrodermic primary cutaneous T-cell lymphoma. Blood 2001; 97:624–630.

11. Koh HK, Charif M, Weinstock MA. Epidemiology and clinical manifestations of cutaneous T-cell lymphoma. Hematol Oncol Clin North Am 1995; 9:943–960.

12. Burg G, Braun-Falco O. Cutaneous Lymphomas, Pseudolymphomas, and Related Disorders. Berlin, Heidelberg, New York, Tokyo: Springer, 1983.

13. Vonderheid EC, Zhang Q, Lessin SR, Polansky M, Abrams JT, Bigler RD, Wasik MA. Use of serum soluble interleukin-2 receptor levels to monitor the progression of cutaneous T-cell lymphoma. J Am Acad Dermatol 1998; 38:207–220.

14. Maeda K, Jimbow K, Takahashi M. Association of vesiculobullous eruptions with mycosis fungoides. Dermatologica 1987; 174:34–38.

15. Lacour JP, Castanet J, Perrin C, Ortonne JP. Follicular mycosis fungoides. a clinical and histologic variant of cutaneous T-cell lymphoma: report of two cases. J Am Acad Dermatol 1993.

16. Goldenhersh MA, Zlotogorski A, Rosenmann E. Follicular mycosis fungoides. Am J Dermatopathol 1994; 16:52–55.

17. Proctor MS, Price NM, Cox AJ, Hoppe RT. Subcutaneous mycosis fungoides. Arch Dermatol 1978; 114:1326–1328.

18. Whitbeck EG, Spiers AS, Hussain M. Mycosis fungoides: subcutaneous and visceral tumors, orbital involvement, and ophthalmoplegia. J Clin Oncol 1983; 1:270–276.

19. Argenyi ZB, Goeken JA, Piette WW, Madison KC. Granulomatous mycosis fungoides.Clinicopathologic study of two cases. Am J Dermatopathol 1992; 14:200–210.

20. Price NM, Fuks ZY, Hoffman TE. Hyperkeratotic and verrucous features of mycosis fungoides. Arch Dermatol 1977; 113:57–60.

21. David M, Shanon A, Hazaz B, Sandbank M. Diffuse, progressive hyperpigmentation: an unusual skin manifestation of mycosis fungoides. J Am Acad Dermatol 1987.

22. Lambroza E, Cohen SR, Phelps R, Lebwohl M, Braverman IM, DiCostanzo D. Hypopigmented variant of mycosis fungoides: demography, histopathology, and treatment of seven cases. J Am Acad Dermatol 1995; 32:987–993.

23. Sezary A, Bouvrain Y. Erythrodermie avecpresence de cellules monstueuses dansle dermeetlesang circulant. Bull Soc Fr Dermatol Syphiligr 1938; 45:254–260.

24. Ralfkiaer E, Wantzin GL, Larsen JK, Andersen V, Geisler C, Plesner T, Thomsen K. Sezary syndrome: phenotypic and functional characterization of the neoplastic cells. Scand J Haematol 1985; 34:385–393.

25. Vonderheid EC, Bernengo MG, Burg G, Duvic M, Heald P, Laroche L, Olsen E, Pittelkow M, Russell-Jones R, Takigawa M, Willemze R. Update on erythrodermic cutaneous T-cell lymphoma: report of the International Society for Cutaneous Lymphomas. J Am Acad Dermatol 2002; 46:95–106.

11

Clinical Staging of Cutaneous Lymphomas

Monika Hess Schmid, Günter Burg, Sonja Michaelis, and Werner Kempf
Department of Dermatology, University Hospital, Zürich, Switzerland

Traditionally, CL are defined as extranodal non-Hodgkin's lymphomas that present in the skin without any signs of extracutaneous disease for a period of at least 6 months after initial staging. Recently, this definition has been criticized. It may be more appropriate to diagnose CL based only on results of initial staging, not on the time course.

Secondary involvement of the skin by primary extracutaneous lymphoma or leukemia, which can be observed in approximately 10% of all B-cell lymphomas, is designated as secondary CL.

Stage of the disease at diagnosis is the most important prognostic factor in CTCL. Various staging protocols have been employed. Because extracutaneous involvement usually occurs late in CTCL, special emphasis has to be placed on the evaluation of skin involvement (e.g., T according to the TNM classification) (Table 1) or the tumor burden index (TBI) (Table 2) to determine the long-term prognosis. We recommend repeating the staging procedures every year after the initial staging to ensure that any extracutaneous involvement is detected (1).

CLASSICAL ALIBERT–BAZIN STAGING

Alibert (2) and Bazin (3) classified MF into three stages: (1) premycotic eczematous stage, not diagnostic on clinical and histologic evaluation, (2) plaque or infiltrate stage, diagnostic on clinical and histologic evaluation, and (3) tumor stage, diagnostic on clinical and histologic evaluation.

TNM STAGING

CTCL may be classified by a modified form of the tumor-node-metastasis (TNM) staging system as devised by the Mycosis Fungoides Co-operative Group and the National Cancer Institute in 1979 (4). Percentage of skin involvement and qualitative (patch, plaque, tumor) assessment of skin involvement (T1–4) in conjunction with the presence or absence of lymph node (N0–3) or visceral organ involvement (M0–1) is the base for this classification (5,6) (Table 1). The T1–4 stages are based

Table 1 TNM Classification

Stage	T	N	M
Ia	1	0	0
Ib	2	0	0
IIa	1,2	1	0
IIb	3	0,1	0
III	4	0,1	0
IVa	1–4	2,3	0
IVb	1–4	0–3	1

T1, limited lesions covering <10% of the skin surface.
T2, generalized lesions covering 10% and more of the skin surface.
T3, tumors, one or more.
T4, generalized erythroderma.
N0, no palpable lymph nodes, pathology negative for CTCL.
N1, palpable peripheral lymph nodes, pathology negative for CTCL.
N2, no palpable peripheral lymph nodes, pathology positive for CTCL.
N3, palpable peripheral lymph nodes, pathology positive for CTCL.
M0, no involvement of visceral organs.
M1, involvement of visceral organs.
Source: From Ref. 4.

on a heterogenous qualitative and quantitative criteria (7,8). Involvement of peripheral blood is not a major criterion in this staging system even though recently
included (9). Zackheim et al. (10) showed in a study with 489 patients that the relative survival of CTCL patients (MF and Sézary) worsens with increasing skin stage.
The 10-year survival in T1 patients is comparable to that of the general population;
in T2 patients, 67.4%; in T3 patients, 39.2%; and in T4 patients, 41%. The great
majority (80–85%) of patients with CTCL do not die from their disease.

TUMOR BURDEN INDEX

An alternative approach for the assessment of prognosis is to determine the tumor
mass using the TBI. The calculation of the TBI is based on the rough clinical estimation of tumor mass obtained by multiplying the percentage of body surface involved
by patches, plaques, and tumors by weighted factors. The procedure for calculating
the TBI is given in Table 2. In a study based on the material collected by the EORTC
between 1975 and 1995, whole body mapping of the skin lesions was performed in
116 patients with CTCL. Both the T stage according to TNM classification and
the TBI were determined. Tumor burden index allowed better discrimination of
survival than TNM staging (11) (Fig. 1).

Table 2 Procedure for Calculation of Tumor Burden Index (TBI) in Cutaneous T-Cell
Lymphomas

$1 + (2 \times 0$ [if patches $< 30\%$] or $\times 1$ [if patches $> 30\%$]) $+ (2 \times 0$ [if no plaques are present]
or $\times 1$ [if plaques are present]) $+ (1.3 \times 0$ [if no tumor present] or $\times 1$ [if any tumor/s present])

[a]According to Hess Schmid et al.(11); range 1–6.3.

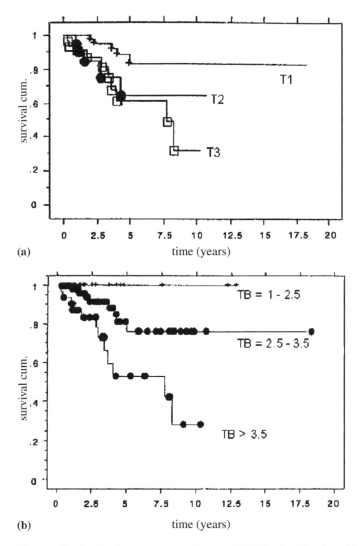

Figure 1 Survival curves according to TNM classification (a) and tumor burden index (TB) (b).

So far, there is no uniformly accepted system for staging of BCL confined to the skin. Attempts have been made according to TNM, taking into account the number of lesions and spread of the disease (7,12). For BCL with secondary skin involvement, the Ann Arbor staging of nodal lymphomas has to be applied (13).

Examples

1. Patient with patches covering about 20% of body surface and two plaques and three tumors has a TBI of $1 + (2 \times 0) + (2 \times 1) + (1.3 \times 1) = 0 + 2 + 1.3 = 4.3$.

2. Patient with patches covering about 40% of body surface and three plaques and four tumors has a TBI of $1 + (2 \times 1) + (2 \times 1) + (1.3 \times 1) = 1 + 2 + 2 + 1.3 = 6.3$.

REFERENCES

1. Dummer R. [Cutaneous lymphomas. Quality Assurance Committee of the German Society of Dermatology and the Professional Organization of German Dermatologists e. V.]. Hautarzt 1998; 48(suppl 1):S49–S55.
2. Alibert JLM. Tableau du pian fongoide. Description des maladies de la peau, observées à l'Hôpital Saint-Louis et exposition des meilleurs méthodes suivies pour leur traitement. Paris: Barrois L'Aîné & Fils, 1806.
3. Bazin A. Leçons sur le traitement des maladies chroniques en général, affections de la peau en particulier, par l'emploi comparé des eaux minérales, de l'hydrothérapie et des moyens pharmaceutiques. Delahaye: Paris, 1870.
4. Bunn PA Jr, Lamberg SI. Report of the Committee on Staging and Classification of Cutaneous T-Cell Lymphomas. Cancer Treat Rep 1979; 63:725–728.
5. Clendenning WE, Rappaport HW. Report of the Committee on Pathology of Cutaneous T Cell Lymphomas. Cancer Treat Rep 1979; 63:719–724.
6. Lamberg SI, Bunn PJ. Proceedings of the Workshop on Cutaneous T-Cell Lymphomas (Mycosis Fungoides and Sezary Syndrome). Introduction. Cancer Treat Rep 1979; 63:561–564.
7. Burg G, Braun-Falco O. Cutaneous Lymphomas, Pseudolymphomas, and Related Disorders. Berlin, Heidelberg, New York,Tokyo: Springer, 1983.
8. Bunn PJ, Huberman MS, Whang PJ, Schechter GP, Guccion JG, Matthews MJ, Gazdar AF, Dunnick NR, Fischmann AB, Ihde DC, Cohen MH, Fossieck B, Minna JD. Prospective staging evaluation of patients with cutaneous T-cell lymphomas. Demonstration of a high frequency of extracutaneous dissemination. Ann Intern Med 1980; 93:223–230.
9. Vonderheid EC, Bernengo MG, Burg G, Duvic M, Heald P, Laroche L, Olscn E, Pittelkow M, Russell-Jones R, Takigawa M, Willemze R. Update on erythrodermic cutaneous T-cell lymphoma: report of the International Society for Cutaneous Lymphomas. J Am Acad Dermatol 2002; 46:95–106.
10. Zackheim HS, Amin S, Kashani-Sabet M, McMillan A. Prognosis in cutaneous T-cell lymphoma by skin stage: long-term survival in 489 patients. J Am Acad Dermatol 1999; 40:418–425.
11. Hess Schmid M, Bird P, Dummer R, Kempf W, Burg G. Tumor burden index as a prognostic tool for cutaneous T-cell lymphoma: a new concept. Arch Dermatol 1999; 135:1204–1208.
12. Burg G, Kerl H, Przybilla B, Braun-Falco O. Some statistical data, diagnosis, and staging of cutaneous B-cell lymphomas. J Dermatol Surg Oncol 1984; 10:256–262.
13. Carbone PP, Kaplan HS, Musshoff K, Smithers DW, Tubiana Mp. Report of the Committee on Hodgkin's Disease Staging Classification. Cancer Res 1971; 31:1860–1861.

12

Laboratory Investigations

Monika Hess Schmid, Günter Burg, and Werner Kempf
Department of Dermatology, University Hospital, Zürich, Switzerland

SKIN BIOPSIES

Multiple skin biopsies for both formalin fixation and paraffin embedding and for snap freezing should be obtained. Immunophenotyping can usually be done on formalin-fixed and parffin-embedded tissue. Fresh frozen tissue is optimal for detection of clonality as well as for other molecular biologic studies.

LYMPH NODE AND BONE MARROW BIOPSIES

Extracutaneous disease must be excluded by a lymph node biopsy if there are palpable lymph nodes. The likelihood of significant node involvement in patients with nonpalpable nodes is low, therefore blind lymph node biopsy is rather not indicated (1).

There is no need for taking bone marrow biopsy in the early stages of low-grade malignant CTCL; however, in advanced stages a bone marrow biopsy is advisable; for B-cell lymphomas a bone marrow biopsy is mandatory.

BLOOD TESTS

A complete blood cell count is performed placing particular emphasis on lymphocyte count, eosinophil count, and pathological evaluation of peripheral smear. Automated evaluation of lymphocyte morphology is often not sufficient for the detection of abnormal lymphocytes in the peripheral blood.

A peripheral blood smear is used to count the number of Sézary cells, but there has been no consensus on the percentage of Sézary cells required for the diagnosis. Circulating Sézary cells were originally identified by Sézary in 1938 as large atypical mononuclear cells (2), many years later the distinctive grooved nuclei were described. Large Sézary cells greater than 14 μm are specific to Sézary syndrome, but smaller cells may also be present in patients with MF or even with certain inflammatory dermatoses (3). Vonderheid et al. (4) reported that a Sézary cell

53

count of greater than 15% was seldom found in benign diseases. Kim et al. (5) have shown that in erythrodermic CTCL, the presence of more than 5% Sézary cells in peripheral blood is an independent prognostic factor for survival. Russell-Jones and Whittaker (6) proposed that the detection of T-cell clonality and the presence of 5% Sézary cells in the peripheral blood are sufficient for the diagnosis of Sézary syndrome.

An absolute Sézary cell count of 1000 cells/mm^3, originally proposed by Winkelmann and Peters (7) as diagnostic criterion, has been recently adopted by the International Society for Cutaneous Lymphoma (ISCL) in their consensus conference on erythrodermic CTCL (8). The hematologic criteria recommended by the ISCL for the diagnosis of Sézary syndrome consist of one or more of the following criteria (9): (1) an absolute Sézary cell count of 1000 cells/mm^3 or more; (2) a CD 4/CD 8 ratio of 10 or higher caused by an increase in circulating T cells and/or an aberrant loss or expression of pan-T-cell markers by flow cytometry; (3) increased lymphocyte counts with evidence of a T-cell clone in the blood by the Southern blot or polymerase chain reaction technique; or (4) a chromosomally abnormal T-cell clone (9).

A *flow cytometry* panel should include CD 4, CD 8, and CD 45 RO. The CD 4/CD 8 ratio can detect disease in the peripheral blood (8,10). The elevated ratio is due to the malignant CD 4 cells entering the peripheral blood (11). Any elevation of the ratio or of CD 45 RO positive cells should be followed by gene rearrangement studies. A CD 4:CD 8 ratio of greater than 10 has been proposed by the EORTC group for defining Sézary syndrome (12).

The peripheral blood should be screened for mononuclear cells with *aberrant T-cell antigen expression* and for *clonal TCR gene rearrangement*. Scarisbrick et al. (8) have shown that the presence of a peripheral blood T-cell clone is an independent factor for survival in patients with T1–T3 stage disease. The presence of a circulating T-cell clone identical to the dominant T-cell clone in the skin provides an additional criterion for CTCL diagnosis. The peripheral blood analysis is most useful when the histologic diagnosis is nonspecific and PCR analysis of the cutaneous biopsy specimen yields positive results (13).

Several studies have shown that the serum concentration of soluble alpha-chain of the *interleukin-2 receptor* (*sIL-2R*) in CTCL correlates well with the disease stage (14–18). The serum *lactate dehydrogenase* level (LDH) increases progressively with stage (8), a rise in serum LDH to more than 10% of the normal value has been found to be a poor prognostic factor in MF and Sézary Syndrome (19). Compared with LDH, sIL-2R seems more sensitive to clinically relevant changes in disease stage (20).

Additional investigations include liver and renal chemistry, electrolytes, and serum electrophoresis. In CBCL cases, an immunoelectropheresis (serum and urine) should be performed (21).

RADIOLOGIC TESTS

Additional investigations include chest x-ray evaluation, sonography of the abdomen, and peripheral lymph nodes. Computed tomography scanning of the abdomen and peripheral lymph nodes is useful in patients with advanced skin disease and palpable lymphadenopathy for accurate baseline assessment and to document disease progression (1).

REFERENCES

1. Foss FM, Sausville EA. Prognosis and staging of cutaneous T-cell lymphoma. Hematol Oncol Clin North Am 1995; 9:1011–1019.
2. Sézary A, Bouvrain Y. Erythrodermie avecpresence de cellules monstueuses dansle dermeetlesang circulant. Bull Soc Fr Dermatol Syphiligr 1938; 45:254–260.
3. Schechter GP, Sausville EA, Fischmann AB, Soehnlen F, Eddy J, Matthews M, Gazdar A, Guccion J, Munson D, Makuchal R. Evaluation of circulating malignant cells provides prognostic information in cutaneous T cell lymphoma. Blood 1987; 69:841–849.
4. Vonderheid EC, Sobel EL, Nowell PC, Finan JB, Helfrich MK, Whipple DS. Diagnostic and prognostic significance of Sézary cells in peripheral blood smears from patients with cutaneous T cell lymphoma. Blood 1985; 66:358–366.
5. Kim YH, Bishop K, Varghese A, Hoppe RT. Prognostic factors in erythrodermic mycosis fungoides and the Sézary syndrome. Arch Dermatol 1995; 131:1003–1008.
6. Russell-Jones R, Whittaker S. T-cell receptor gene analysis in the diagnosis of Sézary syndrome. J Am Acad Dermatol 1999; 41:254–259.
7. Winkelmann RK, Peters MS. Absolute number of circulatory Sézary cells. Arch Dermatol 1981;117.
8. Scarisbrick JJ, Whittaker S, Evans AV, Fraser-Andrews EA, Child FJ, Dean A, Russell-Jones R. Prognostic significance of tumor burden in the blood of patients with erythrodermic primary cutaneous T-cell lymphoma. Blood 2001; 97:624–630.
9. Vonderheid EC, Bernengo MG, Burg G, Duvic M, Heald P, Laroche L, Olsen E, Pittelkow M, Russell-Jones R, Takigawa M, Willemze R. Update on erythrodermic cutaneous T-cell lymphoma: report of the International Society for Cutaneous Lymphomas. J Am Acad Dermatol 2002; 46:95–106.
10. Duvic M. Current treatment of cutaneous T-cell lymphoma. Dermatol Online J 2001; 7:3.
11. Yan SL, Heald PW. Flow cytometry in the evaluation of dermatology patients. Clin Dermatol 1991; 9:149–156.
12. Willemze R, Kerl H, Sterry W, Berti E, Cerroni L, Chimenti S, Diaz Perez JL, Geerts ML, Goos M, Knobler R, Ralfkiaer E, Santucci M, Smith N, Wechsler J, van Vloten WA, Meijer CJ. EORTC classification for primary cutaneous lymphomas: a proposal from the Cutaneous Lymphoma Study Group of the European Organization for Research and Treatment of Cancer. Blood 1997; 90:354–371.
13. Delfau-Larue MH, Laroche L, Wechsler J, Lepage E, Lahet C, Asso-Bonnet M, Bagot M, Farcet JP. Diagnostic value of dominant T-cell clones in peripheral blood in 363 patients presenting consecutively with a clinical suspicion of cutaneous lymphoma. Blood 2000; 96:2987–2992.
14. Burg G, Kempf W, Heaeffner AC, Nestle FO, Hess Schmid M, Doebbeling U, Mueller B, Dummer R. Cutaneous lymphomas. Curr Problems Dermatol 1997; 9:137–204.
15. Dummer R, Posseckert G, Nestle F, Witzgall R, Burger M, Becker JC, Schafer E, Wiede J, Sebald W, Burg G. Soluble interleukin-2 receptors inhibit interleukin 2-dependent proliferation and cytotoxicity: explanation for diminished natural killer cell activity in cutaneous T-cell lymphomas in vivo? J Invest Dermatol 1992; 70:2338–2341.
16. Dummer R, Nestle F, Wiede J, Schäfer E, Röger J, Erhard H, Hefner H, Burg G. Coincidence of increased soluble interleukin-2 receptors, diminished natural killer cell activity and progressive disease in cutaneous T-cell lymphomas. Eur J Dermatol 1991; 1:135–138.
17. Szeimies RM, Rueff F, Kaudewitz P. Soluble interleukin-2 receptor serum levels in mycosis fungoides. Correlation with clinical stage. Cancer 1992; 98:50–54.
18. Neish C, Charlry M, Jegasothy B, Tharp M, Deng JS. Proliferation cell nuclear antigen, soluble interleukin 2 receptor levels in cutaneous T cell lymphoma: correlation with advanced clinical diseases. J Dermatol Sci 1994; 8:11–17.
19. Diamandidou E, Colome M, Fayad L, Duvic M, Kurzrock R. Prognostic factor analysis in mycosis fungoides/Sézary syndrome. J Am Acad Dermatol 1999; 40:914–924.

20. Vonderheid EC, Zhang Q, Lessin SR, Polansky M, Abrams JT, Bigler RD, Wasik MA. Use of serum soluble interleukin-2 receptor levels to monitor the progression of cutaneous T-cell lymphoma. J Am Acad Dermatol 1998; 38:207–220.
21. Dummer R. Cutaneous lymphomas. Quality Assurance Committee of the German Society of Dermatology and the Professional Organization of German Dermatologists e. V. Hautarzt 1998; 48(suppl 1):S49–S55.

13

Immunohistochemistry and Phenotypic Features

Werner Kempf, Dmitry V. Kazakov, and Günter Burg
Department of Dermatology, University Hospital, Zürich, Switzerland

INTRODUCTION

In respect to the concept of nosologic entities as defined by recent lymphoma classifications the diagnostic evaluation of primary cutaneous lymphomas includes the integration of clinical, morphological, phenotypic, and molecular characteristics. Several studies have demonstrated that the diagnostic accuracy employing clinical and histological features alone ranges from 50% to 75%, but reaches 80% when morphologic features are combined with the immunophenotypic or genotypic characterization of tumor cells (1). Immunohistochemical (IHC) identification of the tumor cell phenotype plays such a crucial and invaluable role in the diagnostic work-up of cutaneous lymphoma (CL) that it can be regarded as a mandatory step in establishing the correct diagnosis (2). Moreover, several forms of CL such as cytotoxic lymphomas can only be correctly identified by phenotyping. On the other hand, identical phenotypes and cytomorphologic changes can be seen in clinically and prognostically different CL. Thus, the final diagnosis has always to be based on integrative synopsis of all clinical, histopathological, IHC, and molecular biological findings.

During the last decade, almost all antibodies necessary for adequate classification of CL became commercially available and applicable for archival, i.e., formalin-fixed and paraffin-embedded tissue (3,4). Performing IHC in CL, one has to be aware of various pitfalls and practical aspects (5). There is a need for standardization of IHC to facilitate comparison between different laboratories and antibodies.

Table 1 lists a set of the antibodies, which are useful for the diagnosis of the vast majority of CL. The diagnostic value of these antibodies and some of the pitfalls of IHC will be discussed in the balance of this section.

TECHNICAL ASPECTS OF IMMUNOPHENOTYPING IN CUTANEOUS LYMPHOMAS

The most commonly used technique for IHC is an immune complex method with an enzyme antibody conjugate. Alternatively, biotin and streptavidine can be used. For

Table 1 Antigens and Antibodies, Respectively, for Diagnostic Work-Up and
Differentiation of Cutaneous Lymphoproliferative Disorder

Antigen (CD)	Antibody	Specificity
CD2	Leu5, OKTll	T-lymphocytes
CD3	Leu4, OKT3	Mature thymocytes, peripheral T-lymphocytes
CD4	Leu3, OKT4	Helper/inducer T-cells, some macrophages
CD5	Leul, OKT1, Lyt2	T-lymphocytes; less than 5% of B-lymphocytes
CD7	Leu9, WTl	T-lymphocytes
CD8	Leu2, OKT8	NK cells, suppressor/cytotoxic T-cells
CD19		B-cells
CD20		B-cells
CD21	CR2	Follicular dendritic cells
CD30	Kil, BerH2	Reed–Sternberg cells, Hodgkin cells, large cell anaplastic lymphoma, plasma cells
CD 43	MT-1	T-lymphocytes, monocytes, myeloid cells
CD45RO	UCHL-1	T-lymphocytes, monocytes, myeloid cells
CD56	NCAM	NK cells
CD79a		B-cells

visualization, chromogens are processed by the enzymes horseradish peroxidase or alkaline phosphatase. In our experience, red products are easier to differentiate from melanin or other brownish pigments often found in skin biopsies. To increase sensitivity and for double staining, additional use of fluorescent probes is of value. When performing IHC, antigen retrieval methods are often needed to get satisfying results. Those methods include preheating (e.g., pressure cooker or microwave heating) in various buffers, or enzymatic predigestion with proteolytic enzymes such as trypsin or protease. If possible, recently cut slides should be used for IHC, since storage of mounted but unstained slides leads to deterioration of tissue and thus of antigens; this may lead to false-negative results.

A PRACTICAL STEPWISE APPROACH TO CUTANEOUS LYMPHOMAS

In the first step, a small panel of antibodies directed against T- and B-cells including CD3, CD45RO (UCHL-1), CD20 (or alternatively CD19 or CD22), CD79a, and CD56 may be applied to confirm the tumor cell lineage, i.e. T-, or B-, or NK-cell origin of the neoplasm.

CTCL AND CYTOTOXIC LYMPHOMAS

The expression of CD3, CD43, and CD45RO points to T-cell lineage. The majority of CTCL such as classic forms of mycosis fungoides (MF) and Sezary syndrome (SS) display a T helper cell-phenotype (CD4+, CD8−, CD56−). Often, loss of some pan-T-cell markers such as CD2, CD7, and CD5 is found in CTCL.

If tumor cells do not express a T helper phenotype, but still do express CD3 as a pan-T-cell marker, one should consider the presence of a cytotoxic lymphoma of either cytotoxic T-cell (CD4−, CD8+, CD56−) or T/NK-cell (CD3+, CD8−, CD56+, CD4±) phenotype. This is of particular importance, since CD8+ epidermotropic CTCL have been described which show a predominantly intraepidermal clone of small CD8+ T-cells, whereas the CD4+ cells represent reactive T-cells mostly located around the upper vascular plexus. Demonstration of cytotoxic molecules such as TIA-1, perforin, and granzyme B are additional useful markers to confirm the cytotoxic phenotype of tumor cells. Occasionally, only reactive small lymphocytes may exhibit a T-cell phenotype, whereas tumor cells seem negative for T- and B-cell markers. Those mostly medium-sized to large-cell pleomorphic CL often are so-called "true natural killer (NK) cell lymphomas" with a CD3−, CD4±, CD8+, but CD56+ or CD57+ phenotype. Often these lesions represent secondary cutaneous involvement. Further differentiation of CL with cytotoxic phenotypes includes evaluation for additional markers such as CD57 and CD16. In addition, CD33 and myeloperoxidase (MPO) should be included in the antibody panel when evaluating skin infiltrates expressing NK-associated molecules. Although CD33 and MPO are associated with myeloid differentiation, they are also expressed on bipotential T/NK precursor cells. Therefore, the evaluation of these markers is important to rule out skin involvement by myeloid leukemia or blastic NK cell lymphoma/leukemia (Table 2).

CD30-POSITIVE LYMPHOPROLIFERATIVE DISEASES

Neoplasms with predominately pleomorphic or anaplastic morphology must be evaluated for CD30 expression, since CD30+ CTCL have a much more favorable prognosis than CD30-negative forms (90% vs. 60% 5-yr-survival rates) (6). Several particular phenotypes can be observed in CD30+ lymphoproliferative disorders of the skin (CD30+ LPD). Lymphomatoid papulosis (LyP) usually has a CD4+, CD8−, but TIA-1+ expression pattern. CD30 expression may be absent in the rare histologic type B of LyP simulating histologically MF. Weak expression of CD3 is found in some cases of anaplastic or pleomorphic large-cell lymphomas. Some variants of CD30+ LPD like neutrophil-rich anaplastic large cell lymphoma (ALCL) or sarcomatoid ALCL can only be identified by immunohistochemistry as lymphoid neoplasms. On the other hand, various inflammatory disorders have been reported to harbor atypical CD30+ lymphoid cells such as scabies, molluscum contagiosum, and herpesvirus infections. Thus, the detection of atypical CD30+ cells in an infiltrate is not by itself diagnostic for LyP or another CD30+ LPD. Moreover, the detection of CD30 antigen strongly depends on the antigen retrieval method. In our experience, the combination of heating and enzymatic digest may result in too strong staining results. Moreover, plasma cells express CD30 constitutively, and should not be confused with the large anaplastic tumor cells in CD30+ LPD. Thus, CD30 expression should always be evaluated in respect to cytomorphology (small or pleomorphic cells) and staining pattern. In CD30+ LPD, tumor cells exhibit a membrane-bound signal and perinuclear dot corresponding to the Golgi apparatus. Strong diffuse cytoplasmic staining may indicate too intense antigen retrieval or even nonspecific staining. Therefore, staining results should be correlated with that from other laboratories. Expression of ALK protein has to be regarded as a strong indicator for a secondary cutaneous large T-cell lymphoma, which usually has an

Table 2 Immunohistochemical Markers in NK Cell Neoplasms

Markers	Extranodal T/NK-cell-lymphoma	Blastic NK lymphoma/leukemia	Aggressive NK cell leukemia	Myeloid leukemia (AML)	Myeloid/NK cell precursor acute leukemia
CD3, CD56, CD57	sCD3−, CD3A+ CD56+, CD57−	CD3−, CD4+ CD56+, CD57−	sCD3−, CD3e++ CD56+, CD57−	sCD3−, CD56+ (20%), CD57−	sCD3−, CD56+, CD57−
CD33, CD16	CD33−, CD16−	CD33−, CD16−	CD33−, CD16±	CD33+, CD 16−	CD33+, CD16−
MPO	Negative	Negative	Negative	Unknown	Positive
Other	CD2+, CD4−, CD5−TdT−, CD7∓	CD123+, TdT± CD34−, MPO−	CD2+, CD15± CD5−, CD11b±	CD34± coexpression of CD43 and CD74	CD34−, CD15±
HLA-DR	HLA-DR−	HLA-DR+	HLA-DR+	HLA-DR−	HLA-DR±
Cytotoxic	Positive	Variable	Positive	Negative	Negative
IL-2R (CD25)	Negative	Negative	Positive	Unknown	Negative

Table 3 Expression of Differentiation and Activation Markers in Various CD30+ LPD

Disorder	CD30	CD15	CD45RO	ALK	EMA	HOXC5
LyP	+	∓ (50%?)	+	−	−	n.a.
1° cut. ALCL	+	−	+	− (rarely +)	−	++
2° cut. ALCL (syst. ALCL)	+	∓ (HD-like ALCL +!)	−	+ (65%)	+	∓
HL	+	+	−	−	−	n.a.

Abbreviations: LyP, lymphomatoid papulosis; ALCL, anaplastic large-cell lymphoma; HL, Hodgkin lymphoma; EMA, epithelial membrane antigen.

unfavorable prognosis. The final diagnosis must also incorporate the results of staging examinations. Table 3 gives an overview on expression of differentiation and activation markers in various CD30+ LPD which should be helpful for differential diagnostic purposes.

CBCL AND B-CELL PSEUDOLYMPHOMA

Lymphoid cells of B-cell lineage express CD20 in most cases. CD19, CD22, and CD79a are also useful to verify the B-cell type. Follicular structures can be easily demonstrated by the presence of CD21-positive follicular dendritic cells (FDC) forming networks engulfing germinal center cells such as centroblasts and centrocytes. CD138 antigen is useful for identification of plasma cell differentiation. Immunophenotypic features of mature B-cell neoplasms are summarized in Table 4. Often, a relatively high number of reactive small T-lymphocytes can be found in CBCL. One of the most vexing problems in dermatopathology is differentiation of B-cell pseudolymphoma (B-PSL) from a low grade malignant B-cell lymphoma. Apart from clinical and histologic features, the presence of irregularly structured- networks of CD21+ FDC, the monoclonal expression of immunoglobulin light chains kappa and lambda, and the coexpression of CD20 and CD43 on tumor cells argues for the presence of CBCL, but does not absolutely exclude B-PSL (Fig. 1A and B). Immunohistochemical markers applied for differentiation of follicular center cell lymphoma from pseudolymphoma are listed in Table 5 .

Although the clinical manifestations and cellular composition are the most important factors in determining the classification of CBCL, IHC is very useful in identifying subtypes. Whereas tumor cells express CD20 in follicle center cell lymphoma (FCCL) and marginal zone lymphoma, they are negative for CD20 in both plasmacytoma and pre-B lymphoblastic lymphoma, which is also positive for TdT. Bcl-2 is often found in nodal FCCL, but only in a minority cases of primary cutaneous FCCL and in a subset of diffuse large B-cell lymphomas (7). CD5 can be found in infiltrates of B-cell chronic lymphocytic leukemia (B-CLL), but not in primary CBCL with the exception for rare cases of diffuse large B-cell lymphoma (DLBCL). KiMlp with its characteristic granular staining pattern is exhibited by monocytoid B-cells in MZL. Occasionally, CD30+ blasts resembling centroblasts are present in the germinal centers of FCCL and 172L. Although IHC provides useful information, the final diagnosis in CBCL must also consider all clinical, histologic, phenotypic, and genotypic features and not rely on one single criterion.

Table 4 Mature B-Cell Neoplasms Involving the Skin

Tumor	CD20, CD79	CD5, CD10, CD23,	CD21	bcl-2, bcl-6	Other
FCCL	CD20+, CD79a+	CD5−, CD10∓, CD23±	NF+, RF∓	GC: bcl-2∓, bcl-6+	sIg+, sIgD±
MZL	CD20+, CD79a+	CD5−, CD10−, CD23−	RF+, NF+ FDC+	RF: bcl-2−, bcl-6+ MZC bcl-2+, bcl-6−	sIg±, KiMlp±
Im	CD20+, CD79a+	CD5−, CD10−, CD23−	CD21−	Unknown	sIgM+
DLBCL	CD20+, CD79a+	CD5∓, CD10−, CD23∓	CD21−	LL: bcl-2+; bcl-6±	sIg+
PI	CD20−, CD79a+	CD5−, CD10∓, CD23−	CD21−	NR	sIg+, CLA−, CK+, CD38+, CD138+
MCL		CD5+, CD 10−, CD23−	FDC~	bcl-6−	sIgM > sIgD+, cyclin DI+, FMC7+, CD43+
BL	CD20+, CD79a+	CD5−, CD10+, CD23−	CD21∓(E)	bcl-2+, bcl-6+	Ki-67 (~100%)
B-CLL	CD20+,CD79 a+	CD5+, CD10−, CD23+	NR	NR	SIgM∓, cyclin DI−, FMC7−
B-PLL	CD20+, CD79a+	CD5∓, CD23−	NR	NR	sIgM+, sIgD+, FMC7+
HCL	CD20+, CD79a+	CD5−, CD10−, CD23−	NR	NR	SIg+ CD11c+, CD25+, FMC7+, CD103+, TRAP+

Abbreviations: FCCL, follicular center cell lymphoma; MZL, marginal zone lymphoma; Im, immunocytoma: DLBCL, diffuse large B-cell lymphoma; Pl, plasmacytoma; MCL, mantle cell lymphoma; BL, Burkitt lymphoma; B-CLL, B-cell chronic lymphacytic leukemia; B-PCL, B cell prolymphocytic leukemia; HCL, hairy cell leukemia; NF, neoplastic follicles; RF, reactive follicles; FDC+, extended networks of follicular dendritic cells; FDC~loose networks of follicular dendritic cells; GC, germinal center; MZC, marginal zone cells; LL, lower leg; EF, endemic form; NR, not relevant.

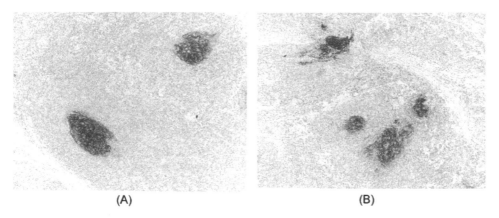

(A)   (B)

Figure 1 CD21 staining in B-cell lymphoproliferative diseases of the skin: regular and well-demarcated networks of CD21-positive FDC in cutaneous B-pseudolymphomas (A) in contrast to irregularly and poorly demarcated networks of FDC in cutaneous B-cell lymphomas (B).

LEUKEMIC INFILTRATES OF THE SKIN

Histologic diagnosis of leukemic infiltrates may be very difficult when based on routine histologic examination and requires IHC phenotyping of tumor cells. Chloroacetate esterase, lysozyme, MPO, CD13, CD33, CD15, CD117, and CD16 are very useful markers, since leukemic infiltrates of monocytic or myelomonocytic origin are variably positive, whereas lymphoid cells are consistently negative for all these markers. The MPO activity in myeloblasts is granular and usually concentrated in the Golgi area. Expression of MPO on monoblasts is variable and seen as scattered fine granules. Lymphoblasts are MPO negative. Further differentiation between AML and acute myelomonocytic leukemia forms required additional staining for various histiocytic/myeloid markers such as CDllb, CDllc, CD14, CD36, CD68, and CD64. Characterization of tumor cells in bone marrow biopsy is crucial to establish diagnosis of the underlying malignancy.

IMMUNOPHENOTYPIC MARKERS AS PROGNOSTIC PARAMETERS

In some cases, there appears to be a correlation between a particular immunophenotype and the prognosis of the associated lymphoma. For example, expression of CD7

Table 5 Immunohistochemistry in Differentiation of Low Grade B-Cell Lymphoma (Marginal Zone Lymphoma, Follicular Center Lymphoma) from B-PSL

Parameters	Low grade B-cell lymphoma	B-PSL
Light chain restriction	Monoclonal, rarely "nonsecreting"	Polyclonal
Bcl-2	Usually negative	Almost always negative
Network of CD21+ FDCs	Irregular	Regular
Proliferation index (Ki-67+)	Low	High (in reactive gemunal centers)
Interfollicular CD10+ cells	Present in 60% of cases	Usually absent

antigen in epidermotropic CD8+ lymphoma is associated with a more favorable prognosis whilst CD8+, CD7– lymphomas run a very aggressive course (8). Expression of CD30 in the group of CD56+ lymphomas is associated with more indolent course.

REFERENCES

1. Burg G, Kempf W, Haeffner AC, Nestle FO, Hess Schmid M, Doebbeling U, Mueller B, Dummer R. Cutaneous lymphomas. Curr Probl Dermatol 1997; 9:137–204.
2. Giannotti B, Pimpinelli N. Modern diagnosis of cutaneous lymphoma. Recent Results Cancer Res 2002; 160:303–306.
3. Cerroni L, Smolle J, Soyer HP, Martinez Aparicio A, Kerl H. Immunophenotyping of cutaneous lymphoid infiltrates in frozen and paraffin-embedded tissue sections: a comparative study. J Am Acad Dermatol 1990; 22:405–413.
4. Ritter JH, Adesokan PN, Fitzgibbon JF, Wick MR. Paraffin section immunohisto-chemistry as an adjunct to morphologic analysis in the diagnosis of cutaneous lymphoid infiltrates. J Cutan Pathol 1994; 21:481–493.
5. Chu PG, Chang KL, Arber DA, Weiss LM. Practical applications of immunohistochem-istry in hematolymphoid neoplasms. Ann Diagn Pathol 1999; 3:104–133.
6. Willemze R, Kerl H, Sterry W, Berti E, Cerroni L, Chimenti S, Diaz Perez JL, Geerts ML, Goos M, Knobler R, Ralfkiaer E, Santucci M, Smith N, Wechsler J, van Vloten WA, Meijer CJ. EORTC classification for primary cutaneous lymphomas: a proposal from the Cutaneous Lymphoma Study Group of the European Organization for Research and Treatment of Cancer. Blood 1997; 90:354–371.
7. Geelen FA, Vermeer MH, Meijer CJ, Van der Putte SC, Kerkhof E, Kluin PM, Willemze R. bcl-2 protein expression in primary cutaneous large B-cell lymphoma is site-related. J Clin Oncol 1998; 16:2080–2085.
8. Agnarsson BA, Vonderheid EC, Kadin ME. Cutaneous T cell lymphoma with suppressor/cytotoxic (CD8) phenotype: identification of rapidly progressive and chronic subtypes. J Am Acad Dermatol 1990; 22:569–577.

14

Genotyping

Udo Döebbeling, Werner Kempf, Antonio Cozzio,
Reinhard Dummer, and Günter Burg
Department of Dermatology, University Hospital, Zürich, Switzerland

Cutaneous T-cell lymphoma (CTCL), especially mycosis fungoides (MF), is often misdiagnosed as eczema or psoriasis. Also in biopsies, T cell infiltrates of early MF are difficult to discern from eczema associated T cell infiltrates. In early stages, CTCL cells have the morphology as normal T-cells and there are no distinctive tumor marker for CTCL cells, which could unambiguously identify the malignant T-cells. Only recently two oncogenes, c-myb and bcl-3, have identified as candidate markers for early CTCL (1), but their expression in T-cells of nonmalignant skin diseases like eczema or psoriasis has not yet been assessed.

A distinctive feature of malignant T-cells is their *clonality*. In an eczematic reaction, the causative antigen is attacked by antigen recognizing T-cells, which derive from many different T-cell clones, as several epitopes of the antigen are recognized and several T-cell clones can recognize an epitope. Malignant T-cells however derive all from a single T-cell clone. In a CTCL, skin infiltrate occur malignant and nonmalignant T-cells, but since the malignant T-cells derive only from one clone, this clone should be the most numerous one.

The malignant clone can be recognized as all its cells express the same T-cell receptor (TCR). During the development of T-cells, the TCR is assembled by V(D)J recombination, i.e., the region coding for the antigen recognizing portion of the TCR is composed by joining different V (variable), D (diversity), and J (joining) DNA-segments. This is one of the main mechanisms, which generate the high diversity of the TCRs of the different T-cells (2). There are four polypeptide chains, which can form a TCR: the alpha, beta, gamma, and delta chain. The alpha and gamma chains are shorter than the beta and delta chains as they contain no D elements (VJ recombination). The alpha chain pairs only with the beta chain, and the gamma chain only with the delta chain. Other combinations do not exist.

The individual members of the V, D, and J segments differ in their DNA sequences and polymerase chain reaction (PCR) with consensus primers can only detect a minority of all combinations. This is especially true for the long beta and delta chains, but also for the alpha chain. Fortunately, the number of V and J elements of the gamma chain is very low, so that depending of the choice of primer sets 90–95% of the possible VJ combinations can be detected (3–5). Since the TCR gamma chain is also rearranged in 90% of T-cells, which display the alpha/beta type

TCR on the surface, these TCR gamma primer sets can also be used for the detection of clonal malignant T-cells, which display the alpha/beta type TCR. Therefore, these primer sets can also be used for the clonality analysis of CTCLs, which mostly display the alpha/beta type TCR on their surface.

THE IDENTIFICATION OF A MALIGNANT T-CELL CLONE BY PCR-DGGE

How can the PCR product from the malignant clone be discerned from the PCR products of nonclonal T-cell after preparation of DNA from suspected CTCL skin lesions and amplification of a portion of the TCR gamma chain? Cutaneous T-cell lymphoma skin lesions contain malignant and nonmalignant cells as well as other cell types like keratinocytes and fibroblasts. The TCR gamma genes of nonlymphoid cells should not yield a PCR product, as the TCR genes are not rearranged in these cell types and the resulting PCR product would be too long to be efficiently synthesized. After gel electrophoresis on a native polyacrylamide gel, a somewhat diffuse band would be found, which consists of the TCR gamma chain products of the malignant and nonmalignant T-cells. However, it is not possible to detect a prominent band that would be diagnostic for the predominant malignant T-cell clone. Thus, an additional step is necessary for its detection and this step is the denaturation and following renaturation of the amplified double-stranded PCR product.

The renaturation products can be separated either by a gel that contains a temperature gradient or denaturing agents like urea and formamide. The resulting methods are therefore called temperature gradient gel electrophoresis (TGGE) and denaturing gradient gel electrophoresis (DGGE). Since the latter method is more popular, we will describe only this method in detail.

For the denaturation of the TCR gamma PCR products, they will be heated at 95°C for 3 min and then slowly cooled down to 60°C. During this time, the denatured single-stranded DNA molecules can renature, however, for the PCR products of the nonclonal T-cells, it will be extremely unlikely to find its original complementary partner. Since all TCR gamma PCR products have some sequences in common, they can partially renature and form partially double-stranded molecules that contain some unpaired single-stranded "bubbles." However, when a TCR gamma PCR reaction contains PCR products from a predominant malignant T-cell clone, a considerable portion of the denatured single strands will find a fully complementary partner. Since these complementary double-stranded molecules are more stable at higher temperatures, they will form during the cooling process before the incompletely complementary molecules appear. Thus, the formation of complementary double-stranded molecules from the malignant T-cell clone is favored over the formation of incompletely double-stranded molecules that derive in their vast majority from nonmalignant T-cells. However, this effect occurs only as long as the malignant clone is significantly more abundant in the biopsy than any other normal T-cell clone.

The completely renatured PCR products are also more resistant to denaturing agents. Thus, in DGGE, gel that contains an increasing gradient of urea and formamide the "bubble" containing PCR products will denature first at lower denaturant concentrations than the fully complementary molecules. Since the latter migrate faster, one will observe on the gel, a distinct band that stems from the fully complementary molecules that is followed by a smear that stems from the "bubble"

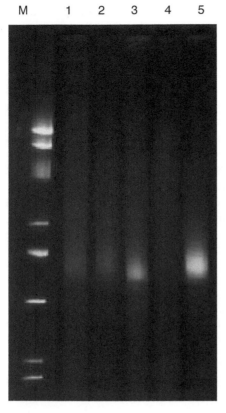

Figure 1 Clonality analysis of different skin biopsies. Lanes 1 and 2: Biopsies from patients with no predominant malignant T-cell clone (no CTCL). Lane 3: Biopsy from a CTCL patient. Lane 4: Peripheral blood lymphocytes from a healthy donor (negative control). Lane 5: MyLa 2059 TCL cell line (positive control).

containing PCR products. In the case that no predominant malignant clone is present in the tested biopsy, only the smear will be visible (Fig. 1).

ADVANTAGES AND LIMITATIONS OF PCR-DGGE

One limitation of this method is that 90% but not all of the alpha/beta TCR type T-cells rearrange their TCR gamma locus during T-cell maturation. Thus, 10% of alpha/beta TCR type T-cell lymphomas cannot be detected by this method. With the initially used consensus primer sets also only 90% of the TCR gamma rearrangements could be detected (4). However, meanwhile new additional primer sets have been developed (5) so that now additional 5% of the TCR gamma rearrangements can be detected.

PCR-DGGE can also detect false positive cases, since it has been shown that 0.5–1% of eczemas prevalent T-clones can be detected, which can mimic the presence of a malignant clone. To see a distinct band on a DGGE gel, a certain minimal amount of the malignant clone is necessary. Dilution experiments with CTCL cell lines and keratinocytes (with a nonrearranged TCR gamma locus) or polyclonal T-cells (with rearranged TCR gamma locus) have shown that to detect the signal of the clonal cells, at least 0.1% of the cells must be monoclonal in the presence of keratinocytes, and at least 1% of the cells must be monoclonal in the presence of polyclonal T-cells (6).

At the beginning, TCR rearrangements have been detected by Southern blotting. In comparison to the Southern blot, PCR-DGGE may have the disadvantage that not all cases may be detectable; however, this method needs 5–10 times less biopsy material (1 μg of extracted DNA for DGGE vs. 5–10 μg DNA for Southern blot) for an analysis and it is at least 2 times faster (1.5 vs. 3–4 days). Since a population of 1% malignant T-cells can be detected in a biopsy, it is approximately 5 times more sensitive. Also older paraffin embedded material, whose DNA is already partially degraded, can be used for PCR-DGGE, since for this method, short DNA fragments of 0.2–0.5 kb have to be detected, whereas for Southern blots, fragments comprising 2–10 kb have to be identified. Shortly, the PCR-DGGE method is faster, less material consuming, and sensitive than the Southern blot, but the Southern blots is still useful for the 10–15% of cases, which cannot be detected by PCR-DGGE.

REFERENCES

1. Qin J-Z, Zhang C-L, Kamarashev J, Dummer R, Burg G, Döbbeling U. IL-7 and IL-15 regulate the expression of the bcl-2 and c-myb genes in cutaneous T cell lymphoma (CTCL) cells. Blood 2001; 98:2778–2783.
2. Tonegawa S. Somatic generation of antibody diversity. Nature 1983; 302:575–581.
3. Bourguin A, Tung R, Galili N, Sklar J. Rapid non-radioactive detection of clonal T-cell receptor gene rearrangements in lymphoid neoplasms. Proc Natl Acad Sci USA 1990; 87:8536–8540.
4. Wood GS, Tung RM, Haeffner AC, Crooks CF, Liao S, Orozco R, Veelken H, Kadin ME, Koh H, Heald P, Barnhill RL, Sklar J. Detection of clonal T-cell receptor gamma gene rearrangements in early mycosis fungoides/Sézary syndrome by polymerase chain reaction and denaturing gradient gel electrophoresis (PCR/DGGE). J Invest Derm 1994; 103: 34–41.
5. Laetsch B, Häffner AC, Döbbeling U, Seifert B, Ludwig E, Burg G, Dummer R. CD4+/ CD7-T-cell frequency and PCR-based clonality assay correlate with stage in CTCL. J Invest Derm 2000; 114:107–111.
6. Meyer C, Hassam S, Dummer R, Muletta S, Döbbeling U, Dommann SNW, Burg G. A realistic approach to the sensitivity of PCR-DGGE and its application as a sensitive tool for the detection of clonality in cutaneous T-cell proliferations. Exp Dermatol 1997; 6:122–127.

15

Cytogenetic Studies in Cutaneous Lymphomas

Werner Kempf, Antonio Cozzio, Dmitry V. Kazakov, and Günter Burg
Department of Dermatology, University Hospital, Zürich, Switzerland

INTRODUCTION

Tumorigenesis is a multistep process during which genetic alterations accumulate resulting in a more aggressive behavior of tumor cells. Chromosomal aberrations can be found even in the early lesions of cutaneous T-cell lymphoma (CTCL). Most lymphomas display multiple structural and numerical chromosomal abnormalities, often involving translocations of genes regulating cell proliferation or programmed cell death (apoptosis). Various methods are now available to study chromosomal alterations (1). They include conventional karyotyping using mitogen-produced metaphases, multicolor fluorescence in situ hybridization (FISH) analysis, and comparative genomic hybridization (CGH).

Genetic instability of T-cells ("genotraumatic cells") may result in chromosomal aberrations. Loss of heterozygosity (LOH) and microsatellite instability (MSI) have recently been identified as factors that may result in genetic instability. In MSI, defects in the DNA mismatch repair genes contribute to the accumulation of genetic defects and thus to neoplastic transformation.

GENETIC ABNORMALITIES IN CUTANEOUS T-CELL LYMPHOMAS

Predisposing genetic factors contributing to the development of cutaneous lymphoma (CL) are suggested by the enhanced risk of CTCL in first-degree relatives of CTCL patients. An association of histocompatibility antigens is frequently found for HLA-DR5 in CTCL patients (31.5% versus 11% in healthy controls). Similar associations have been reported for HLA-DQB1*03 (72% versus 49% in healthy controls).

Mycosis Fungoides and Sézary Syndrome

It seems likely that chromosomal aberrations are involved in the onset of CTCL. Most tumors or tumor cells in peripheral blood of patients with Sézary syndrome display multiple chromosomal abnormalities with translocations of genes regulating cell proliferation or apoptosis. Statistically increased numbers of aberrations have been found in chromosomes 3, 6, 8, 9, 11, 13, and 17, all of them carrying oncogenes and/or tumor suppressor genes/regions (2,3). Structural abnormalities in chromosome 1 are also frequent (4). In addition to structural abnormalities, numerical abnormalities such as trisomies can be found, but are less frequent. By CGH, losses (chromosomes 10q and 13q) and gains (chromosomes 8q and 17q) of chromosomes were found in the majority of Sezary syndrome patients, but not in those with mycosis fungoides (2).

Abnormal expression of p53, which may be due to mutational gene inactivation or overexpression of wild-type protein, has been shown in advanced stages of CTCL, but not in early-stage disease, suggesting that abnormalities in p53 may contribute to disease progression (5–7). Loss of heterozygosity on chromosome 10q was identified in 23% of patients with mycosis fungoides and was associated with disease progression, suggesting that alterations of the PTEN tumor suppressor gene may be of prognostic significance (8).

One limitation of cytogenetic studies in CTCL is the inability to culture tumor cells from CTCL over a long time period. Moreover, tumor cells and reactive lymphocytes are always intermingled in tissue samples. Thus, most studies have been done on circulating tumor cells from peripheral blood samples, which may not be fully representative of tumor cells in skin infiltrates.

CD30+ Lymphoproliferative Disorders

A high percentage of nodal CD30+ anaplastic large-cell lymphomas carry a specific chromosomal translocation, t(2;5) (p23;q35), which causes the nucleophosmin gene (*npm*) located at 5q35 to fuse with the tyrosine kinase anaplastic lymphoma kinase receptor gene (*alk*) at 2p23. As a consequence, the *alk* gene comes under the influence of the *npm* promoter, resulting in a fusion protein NPR–ALK or p80. The activated ALK domain has oncogenic properties. Transfection of hematopoietic cells with the *npm–alk* fusion gene results in lymphoid tumors. The expression of ALK can be detected either by IHC, or the *alk–npm* gene can be demonstrated by FISH. The t(2;5) translocation is found in 65% of systemic CD30+ anaplastic large-cell lymphoma, but it is not, or only very rarely, found in primary cutaneous CD30+ lymphoproliferative disorders (9,10).

Loss of heterozygosity of the tumor suppressor protein p16 was recently described in cutaneous CD30+ large-cell lymphomas (LTCL), which indicates that alterations of this tumor suppressor gene may be involved in the pathogenesis of primary cutaneous CD30 LTCL (11). In contrast, no allelic deletions of the p53 tumor suppressor gene (chromosomal region 17p13), which occur in a wide variety of neoplasms, could be detected by LOH analysis in CD30+ LTCL.

GENETIC ABNORMALITIES IN CUTANEOUS B-CELL LYMPHOMAS

A variety of translocations, and their associations with distinct types of nodal and extranodal B-cell lymphomas, have been extensively investigated and described. Conversely, information regarding chromosomal abnormalities and possible pathogenic implications in the field of primary cutaneous B-cell lymphoma (CBCL) is very scanty.

The translocation t(14;18) (q32;q21), which results in fusion of the IgH locus on chromosome 14q32 with the bcl-2 locus, results in overexpression of Bcl-2. The anti-apoptotic effect of Bcl-2 results in a prolonged life span. Bcl-2 expression is not always caused by an underlying translocation, but may also be triggered by cytokines. Bcl-2 expression has been found in the vast majority (> 95%) of nodal follicle center cell lymphomas and in 20–30% of nodal large-B-cell lymphomas (12). In contrast, the majority (75%) of primary cutaneous low-malignant CBCL are negative for bcl-2. Site-related expression of bcl-2 has been described in diffuse large-B-cell lymphomas, which are bcl-2 positive in 40% in general, whereas all of those located on the lower legs are bcl-2 positive (13).

Overexpression of cyclin D1 due to t(11;14) (q32;q13) involving the IgH locus and bcl-1 locus leads to proliferation via cell cycle deregulation. Cyclin D1 expression has been described in nodal and cutaneous mantle cell lymphoma (14).

CONCLUSIONS

The genetic defects in CL are quite heterogeneous. Thus, the detection of chromosomal abnormalities has limited diagnostic or prognostic value in CTCL and CBCL. Differences in specific genetic alterations such as translocations and expression of oncogenes (e.g., *bcl-2*) between CLs and their nodal counterparts indicate that primary CLs represent, in fact, a distinctive group of lymphomas in clinical and biological aspects.

REFERENCES

1. Roylance R. Methods of molecular analysis: assessing losses and gains in tumours. Mol Pathol 2002; 55:25–28.
2. Karenko L, Kahkonen M, Hyytinen ER, Lindlof M, Ranki A. Notable losses at specific regions of chromosomes 10q and 13q in the Sezary syndrome detected by comparative genomic hybridization [letter]. J Invest Dermatol 1999; 112:392–395.
3. Scarisbrick JJ, Woolford AJ, Russell-Jones R, Whittaker SJ. Allelotyping in mycosis fungoides and Sezary syndrome: common regions of allelic loss identified on 9p, 10q, and 17p. J Invest Dermatol 2001; 117:663–670.
4. Mao X, Lillington D, Scarisbrick JJ, Mitchell T, Czepulkowski B, Russell-Jones R, Young B, Whittaker SJ. Molecular cytogenetic analysis of cutaneous T-cell lymphomas: identification of common genetic alterations in Sezary syndrome and mycosis fungoides. Br J Dermatol 2002; 147:464–475.
5. Lauritzen AF, Vejlsgaard GL, Hou-Jensen K, Ralfkiaer E. p53 protein expression in cutaneous T-cell lymphomas. Br J Dermatol 1995; 133:32–36.
6. McGregor JM, Crook T, Fraser-Andrews EA, Rozycka M, Crossland S, Brooks L, Whittaker SJ. Spectrum of p53 gene mutations suggests a possible role for ultraviolet radiation in the pathogenesis of advanced cutaneous lymphomas. J Invest Dermatol 1999; 112:317–321.
7. Whittaker S. Molecular genetics of cutaneous lymphomas. Ann N Y Acad Sci 2001; 941:39–45.
8. Scarisbrick JJ, Woolford AJ, Russell-Jones R, Whittaker SJ. Loss of heterozygosity on 10q and microsatellite instability in advanced stages of primary cutaneous T-cell lymphoma and possible association with homozygous deletion of PTEN. Blood 2000; 95:2937–2942.

9. Kadin ME, Morris SW. The t(2;5) in human lymphomas. Leuk Lymphoma 1998; 29: 249–256.
10. Wellmann A, Thieblemont C, Pittaluga S, Sakai A, Jaffe ES, Siebert P, Raffeld M. Detection of differentially expressed genes in lymphomas using cDNA arrays: identification of clusterin as a new diagnostic marker for anaplastic large-cell lymphomas. Blood 2000; 96:398–404.
11. Boeni R, Xin H, Kamarashev J, Utzinger E, Dummer R, Kempf W, Kutzner H, Burg G. Allelic deletion at 9p21–22 in primary cutaneous CD30(+) large cell lymphoma. J Invest Dermatol 2000; 115:1104–1107.
12. Kramer MH, Hermans J, Wijburg E, Philippo K, Geelen E, van Krieken JH, de Jong D, Maartense E, Schuuring E, Kluin PM. Clinical relevance of BCL2, BCL6, and MYC rearrangements in diffuse large B-cell lymphoma. Blood 1998; 92:3152–3162.
13. Geelen FA, Vermeer MH, Meijer CJ, Van der Putte SC, Kerkhof E, Kluin PM, Willemze R. Bcl-2 protein expression in primary cutaneous large B-cell lymphoma is site-related. J Clin Oncol 1998; 16:2080–2085.
14. Raffeld M, Jaffe ES. bcl-1, t(11;14), mantle cell-derived lymphomas. Blood 1991; 78: 259–263.

16

Functional Profiling by Microarray Technology

Antonio Cozzio, Werner Kempf, Reinhard Dummer, and Günter Burg
Department of Dermatology, University Hospital, Zürich, Switzerland

Analysis of tissue-specific gene expression is the modern standard procedure to elucidate and define the normal and pathologic state of a cell or tissue type. In oncology, the use of microarray technology at the nucleic acid or protein level can provide useful information concerning tumor classification, prognosis, and response to drug treatment. A particular focus has been on elucidation of cancer etiology and identification of critical signal transduction pathways relevant to cancer drug development. This short chapter reviews current applications of nucleic acid- and protein-based microarray technology (Fig. 1).

One major focus of research in oncology is the identification of initiating signaling events that lead to the induction of cancer. It is widely accepted that cancer is a multistep process (1). Thus, it is of keen interest to find early stages of tumor development. The skin offers a unique chance to find those early, asymptomatic forms of epithelial, melanocytic, and even lymphoproliferative disorders. The expression analysis of lymphoproliferative diseases such as lymphomatoid papulosis in patients developing CTCL later on in their life may shed more light on those early oncogenic metabolic events. Thus, cutaneous lymphoma may represent an ideal study system for tumorigenesis. There is hope that based on microarray data, we will be able to improve the existing lymphoma classifications, and predict appropriate treatment regimens based on metabolic peculiarities of the neoplastic tissues. One problem is that genes of parenchymal and stromal cells contribute to the mRNA pool of an excised tumor. This stromal contamination may hamper the detection of relevant tumor-specific gene expression. Therefore, much effort has been directed towards using microdissected cell populations, which in turn have their own advantages and disadvantages (2). As more and more investigators start to use the technology, we must address specificity of the results, search for the biological relevance of tumor systems, and discern between causative and epiphenomenal changes in gene expression patterns. Classic molecular biological methods, such as expression analysis by northern and western blot, reverse genetic approaches such as in vitro transgenic systems or in vivo knockin, knockout, or knockoff studies will be indispensable to clarify these questions.

73

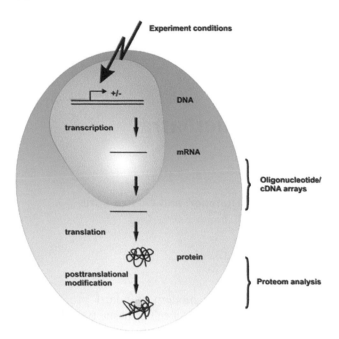

Figure 1 Expression analysis in eukaryotes. Expression levels of known and unknown genes can be influenced by a variety of controlled experimental conditions. Subsequently, alterations of mRNA levels can be detected using oligonucleotide- or cDNA-based arrays. Alternatively, expression levels of native and post-translationally modified proteins at the whole-cell or tissue level are analyzed by proteom profiling technologies.

TYPES OF MICROARRAY EXPERIMENTS

The objectives of DNA microarray experiments can be described as either class comparison, class prediction, or class discovery (3). For example, a typical class comparison study tries to reveal differences in gene expression between tumor tissue from patients who respond to a given treatment and those with the diagnosis who do not respond to the same therapy (4). Thus, the definition of the classes in class comparison studies is independent of the expression data. The objective is to see how the expression patterns differ among the various classes. Class comparison studies also are useful in analyzing metabolic pathways involved in reaction of cells and tissue to various external stimuli.

Class prediction experiments, too, consist of classes whose definition is independent of the expression data. The goal of a class prediction experiment is to define a set of gene markers whose presence or absence define the reaction of cells or tissue to specific stimuli. Analogous to the experiment described in the previous paragraph, class prediction attempts to define a subset of marker genes as a formula that can be applied to predict whether a new patient will respond to that therapy based on their tumor's gene expression profile.

A third set of experiments is described as class discovery. In contrast to the two classes described previously, class discovery discerns between individual members of an otherwise homogenous group of tissue sample solely based on their expression profile. The objective is to define subsets, or clusters, of the cases based on differences of gene expression. This approach has been successfully used to subclassify advanced melanoma where no clinical classification existed (5). Subsequently, this approach proofed to be useful to discern between clusters in diffuse large B-cell lymphoma (DLBCL) (6), breast tumors (7), and small round blue cell tumors such as lung carcinomas (SRBCTs) (8), among others.

DNA MICROARRAY EXPERIMENTS

Microarray technology was initially developed to study differential gene expression using complex populations of RNA (9–13). Further refinement of the technology now allows the analysis of copy number imbalances and gene amplification of DNA (14), and the detection of small deletions and insertions in tumor suppressor genes (15). Two different techniques are available: the spotted microarrays, and the oligonucleotide GeneChip, where DNA oligos are synthesized in situ on glass wafers.

Spotted Arrays

Spotted arrays are manufactured using robots with x–y–z arms that use hollow pins to deposit an aliquot of nucleic acid on a specifically processed glass slide (for an example of glass slide preparation, visit Pat Brown's home page at http://cmgm.stanford.edu/pbrown/). Each element of the two dimensional matrix has a defined address and sequence. The density of spotted elements varies from 100 elements per cm^2 to as many as 25,000 elements per cm^2, and depends on the type of pins used for printing the array. The nucleic acid sequences to be arrayed are derived from public databases (e.g. NCBI's GenBank http://www.ncbi.nlm. nih.gov/Genbank/index.html). DNA to be spotted is amplified by PCR and purified before spotting (for a comprehensive guide, see http://cmgm.stanford.edu/pbrown/protocols/index.html).

This technology has two nice features: it is flexible, and relatively cheap. Microarrays can be fabricated for a specific set of experiments in low numbers with various numbers of spotted DNA (oligo or cDNA). The use of glass as a flat surface allows hybridization with low amounts of labeled target samples (in contrast to the membrane filters with porous surfaces, which need much larger volumes), Furthermore, simultaneous hybridization of differentially labeled probes (Cy3 and Cy5 labeled RNA samples, see http://cmgm.stanford.edu/pbrown/protocols/index.html), such as untreated cells compared with treated cells or healthy tissue compared with cancer cells, allows direct pairwise analysis (for further reading about experimental design of DNA microarray experiments, see Ref. 16). In addition, by using EST derived sequences, spotted arrays can help defining the pathophysiologic role of newly discovered genes. A drawback of the technology is the variability in spot quality from slide to slide and among different printing rounds. Also, a direct quantification of RNA expression is not possible on spotted arrays using competing differentially labeled samples.

Affymetrix GeneChips™

GeneChips are produced in situ by using a combination of photolithography and light-directed solid-phase DNA synthesis on the glass wafers. Typically, a combination of 25-mers represents each gene on the array. A clever use of various internal controls allows differentiation of specific from nonspecific hybridization. An advantage of GeneChips is the generally high quality standard of each chip. Also, their ability to measure the absolute expression of genes in cells or tissues, coupled with a high sensitivity, enabling the detection of mRNAs present at levels as low as 1 transcript in 100,000 to 1 in 1,000,000 (11) is a very useful feature. Their disadvantages include their generally higher costs per chip, and the inability of pairwise direct comparison of differentially labeled probes (for more details, see http://www. affymetrix.com/technology/ge_analysis/index.affx). Recently, microarray fabrication using bubble jet technology appears to combine some of advantages of both the glass arrays and the GeneChip technology (17).

PROTEIN-BASED GENE EXPRESSION ANALYSIS

Within the cells, metabolic changes and adaptive efforts to environmental alterations are largely accomplished through the action of proteins. By applying nucleic acid microarray for the description of gene expression alteration, we assume that changes in transcript levels reflect changes in protein levels. Analyses performed mainly in yeast indicate that large changes in mRNA levels are generally paired with much lower levels of change in protein levels (18–20). In some cases, small transcript levels even correlated with changes of matching protein levels in the opposite direction (19). Furthermore, activation and inactivation of metabolic pathways often occur via modification of proteins, e.g., (de-)phosphorylation that cannot be detected by nucleic acid based expression analysis. If proteome alterations in disease may occur in many different ways that are not predictable from genomic analysis, and if post-transcriptional control is of such importance, one might ask the question whether itwould not be more appropriate to focus on the effector molecules, hence the proteins, from the very beginning. Unfortunately, the development for methods for global analysis of the cell's proteome is still in its infancy. Other problems are the lack of an amplifying method for proteins analogous to PCR, the lack of a protein detection system that covers the dynamic range of protein expression levels in a cell, and problems in getting specific, non-cross-reacting antibodies not only against the proteins, but also against their isoforms. Much work needs to be done also on the surface chemistry of the slides, in terms of attachment chemistries and providing an environment in which the proteins are stable and do not denature by unfolding onto the surface. Thus, although proteomics holds many promises, the daunting physico-chemical problems have limited its widespread use so far (for a review, see Ref. 21).

CUTANEOUS LYMPHOMA

In the field of cutaneous lymphomas, at present, at least two classification schemes are in use. One system was devised by the European Organization for Research and Treatment of Cancer (EORTC) and pertains only to primary lymphomas of the skin, whereas the system by the World Health Organization (WHO) was derived from the Revised European-American Classification of Lymphoid Neoplasms for hematological malignancies and covers nodal as well as extranodal lymphomas (see Chapters 18 and 19). Both classification systems take into account a constellation of morphologic, immunologic, genetic, and clinical criteria. This classification scheme is still under debate.

Few expression analysis studies of cutaneous lymphoma by a massive parallel approach such as microarray analysis have been performed. Based on the seminal study of Alizadeh et al. (6) using genes that define germinal center B-cell signatures, Storz et al. (22) published a study in which they compared 17 cutaneous B-cell lymphomas using punch biopsy material without further purification of the lympho-proliferative cells. Using a hierarchical cluster algorithm, two specific B-cell differentiation stage signatures of germinal center B cells and plasma cells could be identified. Importantly, duplicate specimens clustered together, demonstrating the reproducibility and reliability of the technique. Primary cutaneous follicular (FCCL) and primary cutaneous diffuse large B-cell lymphomas (DLCL) had a germinal center B-cell signature, whereas a subset of marginal zone lymphomas demonstrated a plasma cell signature. This corresponds well with recent reports of Hofbauer et al. (23) showing a responsiveness of DLCL and FCCL to antibiotic treatment, and suggest that DLCL and FCCL are more closely related that expected from immunohistological analysis. Primary diffuse large cell cutaneous lymphoma was distinct in its molecular fingerprint from secondary DLCL, underlining a biological distinctiveness of the two tumor entities. Mao et al. (24) showed by metaphase comparative genomic hybridization (CGH) and array-CGH that in CD30+, primary cutaneous anaplastic large cell cutaneous lymphoma (ALCL), 50% of the cases had gains of chromosome 1/1p, and 38% of cases had gains of chromosomes 6,7, 8/8p, and 19. Unanswered questions include whether the described alterations in oncogene expression are causative or epiphenomenal, and which genes on the chromosomes in question are necessary and sufficient for the formation of primary cutaneous ALCL.

The sequencing of the human genome has opened the doors for genomics and proteomics by providing a sequence-based framework. Based on the tools described previously, and on concomitant massive use of powerful information technology, it seems possible to tackle the problem of understanding tumorigenesis, describe more relevant tumor classifications, and to develop biomarkers and drugs for detection and treatment of cutaneous lymphoma and many other neoplasms.

REFERENCES

1. Vogelstein B, Kinzler KW. The multistep nature of cancer. Trends Genet 1993; 9: 138–141.
2. Paweletz CP, Liotta LA. Tumor classification: gene analysis using DNA microarrays. In: Warrington JA, Todd CR, Wong D, eds. Microarrays and Cancer Research. Westborough, MA: Eaton Publishing, 2002:61–77.
3. Golub TR, Slonim DK, Tamayo P, Huard C, Gaasenbeek M, Mesirov JP, Coller H, Loh ML, Downing JR, Caligiuri MA, Bloomfield CD, Lander ES. Molecular classification of cancer: class discovery and class prediction by gene expression monitoring. Science 1999; 286:531–537.
4. Rosenwald A, Wright G, Chan WC, Connors JM, Campo E, Fisher RI, Gascoyne RD, Muller-Hermelink HK, Smeland EB, Giltnane JM, Hurt EM, Zhao H, Averett L, Yang L, Wilson WH, Jaffe ES, Simon R, Klausner RD, Powell J, Duffey PL, Longo DL, Greiner TC, Weisenburger DD, Sanger WG, Dave BJ, Lynch JC, Vose J, Armitage JO, Montserrat E, Lopez-Guillermo A, Grogan TM, Miller TP, LeBlanc M, Ott G, Kvaloy S, Delabie J, Holte H, Krajci P, Stokke T, Staudt LM. The use of molecular profiling to predict survival after chemotherapy for diffuse large-B-cell lymphoma. N Engl J Med 2002; 346:1937–1947.
5. Bittner M, Meltzer P, Chen Y, Jiang Y, Seftor E, Hendrix M, Radmacher M, Simon R, Yakhini Z, Ben-Dor A, Sampas N, Dougherty E, Wang E, Marincola F, Gooden C, Lueders J, Glatfelter A, Pollock P, Carpten J, Gillanders E, Leja D, Dietrich K, Beaudry

C, Berens M, Alberts D, Sondak V. Molecular classification of cutaneous malignant melanoma by gene expression profiling. Nature 2000; 406:536–540.

6. Alizadeh AA, Eisen MB, Davis RE, Ma C, Lossos IS, Rosenwald A, Boldrick JC, Sabet H, Tran T, Yu X, Powell JI, Yang L, Marti GE, Moore T, Hudson J Jr, Lu L, Lewis DB, Tibshirani R, Sherlock G, Chan WC, Greiner TC, Weisenburger DD, Armitage JO, Warnke R, Staudt LM, et al. Distinct types of diffuse large B-cell lymphoma identified by gene expression profiling. Nature 2000; 403:503–511.

7. Perou CM, Sorlie T, Eisen MB, van de Rijn M, Jeffrey SS, Rees CA, Pollack JR, Ross DT, Johnsen H, Akslen LA, Fluge O, Pergamenschikov A, Williams C, Zhu SX, Lonning PE, Borresen-Dale AL, Brown PO, Botstein D. Molecular portraits of human breast tumours. Nature 2000; 406:747–752.

8. Khan J, Wei JS, Ringner M, Saal LH, Ladanyi M, Westermann F, Berthold F, Schwab M, Antonescu CR, Peterson C, Meltzer PS. Classification and diagnostic prediction of cancers using gene expression profiling and artificial neural networks. Nat Med 2001; 7:673–679.

9. DeRisi JL, Iyer VR, Brown PO. Exploring the metabolic and genetic control of gene expression on a genomic scale. Science 1997; 278:680–686.

10. Lashkari DA, DeRisi JL, McCusker JH, Namath AF, Gentile C, Hwang SY, Brown PO, Davis RW. Yeast microarrays for genome wide parallel genetic and gene expression analysis. Proc Natl Acad Sci USA 1997; 94:13057–13062.

11. Lipshutz RJ, Fodor SP, Gingeras TR, Lockhart DJ. High density synthetic oligonucleotide arrays. Nat Genet 1999; 21:20–24.

12. Lockhart DJ, Winzeler EA. Genomics, gene expression and DNA arrays. Nature 2000; 405:827–836.

13. Schena M, Shalon D, Davis RW, Brown PO. Quantitative monitoring of gene expression patterns with a complementary DNA microarray. Science 1995; 270:467–470.

14. Pollack JR, Perou CM, Alizadeh AA, Eisen MB, Pergamenschikov A, Williams CF, Jeffrey SS, Botstein D, Brown PO. Genome-wide analysis of DNA copy-number changes using cDNA microarrays. Nat Genet 1999; 23:41–46.

15. Frolov A, Prowse AH, Vanderveer L, Bove B, Wu H, Godwin AK. DNA array-based method for detection of large rearrangements in the BRCA1 gene. Genes Chromosomes Cancer 2002; 35:232–241.

16. Simson RM, Dobbin K. Experimental design of DNA microarray experiments. Biotechniques 2003; (supply:):16–21.

17. Okamoto T, Suzuki T, Yamamoto N. Microarray fabrication with covalent attachment of DNA using bubble jet technology. Nat Biotechnol 2000; 18:438–441.

18. Gygi SP, Rochon Y, Franza BR, Aebersold R. Correlation between protein and mRNA abundance in yeast. Mol Cell Biol 1999; 19:1720–1730.

19. Griffin TJ, Gygi SP, Ideker T, Rist B, Eng J, Hood L, Aebersold R. Complementary profiling of gene expression at the transcriptome and proteome levels in *Saccharomyces cerevisiae*. Mol Cell Proteomics 2002; 1:323–333.

20. Kuruvilla FG, Shamji AF, Sternson SM, Hergenrother PJ, Schreiber SL. Dissecting glucose signalling with diversity-oriented synthesis and small-molecule microarrays. Nature 2002; 416:653–657.

21. Hanash S. Disease proteomics. Nature 2003; 422:226–232.

22. Storz MN, van de Rijn M, Kim YH, Mraz-Gernhard S, Hoppe RT, Kohler S. Gene expression profiles of cutaneous B cell lymphoma. J Invest Dermatol 2003; 120:865–870.

23. Hofbauer GF, Kessler B, Kempf W, Nestle FO, Burg G, Dummer R. Multilesional primary cutaneous diffuse large B-cell lymphoma responsive to antibiotic treatment. Dermatology 2001; 203:168–170.

24. Mao X, Orchard G, Lillington DM, Russell-Jones R, Young BD, Whittaker S. Genetic alterations in primary cutaneous CD30+ anaplastic large cell lymphoma. Genes Chromosomes Cancer 2003; 37:176–185.

17

Classification of Nodal Lymphomas in Historical Perspective

Marshall E. Kadin

Beth Israel Deaconess Medical Center, Harvard Medical School, Boston, Massachusetts, U.S.A.

Considerable progress has been made in the classification of nodal lymphomas. The earliest classification schemes were based strictly on morphology. The Jackson and Parker classification included lymphosarcoma, reticulum cell sarcoma, and giant follicle lymphoma (Brill–Symmer disease) corresponding to small lymphocytic lymphoma, large cell lymphoma, and follicular lymphoma, respectively. Other rare types were lymphoblastoma and plasmacytoma. Hodgkin disease (HD) [for historical purposes, we have retained this term; today the preferred designation is Hodgkin lymphoma (HL)] was initially subdivided into paragranuloma, granuloma, and sarcoma subtypes, corresponding to modern classifications of lymphocyte predominance, mixed cellularity, and lymphocyte depletion types.

In 1956, Rappaport (1) emphasized the important distinction between follicular (nodular) and diffuse non-Hodgkin lymphomas. Even a small area of nodular architecture was sufficient to classify the tumor as nodular lymphoma, with a generally better prognosis than diffuse lymphomas. Both nodular and diffuse lymphomas were divided into well differentiated, poorly differentiated, mixed lymphocytic and histiocytic, histiocytic, and undifferentiated forms, as well as HD. This was an entirely morphological classification in which well and poorly differentiated lymphomas corresponded to small lymphocytic lymphomas, histiocytic to large cell lymphomas, and undifferentiated to Burkitt and lymphoblastic lymphomas.

Nodular lymphomas can present as primary cutaneous lymphomas, frequently on the scalp, face, or back. Large B-cell lymphomas often present as primary cutaneous lymphomas of the lower leg. Burkitt and lymphoblastic lymphomas in the skin usually represent secondary manifestations of systemic lymphoma, except for rare presentations of primary cutaneous B lymphoblastic lymphomas, usually occurring in children. Anaplastic large cell lymphomas can be of primary cutaneous or systemic origin. In the latter case, lymphadenopathy is detected in most cases.

In 1966, Lukes and Butler (2) published a new classification of HD. They recognized the distinct nodular sclerosing type in which broad bands of birefringent collagen circumscribe abnormal lymphoid nodules containing Reed–Sternberg cell variants in lacunar spaces; nodular sclerosis is now recognized to be the most common type of HD, with a predilection for mediastinal disease. Mixed cellularity type was recognized as a classical form of HD with frequent diagnostic Reed–Sternberg cells in a mixed inflammatory infiltrate without significant sclerosis.

Both nodular sclerosis and mixed cellularity subtypes were derived from the former granuloma subtype. Both nodular sclerosing and mixed cellularity subtypes have been reported in primary cutaneous HD.

Recognized as less frequent subtypes of HD were the lymphocyte depletion and lymphocyte predominance forms. Lymphocyte depletion contains relatively few small lymphocytes and frequent Reed–Sternberg cells in a background of diffuse fibrosis. This subtype occurs most often in elderly male patients with retroperitoneal lymphadenopathy, bone marrow involvement, and systemic B symptoms. Lymphocyte predominance is a usually localized form of HD without systemic symptoms, showing a peak incidence in children and male patients in the 4th decade.

Recently, lymphocyte predominance type HD has been subdivided into nodular lymphocyte predominance and lymphocyte-rich classical HD. Nodular LPHD has a distinctive biology with a clinically indolent but frequently relapsing clinical course. The lymphoid nodules are comprised of small B lymphocytes with infrequent large B cells known as L&H or popcorn cells, a special variant of Reed–Sternberg cells with a B-cell phenotype (CD20+, CD45+, EMA+, CD15–, CD30–). L&H cells are surrounded by rosettes of CD4+, CD57+ lymphocytes. The Reed–Sternberg cells in lymphocyte rich classical HL have the same phenotype as Reed–Sternberg cells in nodular sclerosis and mixed cellularity (CD30+, CD15+, CD45–, EMA–), usually negative for B- and T-cell antigens. In some studies, a minority of Reed–Sternberg cells stain positive for B-cell antigens CD20 and CD79a corresponding to their origin from germinal center B cells. In 1–2% of classical HD, the Reed–Sternberg cells have a T-cell phenotype/genotype. These T-cell variant cases are more frequently associated with cutaneous T-cell lymphomas including lymphomatoid papulosis.

In 1974, Lukes and Collins published an immunologically based classification of lymphomas. This approach required primary division of lymphomas into B- and T-cell lineages (3). This classification scheme favored cell type at the expense of histologic pattern. Emphasis was placed on the different follicular center cells (small and large cleaved and noncleaved cells) from which most lymphomas arise.

Also in 1974, Lennert and coworkers published the Kiel classification, derived from the concept that most lymphomas corresponded to a stage of normal lymphocyte differentiation/maturation (4). The various neoplasms were grouped according to histologic features into low-grade reflecting a predominance of small cells or "cytes" and high-grade representing a high proportion of large cells or "blasts." Follicular lymphomas were recognized as tumors of germinal center centroblasts and centrocytes. Neither the Lukes–Collins nor Kiel classifications emphasized the distinction of nodular versus diffuse lymphomas.

The International Working Formulation for Clinical Usage of 1982 was a consensus classification reached by pathologists and clinicians in which the major goal was to identify clinically prognostic groups of low-, intermediate-, and high-grade lymphomas (5). Low-grade lymphomas includes small lymphocytic, nodular small cleaved and mixed small cleaved, cell types. Intermediate-grade included nodular and diffuse large cell lymphomas, diffuse small cleaved, diffuse mixed small and large cell, and diffuse large cell lymphomas. High-grade included immunoblastic, lymphoblastic, and small noncleaved cell lymphomas. The classification gained wide acceptance for use by clinicians in North America and formed the basis of cooperative trials supported by the National Cancer Institute.

Table 1 WHO Classification of Tumors of the Haematopoietic and Lymphoid Tissues[a] —
T-, B-, NK-cell Neoplasms and Hodgkin Lymphoma

T-cell and NK-cell neoplasms
  Precursor T-cell neoplasm
    Precursor T lymphoblastic leukemia/lymphoma
    Blastic NK-cell lymphoma
  Mature T-cell and NK-cell neoplasms
    T-cell prolymphocytic leukemia
    T-cell large granular lymphocytic leukemia
    Aggressive NK cell leukemia
    Adult T-cell leukemia/lymphoma
    Extranodal NK/T-cell, nasal type
    Enteropathy-type T-cell lymphoma
    Hepatosplenic T-cell lymphoma
    Subcutaneous panniculitis like T-cell lymphoma
    Mycosis fungoides
    Sézary syndrome
    Primary cutaneous anaplastic large cell lymphoma
    Peripheral T-cell lymphoma, unspecified
    Angioimmunoblastic T-cell lymphoma
    Anaplastic large cell lymphoma
  T-cell proliferation of uncertain malignant potential
    Lymphomatoid papulosis
B-cell neoplasms
  Precursor B-cell neoplasm
    Precursor B lymphoblastic leukemia/lymphoma
  Mature B-cell neoplasms
    Chronic lymphocytic leukemia/small lymphocytic lymphoma
    B-cell prolymphocytic leukemia
    Lymphoplasmacytic lymphoma
    Splenic marginal zone lymphoma
    Hairy cell leukemia
    Plasma cell leukemia
    Solitary plasmacytoma of bone
    Extraosseous plasmacytoma
    Extranodal marginal zone B-cell lymphoma of mucosa-associated lymphoid
      tissue (MALT
    lymphoma)
    Nodal marginal zone B-cell lymphoma
    Follicular lymphoma
    Mantle cell lymphoma
    Diffuse large B-cell lymphoma
    Mediastinal (thymic) large B-cell lymphoma
    Intravascular large B-cell lymphoma
    Primary effusion lymphoma
    Burkitt lymphoma
  B-cell proliferations of uncertain malignant potential
    Lymphomatoid granulomatosis
    Post-transplant lymphoproliferative disorder, polymorphic

[a] The lymphoma entities that are primary cutaneous lymphoma or that often involve the skin secondarily
  are highlighted in italics.
Source: From Ref. 7.

REVISED EUROPEAN–AMERICAN (REAL) CLASSIFICATION

A group of 19 hematopathologists developed a new approach to lymphoma classification emphasizing for the first time all available information, including morphology, immunophenotype, genetic, and clinical features (6). Some diseases such as follicular lymphoma and nodular sclerosing HL remain primarily morphologic entities, whereas other disease such as mantle cell lymphoma and anaplastic large cell lymphoma are recognized equally by immunophenotype and genetic markers. Clinical features such as site of presentation at nodal or specific extranodal sites are also incorporated into the classification.

WORLD HEALTH ORGANIZATION (WHO) CLASSIFICATION OF HEMATOLOGIC MALIGNANCIES

The most recent classification scheme is the WHO classification (Table 1) which incorporates the principles of the REAL classification and extends them to myeloid and histiocytic neoplasms (7). The WHO classification was formulated with the assistance of a clinical advisory committee and is based on histopathological and genetic features. It aims to define specific clinicopathologic entities for optimal treatment. Lymphoid neoplasms are divided into precursor and mature B- and T-cell neoplasms. Most cutaneous lymphomas belong to the group of T-cell and NK-cell neoplasms. Precursor B-cell neoplasms can also present with skin involvement. The remainder of cutaneous B-cell neoplasms arise from mature B-cells.

REFERENCES

1. Rappaport H. Tumors of the hematopoietic system. Armed Forces Institute of Pathology, Washington, 1966.
2. Lukes RJ, Butler JJ. The pathology and nomenclature of Hodgkin's disease. Cancer Res 1966; 26:1063–1083.
3. Lukes RJ, Collins RD. A functional approach to the classification of malignant lymphoma. Recent Results Cancer Res 1974; 46:18–30.
4. Lennert K, Feller A. Histopathology of non-Hodgkin's Lymphomas. Heidelberg: Springer, 1992.
5. Working Formulation. The non-Hodgkin's lymphoma pathologic classification project. National Cancer Institute sponsored study of classification of non-Hodgkin's lymphoma. Summary and description of Working Formulation for clinical usage. Cancer 1982; 49: 2112–2135.
6. Harris NL, Jaffe ES, Stein H, Banks P, Chan J, Cleary M, Delsol G, deWolf-Peeters C, Falini B, Gatter K, Grogan K, Isaacson P, Knowles D, Mason D, Müller-Hermelink H-K, Pileri S, Piris M, Ralfkiaer E, Warnke R. A revised European–American classification of lymphoid neoplasms: a proposal from the international lymphoma study group. Blood 1994; 84:1361–1392.
7. Jaffe ES, Harris NL, Stein H, Vardiman JW, eds. World Health Organization Classification of Tumors. Pathology and Genetics of Tumours of Haematopoietic and Lmyphoid Tissues. Lyon: IARC Press, 2001.

18

Classification of Cutaneous Lymphomas in Historical Perspective

Christian A. Sander and Michael J. Flaig
Department of Dermatology, LMU, Munich, Germany

Werner Kempf and Günter Burg
Department of Dermatology, University Hospital, Zürich, Switzerland

Going back in history, classification of cutaneous lymphomas began with the introduction of mycosis fungoides by Alibert in the last century (1) and was extended by the description of the d'emblée form by Vidal and Brocq in 1885 (2).

In 1924, Letterer (3) introduced the term malignant reticulosis, which defined a proliferation of either benign or malignant reticulum cells. This term was used for decades as a collective term synonymous with malignant lymphoma (4). The cutaneous reticuloses were classified into four groups: infectious granulomas (tuberculosis, syphilis), storage diseases (xanthomatoses, histiocytosis X group), benign neoplasias of connective tissue (histiocytoma, nevoxanthoendothelioma), and malignant reticulosis (5).

With the description of Sézary syndrome by Sézary and Bouvrain in 1938 (6), another clinicopathologic entity was added to the spectrum of cutaneous lymphomas. Up until the late 1960s, cutaneous lymphomas were divided in mycosis fungoides and Sézary syndrome. For other lymphomas, the terms malignant reticulosis or reticulum cell sarcoma were used. An extensive classification scheme including these terms was proposed by Keining and Braun-Falco in 1961 (Table 1) (7).

The next major change in lymphoma classification was the gradual linkage of cutaneous lymphomas with the classification of nodal lymphomas. For many years, malignant lymphomas had been categorized in three basic categories: Hodgkin disease, lymphosarcoma, and reticulum cell sarcoma. There was great confusion among pathologists over the use of these terms, as it was evident that other types of lymphomas existed. Thus, the necessity for a new lymphoma classification was obvious (Table 2) (8).

In 1966, Rappaport (9) proposed his classification for the tumors of the hematopoietic system. The Rappaport classification was the first classification which divided lymphomas by pattern (nodular or diffuse) and by cytologic subtypes (Table 3).

The Rappaport classification was published at a time when very little was known about our immune system. As a consequence, in the 1970s, several schemes

Table 1 Lymphoplasias of the Skin

Lymphadenosis benigna cutis (*Lymphadenosis benigna cutis*)
  Spiegler-Fendt sarcoid (*Spiegler-Fendtsches Sarkoid*)
  Lymphocytic infiltration Jessner-Kanof (*Lymphocytic infiltration Jessner-Kanof*)
Reticuloses (*Retikulosen*)
  Monomorphous reticuloses (*monomorphe Retikulosen*)
    Primary reticuloses (*primäre Retikulosen*)
    Secondary reticuloses (*sekundäre Retikulosen*)
    Lipomelanotic reticulosis (*lipomelanotische Retikulose*)
    Large follicular lymphoblastoma (*großfollikuläres Lymphoblastom*)
    Senile erythroderma (*Alterserythrodermie*)
Mastocytoses (*Mastozytosen*)
Granulomatous reticuloses (*granulomatöse Retikulosen*)
  Mycosis fungoides (*Mykosis fungoides*)
  Hodgkin's disease (*Lymphogranulomatosis maligna*)
Malignant tumors of the reticular connective tissue of the skin (*Maligne Tumoren des reticulären Bindegewebes der Haut*)
  Retothelial sarcoma/retothelial sarcomatosis (*Retothelsarkom/-sarkomatose*)
  Reticulosarcomatosis (*Retikulosarkomatose*)
Cutaneous signs in hematopoietic disorders (*Hautveränderungen bei Leukosen*)
  Chronic lymphatic leukemia (*chronisch lymphatische Leukämie*)
  Lymphosarcoma/lymphosarcomatosis (*Lymphosarkom/-sarkomatose*)
  Myeloid leukemia (*myeloische Leukämie*)
  Agranulocytosis (*Agranulozytose*)

Source: From Refs. 4, 7.

such as the Kiel classification, Lukes–Collins classification, and the Working Formulation were proposed in an attempt to incorporate the highly relevant new information about the immune system (10–12). While the Working Formulation was proposed as an interim compromise approach, it became the de facto classification system in the United States. It was proposed as an alternative approach to the multitude of classification schemes in the 1970s. The categories of the Working Formulation were defined by survival data of patients treated on chemotherapy protocols used in the 1970s. The Kiel classification gained widespread use in Europe and Asia. This classification and the Lukes–Collins scheme were based on an attempt to relate the malignant lymphomas to the normal immune system. Lymphomas were diagnosed by morphology in the Working Formulation, but by a combination of morphologic and immunophenotypic criteria in the Kiel classification.

Table 2 Historical Overview of Lymphoma Classifications

1966	Rappaport classification
1974	Kiel classification, Lukes and Collins classification
1982	Working Formulation
1988	Updated Kiel classification
1994	REAL classification
1997	EORTC classification
2001	WHO classification

Table 3 Classification of Rappaport

Nodular or diffuse
Lymphocytic, well differentiated
Lymphocytic, poorly differentiated
Mixed lymphocytic–histiocytic
Histiocytic
Undifferentiated

Source: From Ref. 9.

Cutaneous lymphomas were classified according to the Kiel classification and the Working Formulation. Additionally, modified classification schemes for cutaneous lymphomas were developed. Kerl et al. (13) reported a new classification for T-cell lymphomas in relation to the cytologic spectrum. They were among the first to distinguish between lymphomas derived from precursor cells and from mature lymphocytes, a principle which was later incorporated in the REAL classification. A few years later, Burg et al. (14) proposed a classification scheme which included all of the current primary and secondary lymphoproliferative diseases involving cutaneous sites (Table 4).

In 1975, Edelson introduced the term *cutaneous T-cell lymphoma* (15) to cover the morphological, immunological, and clinical similarities between mycosis fungoides, Sézary syndrome, and related lymphoproliferative malignancies; the term has gained broad acceptance. A major disadvantage of this concept is that differences in the clinical presentation and prognosis between mycosis fungoides, Sézary syndrome, and other T-cell lymphomas are not considered. Because of this failure, the term cutaneous T-cell lymphoma should no longer be used in classification schemes of cutaneous T-cell lymphomas.

In the early 1990s, the Working Formulation as well as the Kiel classification, although recently updated, were completely outdated (16). The basis for the categories of the Working Formulation were survival data of patients treated on chemotherapy protocols used in the 1970s. Since our knowledge for therapy had dramatically improved in the intervening 20 years, the classification was flawed. The same was true for the Kiel classification which was a cytologically based scheme, which did not rely on clinical data. Additionally, both classification systems did not consider immunologic and molecular genetic findings which have dramatically increased our understanding of malignant lymphomas and did not address new entities which had been recently described as MALT lymphomas, NK/T-cell lymphomas and others.

Regarding cutaneous lymphomas, in retrospect, both classifications were inappropriate since the Kiel classification excluded "extranodal" skin lymphomas with the exception of mycosis fungoides/Sézary syndrome. Additionally, the clinical behavior of cutaneous lymphomas is different compared with their nodal counterparts—a fact which both classifications did not consider.

Furthermore, since the Working Formulation was the classification system in the United States, while the Kiel classification was used in Europe and Asia, there was a lack of a standardized internationally accepted classification system. Since the two classification schemes had major differences, neither clinical data nor basic laboratory studies could be readily compared among institutions not employing the same system.

As a result, there was a need for a new, modern, internationally accepted lymphoma classification system. In 1994, the International Lymphoma Study Group (ILSG) proposed a new classification termed Revised European-American Classifi-

Table 4 Non-Hodgkin's Lymphomas and Related Disorders Occurring in the Skin and their Corresponding Entities in the Working Formulation

T-cell lymphomas	Working Formulation
Lymphomas of T-precursor cells	
T-lymphoblastic lymphoma/leukemia[a]	ML, lymphoblastic (I)
Lymphomas of peripheral T cells	
T-chronic lymphocytic leukemia[a]	ML, small lymphocytic, consistent with CLL (A)
Mycosis fungoides	Mycosis fungoides (A)
Sézary syndrome	Sézary syndrome (A)
Pagetoid reticulosis, circumscribed, disseminated	–
Pleomorphic T-cell lymphoma, HTLV-1 ± small, medium, large	ML, polymorphous (H)
Immunoblastic lymphoma, T-cell type (Ki-1+)	ML, large cell, immunoblastic (H)
Large cell anaplastic lymphoma, T-cell type (Ki-1+)	–
B-cell lymphomas	
B-chronic lymphocytic leukemia[a]	ML, small lymphocytic, consistent with CLL (A)
Lymphoplasmacytoid immunocytoma	ML, small lymphocytic plasmacytoid (A)
Plasmacytoma	Extramedullary plasmacytoma
Centroblastic/centrocytic lymphoma	ML, mixed small cleaved and large (B–G)
Skin associated lymphoid tissue' lymphoma (SALT)	
Centrocytic (mantle cell) lymphoma	ML, small cleaved (E, G)
Centroblastic lymphoma	ML, large cell, non-cleaved (D, G)
Immunoblastic lymphoma	ML, large cell, immunoblastic (H)
Burkitt's lymphoma	ML, small non-cleaved, Burkitt (J)
Rare and distinct forms of lymphoproliferative and related disorders	
Granulomatous slack skin disease (mycosis fungoides)	
Lymphoepithelioid lymphoma (Lennert)[a]	
Midline granuloma[a]	
Lymphomatoid papulosis	
Systemic angioendotheliomatosis (angiotropic lymphoma) (B > T)	
Lymphomatoid granulomatosis (Liebow)[a], angiocentric, angiodestructive	
Angiolymphoid hyperplasia with eosinophilia (Kimura)	
Syringolymphoid hyperplasia with alopecia (10)	
Subcutaneous (lipotropic) T-cell lymphomas (5,20)	
Sinus histiocytosis with massive lymphadenopathy (Rosai–Dorfman)[a]	

(*Continued*)

Table 4 Non-Hodgkin's Lymphomas and Related Disorders Occurring in the Skin and their Corresponding Entities in the Working Formulation (*Continued*)

Peripheral T-cell lymphoma of the AILD-type
T-cell rich large B-cell lymphoma
B-cell rich T-cell lymphoma
Large cell lymphoma of the multilobulated cell type (B or T)
T-cell lymphoma expressing delta T-cell receptor (5)

[a] Usually secondary skin involvement. HTLV-1 = human T-cell leukemia virus; ML = malignant lymphoma; CLL = chronic lymphocytic leukemia; A to J = categories indicating grade of malignancy (A–C, low; D–G, intermediate; H–J, high); AILD = angioimmunoblastic lymphadenopathy with dysproteinemia.
Source: From Ref. 14.

cation of Lymphoid Neoplasms (REAL) (17). The REAL classification proposed that lymphomas should be viewed as a group of individual diseases, and that each disease could be defined by a constellation of morphological, biological, and clinical features. Several reports demonstrated the application of the REAL classification for primary and secondary cutaneous lymphomas (18–20).

Primary cutaneous lymphomas in many instances are distinct from their nodal counterparts. The REAL classification departed from prior classification systems by utilizing clinical features in the definition of entities. It recognized that the site of involvement was often an indication of underlying biological differences. This is in contrast to the Working Formulation or the Kiel classification, both of which had considered the site of involvement as irrelevant to the diagnosis. We have learned that

Table 5 EORTC Classification of Primary Cutaneous Lymphoma

Primary CTCL	Primary CBCL
Indolent	*Indolent*
Mycosis fungoides (MF)	Follicle center cell lymphoma
MF + follicular mucinosis	
Pagetoid reticulosis	Immunocytoma (marginal zone B-cell
Large cell CTCL, CD30+	lymphoma)
Immunoblastic	
Pleomorphic	
Anaplastic	
Lymphomatoid papulosis	
Aggressive	*Intermediate*
Sezary syndrome	Large B-cell lymphoma of the leg
Large cell CTCL, CD30–	
Immunoblastic Pleomorphic	
Provisional	*Provisional*
Granulomatous slack skin CTCL,	Intravascular large B-cell lymphoma
pleomorphic small/medium	Plasmacytoma
Substaneous panniculitis like T-cell	
lymphoma	

Source: From Ref. 24.

the prognosis of primary cutaneous lymphomas is often distinct from their nodal counterpart. They frequently have an indolent natural history, and for that reason, they often require different therapeutic approaches (21). This situation was also recognized by the Dutch Cutaneous Lymphoma Working Group. In 1994, Willemze et al. (22) proposed a new classification, which was the basis for the EORTC classification for primary cutaneous lymphomas introduced in 1997 (Table 5) (22–24).

By definition, the EORTC classification (Table 5) considers only primary cutaneous lymphomas and excludes lymphomas with secondary involvement of the skin. It employs a combination of clinical, histologic, immunohistochemical, and genetic criteria.

In conclusion, in the past decades our knowledge and understanding of the biology and genetics of nodal and also cutaneous lymphomas has dramatically improved. As a result schemes suitable for classification of cutaneous lymphomas which facilitate recognition of the individual disease entities have been developed.

REFERENCES

1. Alibert J. Tableau du pian fongoide. Description des maladies de la peau, observées à l'Hopital Saint-Louis et exposition des meilleurs méthodes suivies pour le traitement. Paris, Barrois L'Aîné & Fils, 1806.
2. Vidal E, Brocq L. Etude sur le mycosis fongoide. La France Méd 1885; 2:946–1019.
3. Letterer E. Aleukämische Retikulose. Frankfurt Z Path 1924; 30:377–394.
4. Burg G, Braun-Falco O. Cutaneous lymphomas, pseudolymphomas, and related disorders. Berlin: Springer Verlag, 1983.
5. Clendenning WE, Brecher G, van Scott E. Mycosis fungoides. Arch Dermatol 1964; 89:785–792.
6. Sézary A, Bouvrain Y. Erythrodermie avec présence de cellules monstrueuses dans le derme et le sang circulant. Bull Soc Fr Dermatol Syphilligr 1938; 45:254–260.
7. Keining E, Braun-Falco O. Dermatologie und Venerologie. München: JF Lehmanns Verlag, 1961:699–715.
8. Jaffe ES. An overview of the classification of non-Hodgkin's lymphomas. In: Jaffe ES, ed. Surgical Pathology of the Lymph Nodes and Related Organs. Philadelphia: WB Saunders Company, 1995:193–204.
9. Rappaport H. Tumors of the Hematopoietic System. Atlas of Tumor Pathology. Sect III, fascicle 8 vol. Washington, DC: Armed Forces Institute of Pathology, 1966:97–161.
10. Gérard-Marchant R, Hamlin I, Lennert K, Rilke F, Stansfeld AG, van Unnik JAM. Classification of non-Hodgkin's lymphomas. Lancet 1974; 2:406–408.
11. Lukes RJ, Collins RD. Immunologic characterization of human malignant lymphomas. Cancer 1974; 34(suppl):1488–1503.
12. National Cancer Institute sponsored study of classifications of non-Hodgkin's lymphomas: summary and description of a working formulation for clinical usage. The Non-Hodgkin's Lymphoma Pathologic Classification Project. Cancer 1982; 49: 2112–2135.
13. Kerl H, Cerroni L, Burg G. The morphologic spectrum of T-cell lymphomas of the skin: a proposal for a new classification. Semin Diagn Pathol 1991; 8:55–61.
14. Burg G, Dummer R, Kerl H. Classification of cutaneous lymphomas. Dermatol Clin 1994; 12:213–217.
15. Edelson R. Cutaneous T-cell lymphomas. Perspective. Ann Intern Med 1975; 83:548–552.
16. Stansfeld AG, Diebold J, Noel H. Updated Kiel classification for lymphomas. Lancet 1988; 1:292–293.

17. Harris NL, Jaffe ES, Stein H. A revised European–American classification of lymphoid neoplasms: a proposal from the International Lymphoma Study Group. Blood 1994; 84:1361–1392.

18. Sander CA, Kind P, Kaudewitz P, Raffeld M, Jaffe ES. The Revised European–American Classification of Lymphoid Neoplasms (REAL): a new perspective for the classification of cutaneous lymphomas. J Cutan Pathol 1997; 24:329–341.

19. Sander CA, Flaig MJ, Kaudewitz P, Jaffe ES. The revised European–American Classification of Lymphoid Neoplasms (REAL): a preferred approach for the classification of cutaneous lymphomas. Am J Dermatopathol 1999; 21:274–278.

20. Duncan LM. Cutaneous lymphoma. Understanding the new classification schemes. Dermatol Clin 1999; 17:569–592.

21. Sander CA, Flaig MJ, Jaffe ES. Cutaneous manifestations of lymphoma: a clinical guide based on the WHO classification. Clin Lymphoma. 2001; 2:86–100.

22. Willemze R, Beljaards RC, Meijer CJ, Rijlaarsdam JR. Classification of primary cutaneous lymphomas. Historical overview and perspectives. Dermatology 1994; 189:8–15.

23. Willemze R, Beljaards RC, Meijer CJ. Classification of primary cutaneous T-cell lymphomas. Histopathology 1994; 24:405–415.

24. Willemze R, Kerl H, Sterry W, Berti E, Cerroni L, Chimenti S, Diaz Perez JL, Geerts ML, Goos M, Knobler R, Ralfkiaer E, Santucci M, Smith N, Wechsler J, van Vloten WA, Meijer CL. EORTC classification for primary cutaneous lymphomas: a proposal from the Cutaneous Lymphoma Study Group of the European Organization for Research and Treatment of Cancer. Blood 1997; 90:354–371.

19

WHO/EORTC Classification of Cutaneous Lymphomas

Günter Burg, Werner Kempf, Dmitry V. Kazakov, Sonja Michaelis, and Reinhard Dummer
Department of Dermatology, University Hospital, Zürich, Switzerland

Over the past decades, each attempt trying to establish a dermatology-specific classification of cutaneous lymphomas (CL) apart from hematopathology has failed. Several attempts have been made to adapt classification of lymphoproliferative skin infiltrates to one of the major nodal lymphoma classifications. There has never been and most probably never will be a nodal-based lymphoma classification, which meets the specific requirements of extranodal, e.g., cutaneous, lymphomas, and is fully sufficient for dermatologic purposes. Nevertheless, in order to be understood by pathologists and hemato-oncologists, it is mandatory to use the same language and to adapt nodal-based lymphoma classifications as far as possible and to supplement them according to organ-specific requirements by adding skin-specific nosologic entities within the category they fit best.

Currently, cutaneous lymphomas can be labeled according to three classifications (REAL, EORTC, or WHO; see also Chapter 18) but each has shortcomings(1). Nonetheless, in an attempt to unify the field, every attempt should be made to categorize these conditions according to the WHO classification for tumours of the haemotopietic and lymphoid tissues (2).

During the preparation of the WHO book for neoplasms of the skin (3), an attempt was made to create a classification for cutaneous lymphoproliferative disorders (4,5), which is compatible with the WHO classification for tumors of hematopoietic and lymphoid tissues (2), and in addition respects additional entities. This attempt which was elaborated in May 2003 by a group of experts—including Günter Burg, MD, Werner Kempf, MD, Elaine Jaffe, MD, Elisabeth Ralfkiaer, MD, and Christian Sander, MD—during a meeting in Zurich. Table 1 shows the WHO/EORCT-consensus classification for cutaneous lymphoproliferative disorders.

Table 1 WHO/EORTC Classification of Cutaneous Lymphomas (Extended Version)

(a) Mature T-cell and NK-cell neoplasms
Mycosis fungoides
  Transformation
Variants of MF
  Pagetoid reticulosis (localized, CD4+)
  Syringotropic
  Granulomatous
  Other variants
Subtype of MF
  Granulomatous slack skin
Sézary syndrome
CD30+ T-cell lymphoproliferative disorders of the skin
  Lymphomatoid papulosis
  Primary cutaneous anaplastic large-cell lymphoma
Subcutaneous panniculitis-like T-cell lymphoma
Peripheral T-cell lymphoma, unspecified
  CD8+ CTCL
  Gamma/delta CTCL
  CD4+ small medium-sized pleomorphic
Extranodal NK/T-cell lymphoma, nasal type
  Hydroa vacciniformia-like lymphoma (variant)
Adult T-cell leukemia/lymphoma
Extracutaneous lymphomas with common skin involvement
  Angioimmunoblastic T-cell lymphoma
  T-zone lymphoma

(b) Mature B-cell neoplasms
Cutaneous marginal zone B-cell lymphoma (MALT type)
Primary cutaneous follicle centre lymphoma
  Variants
    Follicular
    Follicular and diffuse
    Diffuse
Cutaneous diffuse large B-cell lymphoma,
  Leg-type
  Others
Intravascular large B-cell lymphoma

(c) Immature hematopoietic malignancies
Blastic NK-cell lymphoma[a]/CD4 + CD56 + hematodermic neoplasia
Precursor lymphoblastic leukemia/lymphoma
  T-cell
  B-cell

---

[a] Recent evidence suggests an origin from a dendritic cell precursor.
Source: From Refs. 4,5.

REFERENCES

1. Prince HM, O'Keefe R, McCormack C, Ryan G, Turner H, Waring P, Baker C. Cutaneous lymphomas: which pathological classification? Pathology 2002; 34:36–45.
2. Jaffe ES, Harris NL, Stein H, Vardiman JW, eds. World Health Organization Classification of Tumors. Pathology and Genetics of Tumours of Haematopoietic and Lymphoid Tissues. Lyon: IARC Press, 2001.
3. LeBoit Ph, Burg G, Weedon D, Sarasin A, eds. World Health Organization Classification of Tumors. Pathology and Genetics of Tumours of the Skin. Lyon: IARC Press. 2005 in preparation.
4. Burg G, Jaffe ES, Kempf W, Berti E, Cerroni L, Chimenti S, Diaz-Perez JL, Duncan L, Harris NL, Kerl H, Knobler R, Kurrer M, Meijer C, Pimpinelli N, Ralfkiaer E, Sander C, Santucci M, Sterry W, Swerdlow S, Wechsler J, Whittaker S, Willenze R. WHO/EORTC-consensus classification of cutaneous lymphomas. In:Leboit PH, Burg G, Weedon D, Sarasin A, eds. World Health Organization Classification of Tumors. Pathology and Genetics of Tumours of the Skin. Classification. Lyon: IARC Press, 2005 in preparation.
5. Willemze R, Jaffe ES, Burg G, Cerroni L, Berti E, Swerdlow SH, Ralfkiaer E, Chimenti S, Diaz-Perez JL, Duncan LM, Grange F, Harris NL, Kempf W, Kerl H, Kurrer M, Knobler R, Pimpinelli N, Sander C, Santucci M, Sterry W, Vermeer MH, Wechsler J, Whittaker S, Meijer JLM. WHO-EORTC classification for cutaneous lymphomas. Blood 2005.

20

Prognostic Categorization of Lymphoproliferative Disorders of the Skin: A New and Clinically Oriented Approach

Günter Burg, Sonja Michaelis, Philippa Golling, and Werner Kempf
Department of Dermatology, University Hospital, Zürich, Switzerland

The continuous increase of knowledge has led to controversies and produced a plethora of new classifications, presenting the clinician with a dilemma. Many cutaneous lymphomas (CL), in particular B-cell lymphomas, share common clinical and prognostic features, but differ in regard to morphology. In contrast, there are CL forms, especially lymphoproliferative disorders of T-cell origin with similar morphologic findings, but distinct clinical and prognostic features which should therefore not lumped together. Since most *classifications* do not provide information about the biologic behavior of CL to the clinician, we propose a new *categorization* for CL based on prognostic and biological features (Table 1). In analogy to the Working Formulation, different clinicopathologic entities are grouped into classes corresponding to their biological behavior, i.e., grade (low, intermediate, or high) of malignancy.

The proposed categories include (a) pseudolymphoma, (b) abortive, and (c) malignant (divided into low-grade and high-grade malignant forms) lymphoproliferative disorders. These categories are defined as follows.

PROGNOSTIC CATEGORIES

Pseudolymphoma

Cutaneous pseudolymphoma is a reactive benign lymphoproliferative process, localized or disseminated, which heals either spontaneously after elimination of the causative factor (e.g., drugs) or after treatment with nonaggressive (no severe side effects to be expected after long term application) modalities, and which does not recur after removal of the causative agent. The following entities represent examples of cutaneous pseudolymphomas: drug-induced T-cell pseudolymphoma with MF-like histologic changes, and lymphadenosis benigna cutis (Baefverstedt) as a B-cell pseudolymphoma.

Table 1 Biologic Categories of Cutaneous Lymphomas—Criteria and Characteristics

Criteria	Pseudolymphoma	Abortive lymphoma	Malignant lymphoma	
			Low-grade	High-grade
Clinical course	Spontaneous healing usual	Spontaneous healing rarely	Slowly progressive, indolent	Rapidly progressive, aggressive
Systemic spread	Never	Never	Possible	Often
Cure	Yes	Usually not	Not in most cases	Not in most cases
Average survival time	Survival not affected	Survival not affected	>5 years	<2–5 years
Potentially fatal course	No	No	Possible	Often
Potential for transformation (to a less differentiated form)	No	Usually not	Yes	Yes
Clonality	No	May be present	Often present	Often present
Chromosomal alterations	No	May be present	Often present, especially in late stages	Often present

Abortive Lymphoma

Clinically, disorders belonging to this category show a chronic long-standing course, no spontaneous regression in most cases, and no extracutaneous spread with involvement of visceral organs. In some cases, clonality of the infiltrate can be demonstrated. However, in most cases, the neoplastic cell clone never overcomes host control mechanisms and cannot expand and therefore never converts into clinically aggressive and spreading lymphoma. This category includes, for example: large plaque parapsoriasis, lymphomatoid clonal dermatitis, pagetoid reticulosis of Woringer–Kolopp type, syringolymphoid hyperplasia with alopecia, pre-Sézary syndrome, actinic reticuloid, and lymphomatoid papulosis.

Definite Malignant Lymphoma
Definite Low-Grade Malignant Lymphoma

This category includes CL that show a slowly progressive course with systemic spread in later stages and have the potential for transformation into more aggressive high-grade malignant lymphomas.

This category of CTCL include mycosis fungoides, Sézary syndrome, granulomatous slack skin, juvenile granulomatous CTCL, primary cutaneous CD30+ large-cell anaplastic T-cell lymphoma (which shows an excellent prognosis in contrast to its nodal counterpart) and most cases of CBCL. Survival is often not affected by the lymphoma or is greater than at least 5 years.

Some cases of CBCL which result from persistent antigen stimulation due to Borrelia infections may show complete regression after therapy with antibiotics, aphenomenon better establish in mucosa-associated lymphoid tissue (MALT) lymphomas. A majority of those cases might rather be considered as pseudolymphomas, or may be very low-grade malignant CBCL from their very beginning. They have also been referred as semimalignant pseudolymphomas (1).

Definite High-Grade Malignant Lymphoma

These diseases are characterized by a more rapid course than the low-grade lymphomas and usually show a fatal outcome after months or years. This category includes: subcutaneous panniculitis-like T-cell lymphoma, most lymphomas with cytotoxic phenotype and some cases of diffuse large B-cell lymphoma, and secondary or disseminated forms of pleomorphic lymphomas. These lymphomas usually exhibit a bad prognosis with survival times less than 2–5 years.

This model is not a new clinicopathologic classification, but represents a new approach for peripheral lymphoproliferative processes. The categorization respects the specific biologic behavior of the various disease entities. It does not contradict, but supplements existing classifications. It is provisional but flexible and can been modified as new knowledge is obtained.

When diagnosing a cutaneous lymphoproliferative process, we suggest identifying both the clinicopathologic entity as given in the classification systems and the biologic category. As an example, a lymphoproliferative process composed predominantly of centroblast and centrocyte-like B cells, confined to the skin would be diagnosed as a "primary cutaneous follicle center cell lymphoma" and "primary cutaneous follicular lymphoma" according to WHO and EORTC classification, respectively, and in addition, categorized as "definite low-grade malignant lymphoma" (see Table 2). This declaration includes the information that the lesion is

Table 2 Prognostic Categories of Primary Cutaneous Lymphomas (CL) and their Relationship to the WHO Classification (2001)

WHO classification (truncated)	Prognostic categories of primary CL		
		Definite malignant lymphoma	
	Abortive lymphoma	Low-grade	High-grade
Mature T-cell and NK-cell neoplasms			
Mycosis fungoides	Pagetoid reticulosis Syringolymphoid hyperplasia (or syringotropic MF)	Mycosis fungoides (MF)	Transformation from MF or SS into high-grade lymphoma
Sézary syndrome		Sézary syndrome (SS)	
Primary cutaneous anaplastic large cell lymphoma		Primary cutaneous anaplastic large cell lymphoma	
Lymphomatois papulosis	Lymphomatoid papulosis		
Subcutaneous panniculitis-like T-cell lymphoma		Subcutaneous panniculitis-like T-cell lymphoma—indolent form	Subcutaneous panniculitis-like T-cell lymphoma—aggressive form
Peripheral T-cell lymphoma, unspecified		Pleomorphic small-cell lymphoma Granulomatous slack skin Juvenile granulomatous CTCL Cytotoxic TCL (CD8+)	Pleomorphic large-cell lymphoma Cytotoxic TCL (CD8+) Gamma/delta T-cell lymphoma
Adult T-cell leukemia/lymphoma		ATLL	ATLL
Extranodal NK/T-cell, nasal type			Extranodal NK-cell lymphoma

Precursor T-cell neoplasms		
Blastic NK-cell lymphoma		Blastic NK-cell lymphoma
Not listed	Precursor lesions (see comments)	
Large plaque parapsoriasis		
Clonal dermatitis		
Peripheral B-cell lymphoma		
Follicular lymphoma	Primary cutaneous follicular center lymphoma	
Extranodal marginal zone B-cell lymphoma	Primary cutaneous marginal zone B-cell lymphoma	
Lymphoplasmacytic lymphoma	Immunocytoma	
Mantle cell lymphoma		Mantle cell lymphoma
Diffuse large B-cell L.	Diffuse large B-cell lymphoma	Diffuse large B-cell lymphoma
		Localization on lower leg
Histiocyte/T-cell rich variant	T-cell rich B-cell variant	
Intravascular lymphoma		
Intravascular large B-cell lymphoma		Intravascular large B-cell lymphoma

Comments: Parapsoriasis may represent a chronic inflammatory disorder rather than a neoplastic process. Clonal dermatitis is not well characterized. Some cases may represent precursor lesions.
Source: From Ref. 2.

a distinct primary cutaneous B-cell lymphoma, but exhibiting an excellent prognosis. This type of lymphoma can therefore be treated with nonaggressive therapeutic modalities such as orthovolt radiotherapy, antibiotics, or steroids. The advantage of such an approach is to provide the diagnosis according to current classifications of lymphomas, and in addition, to include essential information about the biologic behavior. These data are crucial for the clinician involved in counseling and treatment of the patient and simplifies the management of patients, even in cases of rare and unusual CL.

The three *categories* and the comprised clinicopathologic entities according to the WHO classification for tumours of haemotopoietic (2) are outlined in Table 2.

REFERENCES

1. Burg G, Dummer R, Kerl H. Classification of cutaneous lymphomas. Derm Clinics 1994; 12:213–217.
2. Jaffe ES, Harris NL, Stein H, Vardiman JW. World Health Organization Classification of Tumors. Pathology and Genetics of Tumours of Haematopoietic and Lymphoid Tissues. Lyon: IARC Press, 2001.

21

Mycosis Fungoides

Dmitry V. Kazakov, Günter Burg, and Werner Kempf
Department of Dermatology, University Hospital, Zürich, Switzerland

CLASSIFICATION

WHO/EORTC Classification (2005): Mycosis fungoides
WHO Classification (2001): Mycosis fungoides
REAL Classification (1997): Mycosis fungoides
EORTC Classification (1997): Mycosis fungoides

DEFINITION

Mycosis fungoides (MF) is a generally indolent peripheral T-cell lymphoma initially and preferentially presenting in the skin and showing distinct clinical, histological (except in early stages), immunophenotypical, and genotypical features. It is the most common cutaneous lymphoma.

CLINICAL FEATURES

Men are more often affected than women (male:female ratio, 2:1) (1). Most frequently, MF affects adults, usually in the 5th–6th decades, although any age group may be involved. In some cases, the disease starts with nonspecific scaly lesions resembling chronic dermatitis, parapsoriasis, tinea corporis, or other inflammatory dermatoses. In other instances, patients present with more distinctive irregular, well-circumscribed, scaling patches varying in size from 2–3 to 10–15 cm (Fig. 1). The number of lesions is also variable. In some cases, only a few patches could be observed, whereas in other instances, the lesions can be numerous and widely distributed. Pruritus is common and often severe. In some cases, the patches show a tendency to partial spontaneous remission that, in combination with peripheral growth, leads to the development of lesions with unusual configurations (annular, semicircular, serpinginous). It usually takes several years until the patches progress into plaques and tumors, which may then ulcerate (Figs. 2–4). A subset of patients have persistent patch-stage disease for many years or even decades. Lymph nodes and internal organs may become involved in the later stages of MF. In the advanced

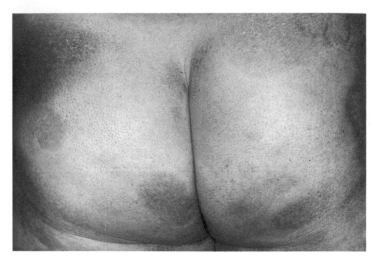

Figure 1 Patch stage: large erythematous and scaling patches on the buttocks, virtually indistinguishable from large plaque parapsoriasis in a patient with proven MF.

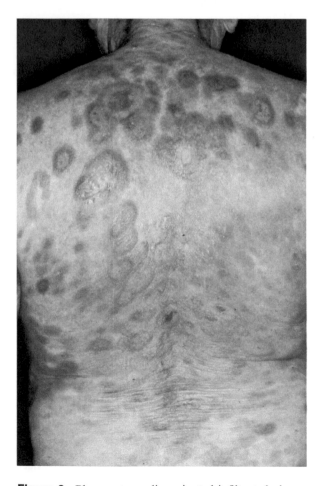

Figure 2 Plaque stage: disseminated infiltrated plaques on the back.

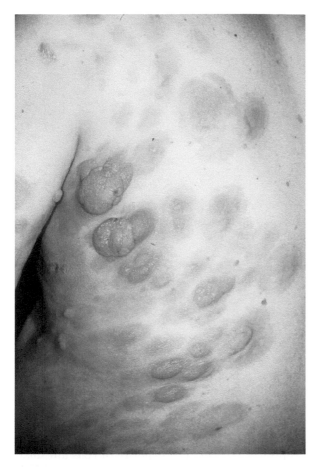

Figure 3 Tumor stage: several large tumors on the background of patches and plaques in advanced MF.

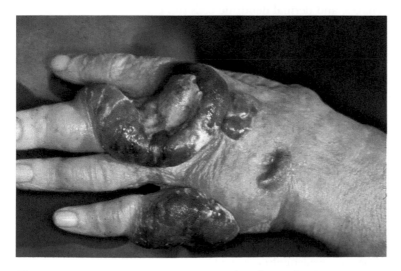

Figure 4 Tumor stage: ulcerated tumor in advanced MF.

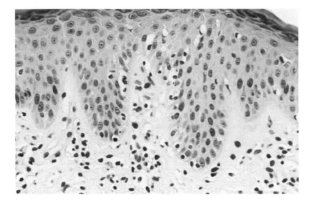

Figure 5 Patch stage: sparse lymphocytic infiltrate with lymphocytes lined up along the junctional zone and scattered throughout the epidermis.

stages, progression to a high-grade T-cell lymphoma (Fig. 4) is observed in approximately 25% of cases and is usually associated with an aggressive clinical course (2–5).

HISTOLOGY

In very early stages, the histological picture is nonspecific, characterized by a mild perivascular infiltrate in the upper dermis containing no atypical lymphocytes and lacking epidermotropism (Figs. 5 and 6). Early MF can produce practically all of the patterns used for diagnosing inflammatory skin disease (6). The histological findings become diagnostic, when a denser infiltrate with lymphocytes lining up in the basal layer and showing single-cell epidermotropism is present. The majority of cells are small, well-differentiated lymphocytes with round or only slightly cerebriform nuclei. In addition, there can be mild acanthosis, hyperkeratosis, signs of basal layer damage (pigment incontinence), edema or fibrosis of the papillary dermis, and proliferation of postcapillary venules. The infiltrate may contain an admixture of eosinophils, plasma cells, macrophages, and dermal dendritic cells (6,7).

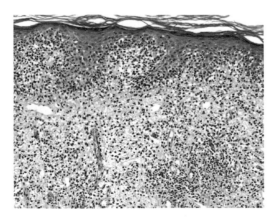

Figure 6 Patch stage: extensive epidermotropism and lining-up of lymphocytes with minimal spongiosis.

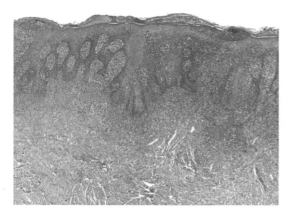

Figure 7 Plaque stage: dense lichenoid lymphocytic infiltrate with epidermotropism and reactive epidermal hyperplasia.

The plaque stage is typified by a dense, subepidermal, usually band-like infiltrate containing a high number of cerebriform cells (Figs. 7 and 8). Epidermotropism is more prominent with small intraepidermal clusters (2–3 cells) of lymphocytes (Fig. 9). Typical Pautrier microabscesses are seen only in approximately one-third of cases. Collections of atypical lymphocytes in the dermis are found in some cases (Fig. 10).

In the tumor stage, the infiltrate is nodular or diffuse and usually demonstrates loss of epidermotropism . In addition to a predominant population of small cerebriform cells, there is a variable admixture of immunoblasts, lymphoblasts, and medium-sized or large pleomorphic or anaplastic cells (Fig. 11). In the transformed cases, the histological picture is identical to that seen in a correspondent primary cutaneous lymphoma arising without preceding MF. The morphological spectrum of the transformation is wide, with CD30– pleomorphic lymphoma being the most common type.

IMMUNOHISTOCHEMISTRY

The typical phenotype of the neoplastic cells is CD2+, CD3+, CD5+, CD4+, CD45RO+, CD8–, TCRβ+, CD30–. As the disease progresses, an aberrant

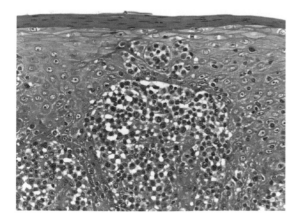

Figure 8 Plaque stage: epidermotropism of lymphocytes forming Pautrier microabscesses.

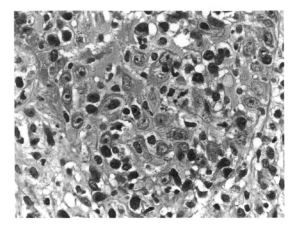

Figure 9   Epidermotropism of atypical lymphocytes with convoluted nuclei in advanced MF.

phenotype with loss of T-cell antigens is a common finding. CD7 is expressed in one-third of the lesions. In rare cases, expression of CD8 and TCRδ can occur. Immunohistochemistry plays a minor role in the diagnosis of MF, since the neoplastic cells in early stages have no immunophenotypical aberrations (9).

Functionally, the neoplastic cells in MF express Th2 phenotype, which accounts for many systemic changes associated with MF due to the production of a Th2-specific cytokine pattern (IL-4, IL-5, IL-10, and others) leading to eosinophilia, increase of IgE or IgA, and impaired delayed type reactivity (10,11).

MOLECULAR BIOLOGY

TCRβ or γ chain genes are clonally rearranged in most cases, including patch-stage disease. Even in early stages of the disease, T-cell clones can be detected in lymph nodes and peripheral blood; the biological significance of this phenomenon remains unclear, since T-cell clones in the extracutaneous compartment are often different

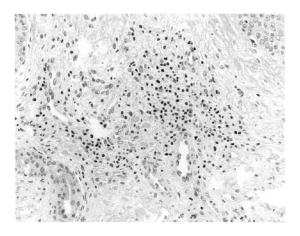

Figure 10   Dermal accumulation of atypical lymphocytes, histologically termed interstitial MF.

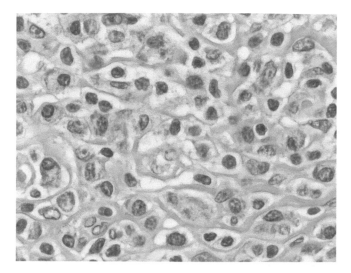

Figure 11 Tumor stage: medium-sized to large atypical lymphocytes with pleomorphic nuclei and abundant cytoplasm. These cytologic features are not seen in early stages of MF. *Source:* From Ref. 8.

from those found in the skin and seem to represent an expanded normal T-cell population rather than circulating neoplastic cells. Two (or more) unrelated clones in the skin are seen in about 20% of cases as demonstrated by cytogenetic analysis and RT-PCR analysis of TCRβ genes. In advanced cases with extracutaneous involvement, the same clone is usually detected in the skin and in the extracutaneous lesions. In transformed cases, the same clone is present in the pre-existing lesions and the high-grade lymphoma (12–16)

CYTOGENETIC ANALYSIS

Complex single cell abnormalities detected by G-banding and interphase cytogenetic methods possibly reflect increased genetic instability as a basic prerequisite for the development of lymphoma.

TREATMENT

Treatment of MF is stage-dependent, with a range of treatment modalities, as discussed in Chapter 47.

CLINICAL COURSE AND PROGNOSIS

The majority of MF patients show an indolent clinical course over years or decades. The prognosis of the disease is defined by its stage. Patients with early stages have an excellent prognosis with survival similar to that of an age-, sex-, and race-matched population. Factors indicating poor prognosis are advanced stage and age above 60 years. When extracutaneous involvement or transformation into high-grade lymphoma occurs, suspected survival is usually less than 1 year (17,18). It has been speculated that expression of CD44v6 may be helpful as a prognostic marker for assessing the potential for extracutaneous spread and homing behavior of the neoplastic cells.

Mycosis fungoides

Clinical features
  Male:female ratio, 2:1
  Mostly adults/elderly patients
  Patches–plaques–tumors
  Pruritus
  Extracutaneous spread in late stages
Histological features
  Early: nonspecific findings
  Later: lining-up of cerebriform lymphocytes in junctional zone
  Admixture of eosinophils and plasma cells
  Edema or fibrosis in the upper dermis
  Transformation into high-grade lymphoma in late stages
Immunophenotype
  CD2+, CD3+, CD5+, CD4+, CD45RO+, CD8–, CD30–
  Some cases CD8+ or TCRγ/δ+
  Not helpful in the diagnosis of early disease
Molecular biology
  Clonal TCR rearrangement in majority of cases including early disease
Laboratory evaluation
  Plays no important role in diagnosis
  Eosinophilia
Treatment
  Topical steroids, PUVA, retinoids, IFN-α, in later stages chemotherapy and
    experimental protocols
Clinical course and prognosis
  Stage-dependent
  Indolent and excellent in early stages
  Aggressive after transformation

DIFFERENTIAL DIAGNOSIS

In very early stages of MF, differentiation from the many inflammatory simulators on clinical and histological grounds is often not possible. Molecular biology can be helpful in such cases, but the detection of a clonal population alone without compatible clinicopathological findings does not suffice for the diagnosis of MF, because of the existence of the so-called "clonal dermatoses." Compatible histology coupled with the evidence of clonal TCR gene rearrangements make the diagnosis of MF very likely. In many cases, both the history (persistency of lesions, resistance to therapy, striking tendency to recur) and the clinical features raise the question of MF. Plaque- and tumor stages of the disease usually pose no diagnostic challenge.

COMMENTS

Along with the above-described classical presentation of the disease, known as the Alibert–Bazin form, there is a number of atypical clinical and histological forms of MF described in Chapter 22.3

The sudden multifocal development of tumors without preceding patches or plaques was previously designated as the d'emblee form of MF. Today, it is agreed that such cases represent primary large T-cell lymphomas, some of them being CD30+. In some cases, patients with patches and plaques are apt to develop erythroderma in the course of the disease — the condition often referred to as erythrodermic MF. The relation of this disorder to Sezary syndrome (Chapter 24) has not yet been clarified.

The relation of MF and small as well as large plaque parapsoriasis (SPP) (Chapter 41) is still the subject of debate. The similarity of histopathological findings in these conditions lead to the speculation that SPP represents a very early stage of MF.

MYCOSIS FUNGOIDES IN CHILDHOOD AND ADOLESCENCE

Mycosis fungoides (MF) is not purely a disease of the elderly. A thorough history taken from an adult patient may reveal the onset of symptoms during childhood or adolescence (younger than age 20). The incidence of MF starting at an early age has been estimated at 1.8–7% (19–23).

CLINICAL FEATURES

In contrast to MF in adults, MF in childhood and adolescence does not favor boys; one recent series even revealed a striking female predominance (24). Features typical for ordinary MF as well as various atypical clinical variants have been reported. Among the latter, the hypopigmented form appears to be over-represented.

HISTOLOGY

The histological features are identical to those seen in adults.

IMMUNOHISTOCHEMISTRY

In many cases, the disease in young patients has immunophenotypical features identical to those seen in the adult population. In a subset of patients (usually with hypopigmented subtype), the neoplastic cells exhibit a cytotoxic phenotype (CD8+, TIA1+).

MOLECULAR BIOLOGY

The findings are similar to those seen in adult patients.

TREATMENT

The same approach is taken as with adult patients.

CLINICAL COURSE AND PROGNOSIS

The vast majority of patients present with stage IA and IB disease and therefore have an excellent prognosis with survival rates similar to those seen in the background population (23). Progression to plaque-stage disease and death from disease have been documented in retrospective studies (22,23). There are no factors which predict tumor progression in young MF patients

DIFFERENTIAL DIAGNOSIS

MF in childhood and adolescence is rare and therefore prone to under-recognition

---

MF in childhood and adolescence

Clinical features
    No male predominance
    Features identical to ordinary MF as well as atypical forms can be seen
    Often hypopigmented
Histological features
    Similar to those in adult MF
Immunophenotype
    Similar to that in adult MF
    Some cases: CD2+, CD7–, CD8+, TIA+
Molecular biology
    Clonal TCR rearrangement in majority of cases
Clinical course and prognosis
Usually indolent and favorable (independent of immunophenotype)

COMMENTS

Cytotoxic phenotype expressed by neoplastic cells in cutaneous lymphoma is usually associated with an unfavorable prognosis. In contrast to most cases of CD8+ epidermotropic lymphoma, which inevitably run an aggressive course, young MF patients with cytotoxic phenotype take an indolent disease. The expression of CD2 and the lack of expression of CD7 by neoplastic cells in these patients may explain the phenomenon; patients with cytotoxic lymphomas with CD2+, CD7– phenotype are more likely to have an indolent course than those with CD2–, CD7+ phenotype (25).

REFERENCES

1. Kim YH, Hoppe RT. Mycosis fungoides and the Sezary syndrome. Semin Oncol 1999; 26:276–289.
2. Burg G, Braun-Falco O. Cutaneous Lymphomas, Pseudolymphomas and Related Disorders. Berlin: Springer-Verlag, 1983.
3. Abel EA, Wood GS, Hoppe RT. Mycosis fungoides: clinical and histologic features, staging, evaluation, and approach to treatment. CA Cancer J Clin 1993; 43:93–115.

4. Burg G, Dummer R, Nestle FO, Doebbeling U, Haeffner A. Cutaneous lymphomas consist of a spectrum of nosologically different entities including mycosis fungoides and small plaque parapsoriasis. Arch Dermatol 1996; 132:567–572.
5. Diamandidou E, Cohen PR, Kurzrock R. Mycosis fungoides and Sezary syndrome. Blood 1996; 88:2385–2409.
6. Shapiro PE, Pinto FJ. The histologic spectrum of mycosis fungoides/Sezary syndrome (cutaneous T-cell lymphoma). A review of 222 biopsies, including newly described patterns and the earliest pathologic changes. Am J Surg Pathol 1994; 18:645–667.
7. Guitart J, Kennedy J, Ronan S, Chmiel JS, Hsiegh YC, Variakojis D. Histologic criteria for the diagnosis of mycosis fungoides: proposal for a grading system to standardize pathology reporting. J Cutan Pathol 2001; 28:174–183.
8. Kazakov DV, Burg G, Kemp W. Clinicopathological spectrum of mycosis fungoides. JEADV 2004; 18: 397–415.
9. Smoller BR. The role of immunohistochemistry in the diagnosis of cutaneous lymphoma. Adv Dermatol 1997; 13:207–234.
10. Vowels BR, Lessin SR, Cassin M, Jaworsky C, Benoit B, Wolfe JT, Rook AH. The cytokine mRNA expression in skin in cutaneous T-cell lymphoma. J Invest Dermatol 1994; 103:669–673.
11. Rook AH, Vowels BR, Jaworsky C, Singh A, Lessin SR. The immunopathogenesis of cutaneous T-cell lymphoma. Abnormal cytokine production by Sezary T cells. Arch Dermatol 1993; 129:486–489.
12. Bakels V, van Oostveen JW, Gordijn RL, Walboomers JM, Meijer CJ, Willemze R. Frequency and prognostic significance of clonal T-cell receptor beta-gene rearrangements in the peripheral blood of patients with mycosis fungoides. Arch Dermatol 1992; 128:1602–1607.
13. Bergman R. How useful are T-cell receper gene rearrangement studies as an adjunct to the histopathologic diagnosis of mycosis? Am J Dermatopathol 1999; 21:498–502
14. Guitart J, Kaul K. A new polymerase chain reaction-based method for the detection of T-cell clonality in patients with possible cutaneous T-cell lymphoma. Arch Dermatol 1999; 135:158–162.
15. Delfau-Larue MH, Laroche L, Wechsler J, Lepage E, Lahet C, Asso-Bonnet M, Bagot M, Farcet JP. Diagnostic value of dominant T-cell clones in peripheral blood in 363 patients presenting consecutively with a clinical suspicion of cutaneous lymphoma. Blood 2000; 96:2987–2992.
16. Dommann SN, Dommann-Scherrer CC, Dours-Zimmermann MT, Zimmermann DR, Kural-Serbes B, Burg G. Clonal disease in extracutaneous compartments in cutaneous T-cell lymphomas. A comparative study between cutaneous T-cell lymphomas and pseudo lymphomas. Arch Dermatol Res 1996; 288:163–167.
17. van Doorn R, Van Haselen CW, van Voorst Vader PC, Geerts ML, Heule F, de Rie M, Steijlen PM, Dekker SK, van Vloten WA, Willemze R. Mycosis fungoides: disease evolution and prognosis of 309 Dutch patients. Arch Dermatol 2000; 136:504–510.
18. Toro JR, Stoll HL Jr, Stomper PC, Oseroff AR. Prognostic factors and evaluation of mycosis fungoides and Sezary syndrome. J Am Acad Dermatol 1997; 37:58–67.
19. Quaglino P, Zaccagna A, Verrone A, Dardano F, Bernengo MG. Mycosis fungoides in patients under 20 years of age: report of 7 cases, review of the literature and study of the clinical course. Dermatology 1999; 199:8–14.
20. Peters MS, Thibodeau SN, White JW Jr, Winkelmann RK. Mycosis fungoides in children and adolescents. J Am Acad Dermatol 1990; 22:1011–1018.
21. Burns MK, Ellis CN, Cooper KD. Mycosis fungoides-type cutaneous T-cell lymphoma arising before 30 years of age. Immunophenotypic, immunogenotypic and clinicopathologic analysis of nine cases. J Am Acad Dermatol 1992; 27:974–978.
22. Crowley JJ, Nikko A, Varghese A, Hoppe RT, Kim YH. Mycosis fungoides in young patients: clinical characteristics and outcome. J Am Acad Dermatol 1998; 38:696–701.

23. Koch SE, Zackheim HS, Williams ML, Fletcher V, LeBoit PE. Mycosis fungoides begin-
     ning in childhood and adolescence. J Am Acad Dermatol 1987; 17:563–570.
24. Whittam LR, Calonje E, Orchard G, Fraser-Andrews EA, Woolford A, Russell-Jones R.
     CD8-positive juvenile onset mycosis fungoides: an immunohistochemical and genotypic
     analysis of six cases. Br J Dermatol 2000; 143:1199–1204.
25. Agnarsson BA, Vonderheid EC, Kadin ME. Cutaneous T cell lymphoma with
     suppressor/cytotoxic (CD8) phenotype: identification of rapidly progressive and chronic
     subtypes. J Am Acad Dermatol 1990; 22:569–577.

21.1. Transformation of CTCL

Werner Kempf, Dmitry V. Kazakov, Sonja Michaelis, and Günter Burg
Department of Dermatology, University Hospital, Zürich, Switzerland

DEFINITION

Mycosis fungoides evolves slowly over years starting with patches, which are followed by plaques and tumors. Only about 10% of patients manifest initially with tumors (so-called d'emblée form). The term "transformation" is commonly used to describe progression of classic CTCL such as MF to large-cell lymphomas. Transformation of low-grade CTCL into a high-grade lymphoma is more often observed in patients with classical MF, but can also be seen in patients with Sézary syndrome (SS) (1).

CLINICAL FEATURES

Between 8% and 55% of patients with CTCL undergo transformation (2,3). The interval between diagnosis of MF and transformation is about 1–2 years (3,4) but can be more than 5–10 years. Clinically, transformation is characterized by occurrence of large tumors, which often become ulcerated (Fig. 1). Those tumors evolve from infiltrated plaques, but can also arise on previously unaffected skin and at any time point in the course of the disease. Superinfection of ulcerated lesions with *Staphylococcus aureus* and *Pseudomonas aeruginosa* is very common. Together with extracutaneous spread, septicemia originating from infected tumors is the major cause of death in patients with advanced stages of MF and SS.

HISTOLOGY

Transformed tumors usually feature dense deep-reaching cohesive infiltrates of large pleomorphic tumor cells, but tumors with immunoblastic, anaplastic, and medium-sized pleomorphic cells are also observed (5) (Fig. 2). Clusters of B-cells can be found

113

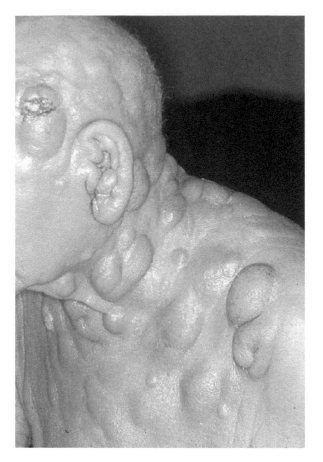

Figure 1 Transformation of Sézary syndrome: multiple large and partly ulcerated nodules in an erythrodermic patient.

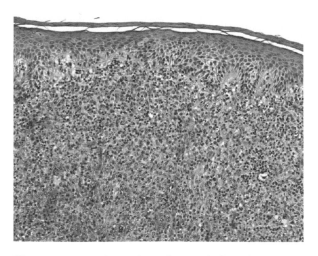

Figure 2 Transformation of mycosis fungoides: dense dermal infiltrate of tumor cells with loss of epidermotropism.

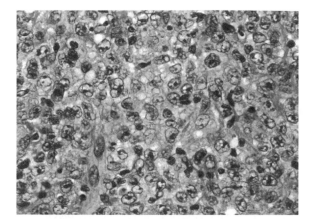

Figure 3 Transformation of mycosis fungoides: cohesive sheets of CD30– large pleomorphic tumor cells.

in about 25% of tumors. Scattered eosinophils and plasma cells may be admixed, while ulceration is a very common finding. Histologic features of transformation may precede the clinical development of tumors (6).

IMMUNOHISTOCHEMISTRY

Loss of pan-T-cell markers is common. CD3 expression may be weak. CD30– pleomorphic lymphoma is the most common type, whereas CD30+ large cell pleomorphic lymphoma is relatively rarely found (Fig. 3). Clonal T-cells can be detected in most cases. The identical gene rearrangement as in pre-existing infiltrates has been identified in the transformed tumors (7).

TREATMENT

Therapy with multiagent chemotherapy (CHOP), radiation therapy, or autologous bone marrow transplantation results in complete remission in only a small percentage (approximately 25–30%) of patients.

CLINICAL COURSE AND PROGNOSIS

Transformation indicates an unfavorable prognosis in most patients with median survival from transformation of 2–27 months versus 53% for patients with nontransformed MF (2–4). Median time from diagnosis of MF to transformation was 6.5 years in one study (6). In this same study, mean survival from transformation to death was 22 months. CD30 expression has no prognostic impact in transformed cases, whereas age (at least 60 years) and extracutaneous spread are associated with a poor prognosis with a 5-year actuarial survival of 8% versus 32% in transformed cases (6). Most patients experience disease progression with fatal outcome (8).

Remarkably, tumors can undergo spontaneous regression as it is seen in 25% of CD30+ ALCL, but systemic spread with involvement of all visceral organs can subsequently follow and result in a fatal outcome.

DIFFERENTIAL DIAGNOSIS

In most cases, the history of early stages of MF or erythroderma of SS allow readily differentiation of transformed MF or SS from pleomorphic large T-cell lymphomas (LTCL) arising de novo. In cases of d'emblée form of MF, in which tumors are the initial presentation, it can be very difficult or even impossible to distinguish between MF d'emblée and multifocal primary or secondary cutaneous LTCL. Staging examinations are mandatory with this clinical scenario.

REFERENCES

1. Diamandidou E, Colome-Grimmer M, Fayad L, Duvic M, Kurzrock R. Transformation of mycosis fungoides/Sézary syndrome: clinical characteristics and prognosis. Blood 1998; 92:1150–1159.
2. Salhany KE, Cousar JB, Greer JP, Casey TT, Fields JP, Collins RD. Transformation of cutaneous T cell lymphoma to large cell lymphoma. A clinicopathologic and immunologic study. Am J Pathol 1988; 132:265–277.
3. Greer JP, Salhany KE, Cousar JB, Fields JP, King LE, Graber SE, Flexner JM, Stein RS, Collins RD. Clinical features associated with transformation of cerebriform T-cell lymphoma to a large cell process. Hematol Oncol 1990; 8:215–227.
4. Dmitrovsky E, Matthews MJ, Bunn PA, Schechter GP, Makuch RW, Winkler CF, Eddy J, Sausville EA, Ihde DC. Cytologic transformation in cutaneous T cell lymphoma: a clinicopathologic entity associated with poor prognosis. J Clin Oncol 1987; 5:208–215.
5. Cerroni L, Rieger E, Hodl S, Kerl H. Clinicopathologic and immunologic features associated with transformation of mycosis fungoides to large-cell lymphoma. Am J Surg Pathol 1992; 16:543–552.
6. Vergier B, de Muret A, Beylot-Barry M, Vaillant L, Ekouevi D, Chene G, Carlotti A, Franck N, Dechelotte P, Souteyrand P, Courville P, Joly P, Delaunay M, Bagot M, Grange F, Fraitag S, Bosq J, Petrella T, Durlach A, De Mascarel A, Merlio JP, Wechsler J. Transformation of mycosis fungoides: clinicopathological and prognostic features of 45 cases. French Study Group of Cutaneous Lymphomas. Blood 2000; 95:2212–2218.
7. Wood GS, Bahler DW, Hoppe RT, Warnke RA, Sklar JL, Levy R. Transformation of mycosis fungoides: T-cell receptor beta gene analysis demonstrates a common clonal origin for plaque-type mycosis fungoides and CD30+ large-cell lymphoma. J Invest Dermatol 1993; 101:296–300.
8. Scarisbrick JJ, Child FJ, Evans AV, Fraser-Andrews EA, Spittle M, Russell-Jones R. Secondary malignant neoplasms in 71 patients with Sézary syndrome. Arch Dermatol 1999; 135:1381–1385.

22

Variants and Subtypes of Mycosis Fungoides

22.1. Pagetoid Reticulosis

Dmitry V. Kazakov, Günter Burg, and Werner Kempf
Department of Dermatology, University Hospital, Zürich, Switzerland

CLASSIFICATION

WHO/EORTC Classification (2005): Variants and subtypes of mycosis fungoides, pagetoid reticulosis
WHO Classification (2001): Not listed
REAL Classsification (1997): Not listed
EORTC Classsification (1997): Pagetoid reticulosis

DEFINITION

Pagetoid reticulosis (PR) in its unilesional form (Woringer–Kolopp disease) is a low-grade malignant variant of mycosis fungoides (MF) with characteristic histologic features, but various phenotypes. The terminology of PR is confusing. Originally, two forms of PR were described, namely disseminated and unilesional PR. In 1931, Ketron and Goodman (1) described multiple lesions of the skin "apparently of epithelial origin" clinically resembling MF, while in 1939, Woringer and Kolopp (2) reported a solitary plaque-like lesion on the arm of a 6–year old boy. The term "pagetoid reticulosis" was proposed by Braun-Falco et al. (3) because of the distinct histological appearance. Most experts today consider disseminated PR a form of MF or cytotoxic epidermotropic T-cell lymphoma. The localized form of PR (Woringer–Kolopp disease) is regarded as a "superficial spreading" form of MF. In our opinion, only the localized form should be referred to as PR sensu strictu.

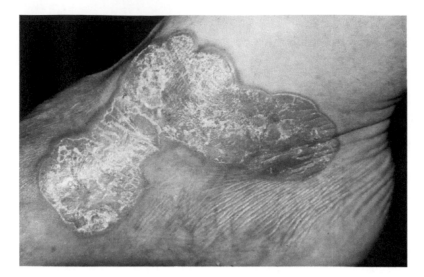

Figure 1 Sharply demarcated erythematous and scaling plaque on the foot.

CLINICAL FEATURES

PR presents as a solitary psoriasiform or bowenoid erythematous, scaling or crusty plaque, exhibiting centrifugal growth (4) (Fig. 1). Acral body areas are the sites of predilection. Rarely, mucosal involvement has been observed (5). In contrast to MF, PR never spreads to other sites of the body: to lymph nodes, peripheral blood, internal organs, or bone marrow.

HISTOLOGY

The epidermis shows marked psoriasiform hyperplasia with para- and orthohyperkeratosis, including small abscess-like formations, containing serum, some neutrophils, and cellular debris (6). A sponge-like disaggregation to the acanthotic

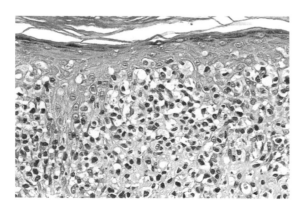

Figure 2 Pagetoid epidermotropism of lymphocytes with abundant cytoplasm (halo cells).

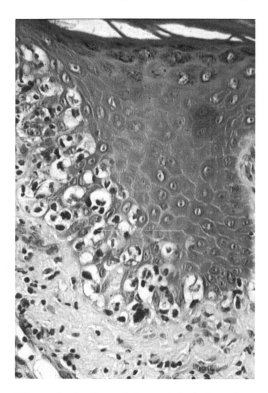

Figure 3   In the periphery of the lesion, the tumor cells are located in the lower third of the epidermis.

epidermis by medium-sized to large atypical lymphoid cells with vacuolated, abundant cytoplasm, arranged singly or in clusters, is the hallmark of PR (7) (Fig. 2). The nuclei are large, sometimes convoluted and hyperchromatic. Mitotic figures are rare. Single cells and small clusters of tumor cells can also be observed within the epithelia of adnexal structures. Towards the center of the lesion, the diffuse band-like infiltrate consisting of small cerebriform lymphocytes increasingly involves the upper dermis. At the margins of the lesion, tumor cells are mostly found in the lower third of the epidermis (Fig. 3).

IMMUNOHISTOCHEMISTRY

Several phenotypes of neoplastic lymphocytes in PR have been reported. The neoplastic cells in PR may express CD4, CD8 or be CD4/CD8 double negative. Most cases of PR express a T helper phenotype: CD3+, CD4+, CD5+, CD8− (8). There are reports on CD8+ cases (5,9) or PR expressing a gamma/delta phenotype (10). The neoplastic cells demonstrate a higher proliferation rate (>30%) in comparison to lymphocytes in the patch or plaque stage MF (<10%). Lastly, in some cases, infiltrates in PR may contain high numbers (>50%) of CD30+ cells, whereas such CD30 reactivity is never observed in nontransformed MF (5,11). Loss of leukocyte common antigen (CD45) on tumor cells was only found in the localized form of PR (12). Only about 10% of tumor cells show proliferative activity (13).

Neoplastic cells in PR strongly express cutaneous lymphocyte antigen, a skin-homing receptor interacting with E-selectin on cutaneous endothelial cells. In addition, tumor cells express the adhesion molecule alpha E beta 7, which interacts with E-cadherin on keratinocytes. These data may explain the pronounced epidermotropism of neoplastic lymphocytes in PR (14).

MOLECULAR BIOLOGY

Clonal T-cell receptor (TCR) gene rearrangement has been demonstrated in some cases of PR (5,15).

TREATMENT

Therapy includes surgical excision, radiotherapy, PUVA, or bath PUVA, and topical application of DNCB.

CLINICAL COURSE AND PROGNOSIS

In contrast to other CTCL, PR exhibits an excellent prognosis. Recurrences seem to be rare. Occasionally, the occurrence of a second lymphoid neoplasm such as CD30+ large-cell NHL in patients with PR has been observed (16).

DIFFERENTIAL DIAGNOSIS

Clinically, the differential diagnosis includes solitary lesions of psoriasis, Bowen disease, or circumscribed forms of chronic dermatitis. Although unilesional MF and PR share common clinical and histologic features, PR is distinguished histolo-

---

Pagetoid reticulosis

Clinical features
  Solitary sharply demarcated plaque
Histological features
  Prominent epidermotropism of lymphocytes with clear cytoplasm
Immunophenotype
  CD2+, CD3+, CD5+, CD4+, CD45RO+, CD8−, CD30−/+
  Some cases: CD8+ or TCRgamma/delta+
Molecular biology
  Clonal TCR rearrangement
Treatment
  Excision or ionizing radiation
Clinical course and prognosis
  Excellent

---

gically from MF by the presence of marked hyperkeratosis, prominent pagetoid epidermotropism of somewhat larger cerebriform cells and paucicellular dermal infiltrate lacking eosinophils (11,17). Histologically, superficial spreading melanoma and Paget disease may mimic PR, but can readily be distinguished by cytomorphologic and immunophenotypic features (S-100; CEA; EMA) (18,19).

COMMENTS

Since some cases of unilesional PR express a cytotoxic phenotype (CD3+, CD8+, or CD56+), these cases could also be classified as cytotoxic T- or NK-cell lymphomas, respectively (10). We prefer to consider them PR because of their characteristic clinical and histological features. So far, no differences in the course between cases of PR with different phenotypes have been delineated.

REFERENCES

1. Ketron LW, Goodman MH. Multiple lesions of the skin apparently of epithelial origin resembling clinically mycosis fungoides. Arch Dermatol 1931; 24:758–777.
2. Woringer F, Kolopp P. Lésion érythématosquameuse polycyclique de l'avant-bras évoluant depuis 6 ans chez un garçonnet de 13 ans. Ann Dermatol Syphilol 1939; 10: 945–958.
3. Braun-Falco O, Marghescu S, Wolff HH. Pagetoide reticulose. Hautarzt 1973; 24:11–21.
4. Braun-Falco O, Schmoeckel C, Burg G, Ryckmanns F. Pagetoid reticulosis. A further case report with a review of the literature. Acta Derm Venereol Suppl (Stockh) 1979; 59:11–21.
5. Haghighi B, Smoller BR, LeBoit PE, Warnke RA, Sander CA, Kohler S. Pagetoid reticulosis (Woringer–Kolopp disease): an immunophenotypic, molecular, and clinicopathologic study. Mod Pathol 2000; 13:502–510.
6. Medenica M, Lorincz AL. Pagetoid reticulosis (Woringer–Kolopp disease). Histopathologic and ultrastructural observations. Arch Dermatol 1978; 114:262–268.
7. Deneau DG, Wood GS, Beckstead J, Hoppe RT, Price N. Woringer–Kolopp disease (pagetoid reticulosis). Four cases with histopathologic, ultrastructural, and immunohistologic observations. Arch Dermatol 1984; 120:1045–1051.
8. Kaudewitz P, Stein H, Klepzig K, Mason DY, Braun-Falco O. Monoclonal antibody patterns in lymphomatoid papulosis. Dermatol Clin 1985; 3:749–757.
9. Mackie RM, Turbitt ML. A case of pagetoid reticulosis bearing the T cytotoxic suppressor surface marker on the lymphoid infiltrate: further evidence that pagetoid reticulosis is not a variant of mycosis fungoides. Br J Dermatol 1984; 110:89–94.
10. Berti E, Cerri A, Cavicchini S, Delia D, Soligo D, Alessi E, Caputo R. Primary cutaneous gamma/delta T-cell lymphoma presenting as disseminated pagetoid reticulosis. J Invest Dermatol 1991; 96:718–723.
11. Burns MK, Chan LS, Cooper KD. Woringer–Kolopp disease (localized pagetoid reticulosis) or unilesional mycosis fungoides? An analysis of eight cases with benign disease. Arch Dermatol 1995; 131:325–329.
12. Sterry W, Hauschild A. Loss of leucocyte common antigen (CD45) on atypical lymphocytes in the localized but not disseminated type of pagetoid reticulosis. Br J Dermatol 1991; 125:238–242.
13. Kaudewitz P, Burg G, Majiewski G, Gerdes J, Schwarting R, Braun-Falco O. Cell populations in pagetoid reticulosis: an immunological study using cell activation associated monoclonal antibodies. Acta Derm Venereol 1987; 67:24–29.

14. Drillenburg P, Bronkhorst CM, van der Wal AC, Noorduyn LA, Hoekzema R, Pals ST. Expression of adhesion molecules in pagetoid reticulosis (Woringer–Kolopp disease). Br J Dermatol 1997; 136:613–616.
15. Wood GS, Weiss LM, Hu CH, Abel EA, Hoppe RT, Warnke RA, Sklar J. T-cell antigen deficiencies and clonal rearrangements of T-cell receptor genes in pagetoid reticulosis (Woringer Kolopp disease). N Engl J Med 1988; 318:164 167.
16. Ralfkiaer E, Thomsen K, Agdal N, Hou-Jensen K, Wantzin GL. The development of a Ki-1-positive large cell non-Hodgkin's lymphoma in pagetoid reticulosis. Acta Derm Venereol 1989; 69:206–211.
17. Jones RR, Chu A. Pagetoid reticulosis and solitary mycosis fungoides. Distinct clinico-pathological entities. J Cutan Pathol 1981; 8:40–51.
18. Burg G. Pagetoide Hautinfiltrate. Pathologe 1986; 7:199–206.
19. Kohler S, Rouse RV, Smoller BR. The differential diagnosis of pagetoid cells in the epidermis. Mod Pathol 1998; 11:79–92.

Syringotropic Cutaneous T-cell Lymphoma

Dmitry V. Kazakov, Günter Burg, and Werner Kempf
Department of Dermatology, University Hospital, Zürich, Switzerland

CLASSIFICATION

WHO/EORTC Classification (2005): Mycosis fungoides, variants and sub-
 types, syringotropic
WHO Classification (2001): Not listed
REAL Classification (1997): Not listed
EORTC Classification (1997): Not listed

DEFINITION

Syringotropic cutaneous T-cell lymphoma (CTCL) originally has been described as "syringolymphoid hyperplesia with alopecia" (1). It is a rare variant of mycosis fungoides (MF) showing a specific histopathological pattern with predominant involvement of eccrine sweat glands by small cerebriform lymphocytes (2).

CLINICAL FEATURES

Remarkably, all patients reported to date have been men. The lesions are usually red-brown patches, slightly infiltrated scaling plaques, or small red or skin-colored papules (Fig. 1). Anhidrosis and hair loss in the affected areas are common.

HISTOLOGY

There is a periadnexal infiltrate composed of small cerebriform lymphocytes invading both the secretory and ductal portions of hyperplastic eccrine glands (Fig. 2 and 3). The irregular proliferation of small eccrine epithelial islands infiltrated by

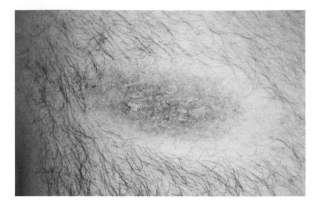

Figure 1 Well-circumscribed erythematous and scaling plaque with alopecia.

lymphocytes may resemble small aggregations of "eccrine spiradenoma en minia-ture" (3). The infiltrate may also invade the epidermis focally, but epidermotropism is not a prominent feature and Pautrier microabscesses are not usually seen. Some-times, hair follicles may be concurrently involved and even destroyed by the neoplastic infiltrate (syringolymphoid hyperplasia with alopecia); follicular mucino-sis is not usually seen.

IMMUNOHISTOCHEMISTRY

The neoplastic lymphocytes are T-helper cells (CD3+, CD4+, CD8–).

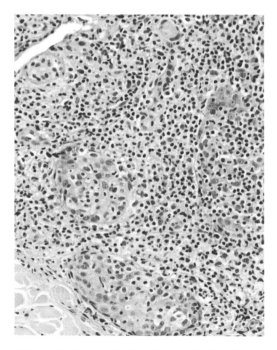

Figure 2 Sweat glands infiltrated by lymphocytes with an admixture of scattered eosinophils.

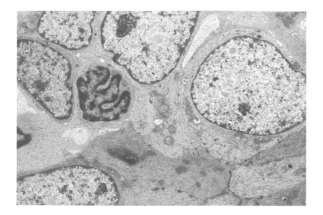

Figure 3 Atypical lymphocyte between epithelial cells of sweat glands (electron microscopy, original magnification 3000×).

MOLECULAR BIOLOGY

Clonal rearrangement of TCR genes is found in most cases.

TREATMENT

The same approaches used for MF are employed.

CLINICAL COURSE AND PROGNOSIS

The data are scarce, but the clinical course and prognosis appear to be similar to those of mycosis fungoides.

DIFFERENTIAL DIAGNOSIS

Syringotropic CTCL should be distinguished from idiopathic forms of syringolymphoid hyperplasia with alopecia. Lesions in the idiopathic disease lack atypical lymphocytes and harbor no dominant T-cell clones. Some suspect that the idiopathic form of the disease may be part of the early spectrum of the lymphoma form (4).

COMMENTS

The clinical presentation, expression of CD4 by the neoplastic cells with small cerebriform cytology, and clonal rearrangement of TCR genes indicate that syringotropic CTCL merely represents a variant of MF.

REFERENCES

1. Vakilzadeh F, Brocker EB. Syringolymphoid hyperplasia with alopecia? Br J Dermatol 1984; 110:95–101.
2. Burg G, Schmoeckel C. Syringolymphoid hyperplasia with alopecia—a syringotropic cutaneous T-cell lymphoma? Dermatology 1992; 184:306–307.

3. Zelger B, Sepp N, Weyrer K, Grunewald K. Syringtropic cutaneous T-cell lymphoma: a variant of mycosis fingoides? Br J Dermatol 1994; 130:765–769.
4. Tannous Z, Baldassano MF, Li VW, Kvedar J, Duncan LM. Syringolymphoid hyperplasia and follicular mucinosis in a patient with cutaneous T-cell lymphoma. J Am Acad Dermatol 1999; 41:303–308.

22.3. Other Variants of Mycosis Fungoides

Dmitry V. Kazakov, Werner Kempf, and Günter Burg
Department of Dermatology, University Hospital, Zürich, Switzerland

Apart from the classical form of mycosis fungoides (MF), there are several variants of this disease with unusual or atypical clinical and/or histopathological features (Table 1).

Follicular MF has been given many names including folliculotropic MF, pilotropic MF, folliculocentric MF, and MF-associated follicular mucinosis (1–6). Some authors believe that the latter should be distinguished from folliculotropic MF, we think that folliculotropic MF and MF-associated follicular mucinosis belong to a spectrum of MF with a predilection for hair follicles. Clinically, the disease manifests itself as erythematous patches or plaques with follicular hyperkeratosis producing comedo-like plugs and often hair loss. The face and upper trunk are the sites of predilection (Fig. 1). Histologically, the disease is typified by dense lymphocytic infiltrates surrounding and infiltrating the hair follicles and sparing interfollicular skin

Table 1 Atypical Clinicopathological Forms of Mycosis Fungoides

Follicular
Bullous
Granulomatous
Hypopigmented
Poikilodermic
Hyperpigmented
Pigmented purpura-like
Unilesional
Palmoplantar
Hyperkeratotic/verrucous
Vegetating/papillomatous
Ichthyosiform
Pustular
Extracutaneous

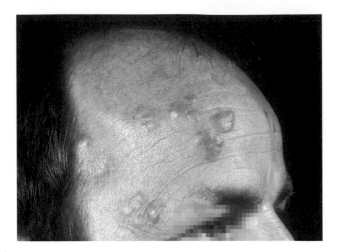

Figure 1 Ulcerated infiltrated plaques on the forehead.

(Fig. 2). The neoplastic cells are small to medium-sized cells with irregular nuclei. In some cases, Pautrier microabscesses can be seen within the follicular epithelium (Fig. 3). The follicles show cystic dilatation, cornified plugging, and, in some cases, mucin deposition. Since some patients experience an aggressive clinical course with large cell transformation and lymph node involvement, folliculotropic MF may carry a worse prognosis than classic MF (7,8). The exact cause of folliculotropism in follicular MF is not known. Changes in intercellular adhesion receptors may account for the phenomenon. In particular, the intercellular adhesion molecule-1 (ICAM-1) receptor has a high affinity for lymphocyte function associated antigen-1 (LFA-1) -positive cells, which are present in high numbers in MF (9). In one study, an increased expression of ICAM-1 was seen in follicular epithelial cells in association with folliculotropic LFA-1 lymphocytes, with concurrent decrease of ICAM-1 expression on epidermal keratinocytes (9).

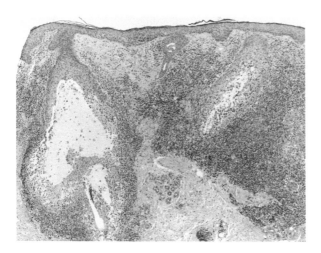

Figure 2 Dense lymphocytic infiltrate involving two hair follicles with mucinous degeneration.

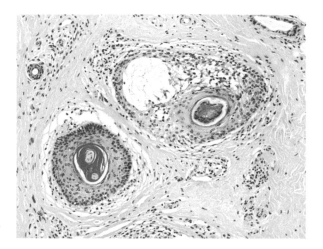

Figure 3 Exocytosis of lymphocytes into follicular epithelium with mucinous degeneration.

Bullous MF is seen in elderly people (average age 66 years) and has no gender predominance (10). It is typified by flaccid or tense, often multiple or even generalized blisters appearing either on normal skin, on an erythematous base, or within typical plaques and tumors of MF (Fig. 4). The trunk and limbs are the site of predilection. Flaccid bullae can sometimes demonstrate a positive Nikolsky sign (11–14). If the bullae are accompanied by other typical lesions of MF or a patient has a previous history suggestive of MF, the diagnosis can be readily established. Otherwise, a patient with bullous MF may pose a diagnostic problem. Histologically, all the common features of MF are seen in the bullous variant (15). Blisters have been found to occur in various locations—subcorneal, intraepidermal, and subepidermal (Fig. 5). The exact mechanism of blister formation is not clear. Negative immunofluorescence studies (both direct and indirect) speak against an autoimmune

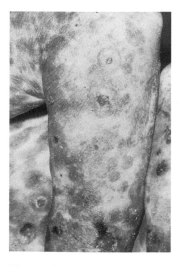

Figure 4 Patches and infiltrated plaques with central blistering. (From Burg G, ed. Cutaneous Lymphomas. Springer, 1983.)

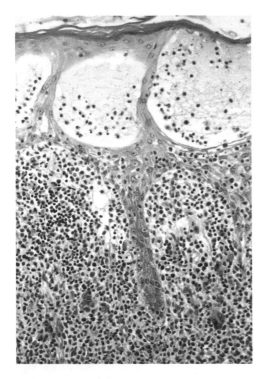

Figure 5 Intraepidermal vesicles harboring atypical lymphocytes.

process although acantholysis may be seen. The following explanations for bulla formation have been proposed (11). (1) An intraepidermal blister may appear as a result of confluence of Pautrier microabscesses. (2) A subepidermal blister may be caused by accumulation of neoplastic cells in the basal layer leading to loss of coherence between the basal keratinocytes and basal lamina. (3) Normal cohesion of keratinocytes may be affected by the release of lymphokines by neoplastic cells. Bullous lesions in MF seem to indicate a poor prognosis, since almost 50% of patients have died within 1 year after the appearance of the blisters (13).

Granulomatous MF is another unusual subtype characterized by the histological presence of a granulomatous reaction. The latter can adopt several patterns, namely (1) sarcoidal pattern, (2) granuloma annulare-like pattern, and (3) granulomatous pattern with multinucleated giant cells (16–19). We regard granulomatous slack skin (see Chapter 23) to be a distinct variant of MF. In the sarcoidal pattern, naked epithelioid granulomas are the hallmarks. In the granuloma annulare-like variant, there is a dermal interstitial infiltrate of lymphocytes with rare histiocytes, producing a pattern which resembles the interstitial form of granuloma annulare or inflammatory morphea. Epidermotropic lymphocytes are present at least focally in all cases. Increased dermal mucin deposition can also be demonstrated. The presence of additional skin lesions with typical MF features and the detection of T cell clones enable one to distinguish this variant from granuloma annulare. The third pattern is typified, as its name implies, by the presence of multinucleated giant cells, usually of the foreign body type. Emperipolesis can be seen. This subtype differs from granulomatous slack skin by the absence of both giant cells with a peculiar and

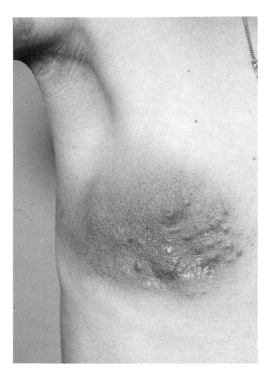

Figure 6 Small nodules arising in a patch of MF, histologically displaying granulomatous features.

characteristic wreath-like arrangement of nuclei and of elastophagocytosis, although elastic fibers may be reduced in number.

When granulomatous changes occur in patients with well-established MF later in the course of the disease, they do not pose any diagnostic problem (Fig. 6). When they are an early sign or when extensive granulomas obscure the underlying cutaneous lymphoma, the diagnosis may be a challenge. The prognostic and clinical significance of a granulomatous reaction in MF remains uncertain. Initially, a protective role was claimed for a granulomatous reaction. Later studies showed that granulomatous MF may have an aggressive course with rapid extracutaneous spread and death (20). A recent analysis of the literature revealed that nearly 40% of the reported patients with granulomatous MF died of the disease, and in half of them, death occurred within 5 years of the onset of the skin lesions (21). The exact cause of granuloma formation in MF is not clear but may be related to treatment with interferon-alpha in some instances.

Hypopigmented MF is often seen in young, dark-skinned patients of Indian or African–American origin who present with asymptomatic or slightly pruritic, non-scaly patches with irregular borders (Fig. 7) (22–28). In some instances, typical patches, plaques, or tumors may accompany the hypopigmented lesions. If this is not the case, MF is rarely suspected, as the differential diagnostic considerations may include pityriasis versicolor, pityriasis alba, vitiligo, leprosy, sarcoidosis, and postinflammatory hypopigmentation. The histological findings as well as clinical course and prognosis in hypopigmented MF are similar to those of classical patch-stage disease. The neoplastic cells in hypopigmented MF often express CD8 (29). The peculiar clinical changes may result from a decreased transfer of melano-

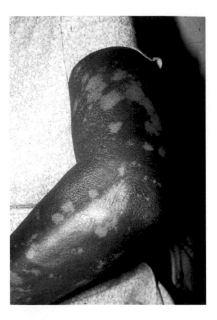

Figure 7 Sharply demarcated patches which are virtually depigmented and resemble vitiligo.

somes from melanocytes to keratinocytes and melanocyte degeneration as evidenced by electron microscopic studies (30,31).

A subset of patients with an otherwise typical clinical picture of MF may also develop *poikilodermic* lesions characterized by alternating hypo- and hyperpigmentation, dryness, atrophy, and telangiectases (poikiloderma vasculare atrophicans [PVA]) (Fig. 8) (32–36). Frequently, these lesions develop slowly at the sites of pre-existing patches, usually in the areas where the skin is chronically rubbed by clothes, and are accompanied by otherwise typical patches and plaques of MF elsewhere. In some patients, the poikilodermic areas can predominate or even be the only finding. A biopsy from these areas will show histological findings similar to those seen in long-standing patch or plaque lesions. Additional pathological changes typical for poikiloderma include atrophy of the epidermis with flattening of rete

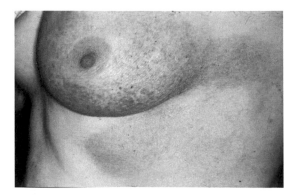

Figure 8 Patch on breast with hypo- and hyperpigmentation, atrophy (wrinkling) and marked telangiectases.

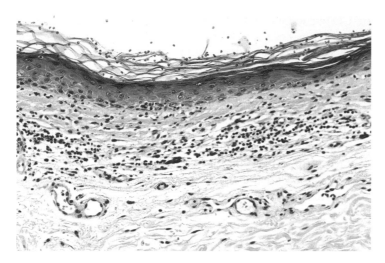

Figure 9 Epidermal atrophy, dilated vessels, and sparse lymphocytic infiltrate with minimal epidermotropism.

ridges, vacuolar alteration of the basal layer with loss of pigment, increased numbers of melanophages in the papillary and upper reticular dermis, and wide dilatation of superficial blood vessels containing erythrocytes (Fig. 9).

The poikilodermic variant of MF should be delineated from the *hyperpigmented* subtype. The latter is characterized by diffuse macular hyperpigmentation as the only clinical feature, not associated with PVA or regression of pre-existing lesions (Fig. 10) (37,38). Lymphadenopathy can be present. Ultrastructural studies have demonstrated the presence of giant melanin granules in neoplastic cells, keratinocytes, and Langerhans cells (37).

Patients with the *pigmented purpura-like* variant of MF present clinically with persistent pigmented purpuric dermatitis. On histological examination, there usually is a lichenoid band-like infiltrate composed mainly of small cerebriform lymphocytes accompanied by substantial numbers of siderophages and extravasated erythrocytes. The lymphocytes invade the epidermis with typical lining-up in the basal layer. The

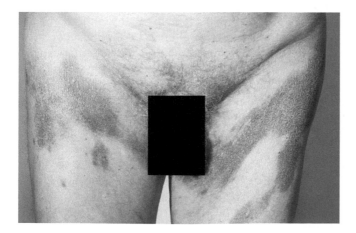

Figure 10 Brown patches on the thighs.

majority of the cells are CD4+; some express CD8. Epidermal changes are variable but spongiosis and apoptosis are not seen. Clonal rearrangement can be demonstrated in a subset of cases. Close follow-up is crucial to distinguish between benign pigmented purpuric dermatoses and this type of MF (39–43).

Unilesional MF is typified by the presence of a single contiguous area of involvement covering less than 5% body surface area. The lesions are usually found on body regions typical for classical MF with breast, axilla, and buttocks being the most common sites (44). Pathological findings are identical to those seen in classical MF. Woringer–Kolopp is distinguished histologically from unilesional MF by the presence of marked hyperkeratosis, prominent pagetoid epidermotropism, and a paucicellular dermal infiltrate (44–46). Patients with unilesional MF demonstrate an excellent response to topical chemotherapy or irradiation.

Involvement of the palms and soles occurring at some time in the course of MF are seen in 11.5% of cases (47). A subset of MF patients [0.6%] present with lesions limited to or predominantly affecting the palms and/or soles, a condition referred to as *mycosis fungoides palmaris et plantaris* (47). Clinical variations include annular and hyperpigmented patches, plaques, hyperkeratotic lesions, vesicles, pustules, dyshidrotic lesions, verrucous changes, psoriasiform plaques, ulceration, and nail dystrophy (47–56). The lesions are either strictly confined to the palms and/or soles or may extend onto the feet, arms, and fingers. If these changes are not accompanied by typical MF lesions elsewhere on the body, the clinical diagnosis is usually challenging. The histological findings are usually compatible with typical MF, and demonstration of clonal rearrangement of TCR genes enable one to reach the correct diagnosis. Differential diagnostic considerations include mycotic infections, dyshidrotic eczema, contact dermatitis, palmoplantar psoriasis, verrucae, hypertrophic lichen planus, and granuloma annulare. The course of this MF subtype is usually indolent. The disease remains confined to the initial area of involvement in most cases but extension of lesions to the limbs and trunk can occur, although no extracutaneous involvement has been reported. The relation of Woringer–Kolopp disease (unilesional pagetoid reticulosis) restricted to acral sites and hyperkeratotic cases of mycosis fungoides palmaris et plantaris has not yet been clarified.

Hyperkeratotic and verrucous changes may be found not only in MF palmaris et plantaris. *Hyperkeratotic/verrucous* MF manifests itself as hyperkeratotic and verrucous plaques which may or may not be accompanied by classical lesions or involvement of palms and soles (57,58).

The lesions of *vegetating/papillomatous* MF (sometimes this subtype is also referred to as acanthosis nigricans-like) arise in flexural areas (axillae, groins), neck, and breast (nipple, areolae) (59–61). They may resemble acanthosis nigricans or seborrheic keratosis, depending on their configuration, size, and color. Histologically, there is papillomatosis, marked acanthosis which may have an appearance similar to that seen in seborrheic keratosis (interconnected rete ridges, horny pseudocysts), and a band-like/diffuse infiltrate of atypical lymphocytes (small convoluted or medium-sized blast-like).

Ichthyosiform MF is a rare subtype, which in a recent series represented 1.8% of MF cases (62). Clinically widespread ichthyosiform lesions are seen, often accompanied by comedo-like lesions and/or follicular keratotic papules. The ichthyosiform skin lesions favor the extremities, but the whole body surface may be involved. Pruritus is prominent and excoriations common. While the ichthyotic changes are usually the only manifestations of MF, the combination of classical MF and acquired ichthyosis (as a paraneoplastic phenomenon) has been documented (63,64). Histologically, the ichthyosiform areas demonstrate compact orthokeratosis, hypogranulosis, and a band-like epidermotropic infiltrate composed of small cerebriform lymphocytes, whereas a biopsy from the follicular papules will display cyst-like dilated ostia of hair follicle with cornified plugging and infiltration of the follicular epithelium by neoplastic cells. No deposition of mucin within the follicular epithelium is found. Oral retinoids, in combination with PUVA or UVA therapy, have been shown to be the most effective treatment for this subtype of MF.

Pustular MF is marked by pustular eruptions which may be limited to palmoplantar areas or generalized. Histologically, there are intraepidermal spaces filled with a mixture of atypical lymphocytes, neutrophils, and eosinophils. The proportions of the above cell types is variable, and the inflammatory cells can outnumber the neoplastic ones (52–54,65).

In addition to all these well-established atypical forms of MF, there are anecdotal reports of the disease presenting as or mimicking keratosis lichenoides chronica, pityriasis lichenoides, and perioral dermatitis (66).

On very rare occasions, MF involves extracutaneous compartments such as oral cavity (tongue, oral mucosae), esophagus, breast, and eyes (Fig. 11). When this occurs before large cell transformation and spread to internal organs, one can speak of extracutaneous MF (67,68). Since typical lesions are also usually present, the diagnosis should be straightforward. In the oral cavity, both the tongue and mucosae may be affected. The incidence of tongue involvement in MF is estimated to be lower than 1%, with approximately 30 cases reported. It is a poor prognostic sign, since all reported patients have died within 3 years after the appearance of their oral lesions (13). Histopathologically, features typical for MF (epitheliotropic infiltrate composed of cerebriform cells) are demonstrable in extracutaneous lesions. In

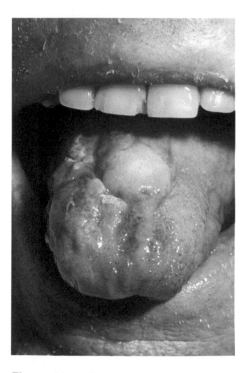

Figure 11 Infiltrated tongue.

advanced stages of the disease, an extracutaneous spread may occur with involvement of internal organs.

REFERENCES

1. Pereyo NG, Requena L, Galloway J, Sangueza OP. Follicular mycosis fungoides: a clinicohistopathologic study. J Am Acad Dermatol 1997; 36:563–568.
2. Hess Schmid M, Dummer R, Kempf W, Hilty N, Burg G. Mycosis fungoides with mucinosis follicularis in childhood. Dermatology 1999; 198:284–287.
3. Flaig MJ, Cerroni L, Schuhmann K, Bertsch HP, Kind P, Kaudewitz P, Sander CA. Follicular mycosis fungoides. A histopathologic analysis of nine cases. J Cutan Pathol 2001; 28:525–530.
4. Mehregan DA, Gibson LE, Muller SA. Follicular mucinosis: histopathologic review of 33 cases. Mayo Clin Proc 1991; 66:387–390.
5. Nickoloff BJ, Wood C. Benign idiopathic versus mycosis fungoides-associated follicular mucinosis. Pediatr Dermatol 1985; 2:201–206.
6. Cerroni L, Fink-Puches R, Back B, Kerl H. Follicular mucinosis: a critical reappraisal of clinicopathologic features and association with mycosis fungoides and Sezary syndrome. Arch Dermatol 2002; 138:182–189.
7. Kanno S, Niizuma K, Machida S, Takahashi M, Ohkido M, Nagura H, Murakosi M, Mori T. Follicular mucinosis developing into cutaneous lymphoma. Report of two cases and review of literature and 64 cases in Japan. Acta Derm Venereol 1984; 64: 86–88.
8. van Doorn R, Scheffer E, Willemze R. Follicular mycosis fungoides, a distinct disease entity with or without associated follicular mucinosis: a clinicopathologic and follow-up study of 51 patients. Arch Dermatol 2002; 138:191–198.
9. Gilliam AC, Lessin SR, Wilson DM, Salhany KE. Folliculotropic mycosis fungoides with large-cell transformation presenting as dissecting cellulitis of the scalp. J Cutan Pathol 1997; 24:169–175.
10. Bowman PH, Hogan DJ, Sanusi ID. Mycosis fungoides bullosa: report of a case and review of the literature. J Am Acad Dermatol 2001; 45:934–939.
11. Franken J, Haneke E. Mycosis fungoides bullosa. Hautarzt 1995; 46:186–189.
12. Lund KA, Parker CM, Norins AL, Tejada E. Vesicular cutaneous T cell lymphoma presenting with gangrene. J Am Acad Dermatol 1990; 23:1169–1171.
13. McBride SR, Dahl MG, Slater DN, Sviland L. Vesicular mycosis fungoides. Br J Dermatol 1998; 138:141–144.
14. Roenigk HH Jr, Castrovinci AJ. Mycosis fungoides bullosa. Arch Dermatol 1971; 104:402–406.
15. Kartsonis J, Brettschneider F, Weissmann A, Rosen L. Mycosis fungoides bullosa. Am J Dermatopathol 1990; 12:76–80.
16. Mainguene C, Picard O, Audouin J, Le Tourneau A, Jagueux M, Diebold J. An unusual case of mycosis fungoides presenting as sarcoidosis or granulomatous mycosis fungoides. Am J Clin Pathol 1993; 99:82–86.
17. Garrie SA, Hirsch P, Levan N. Granuloma annulare-like pattern in mycosis fungoides. Arch Dermatol 1972; 105:717–719.
18. LeBoit PE, Zackheim HS, White CR Jr. Granulomatous variants of cutaneous T-cell lymphoma. The histopathology of granulomatous mycosis fungoides and granulomatous slack skin. Am J Surg Pathol 1988; 12:83–95.
19. Ackerman AB, Flaxman BA. Granulomatous mycosis fungoides. Br J Dermatol 1970; 82:397–401.
20. Gomez-De La Fuente E, Ortiz PL, Vanaclocha F, Rodriguez-Peralto JL, Iglesias L. Aggressive granulomatous mycosis fungoides with clinical pulmonary and thyroid involvement. Br J Dermatol 2000; 142:1026–1029.

21. Chen KR, Tanaka M, Miyakawa S. Granulomatous mycosis fungoides with small intestinal involvement and a fatal outcome. Br J Dermatol 1998; 138:522–525.
22. Akaraphanth R, Douglass MC, Lim HW. Hypopigmented mycosis fungoides: treatment and a 6(1/2)-year follow-up of 9 patients. J Am Acad Dermatol 2000; 42:33–39.
23. Di Landro A, Marchesi L, Naldi L, Motta T, Cainelli T. A case of hypopigmented mycosis fungoides in a young Caucasian boy. Pediatr Dermatol 1997; 14:449–452.
24. el-Hoshy K, Hashimoto K. Adolescence mycosis fungoides: an unusual presentation with hypopigmentation. J Dermatol 1995; 22:424–427.
25. Lambroza E, Cohen SR, Phelps R, Lebwohl M, Braverman IM, DiCostanzo D. Hypopigmented variant of mycosis fungoides: demography, histopathology, and treatment of seven cases. J Am Acad Dermatol 1995; 32:987–993.
26. Moulonguet I, Robert C, Baudot N, Flageul B, Dubertret L. Hypopigmented mycosis fungoides in a light-skinned woman. Br J Dermatol 1998; 139:341–343.
27. Neuhaus IM, Ramos-Caro FA, Hassanein AM. Hypopigmented mycosis fungoides in childhood and adolescence. Pediatr Dermatol 2000; 17:403–406.
28. Stone ML, Styles AR, Cockerell CJ, Pandya AG. Hypopigmented mycosis fungoides: a report of 7 cases and review of the literature. Cutis 2001; 67:133–138.
29. El-Shabrawi-Caelen L, Cerroni L, Medeiros LJ, McCalmont TH. Hypopigmented mycosis fungoides: frequent expression of a CD8+ T-cell phenotype. Am J Surg Pathol 2002; 26:450–472.
30. Breathnach SM, McKee PH, Smith NP. Hypopigmented mycosis fungoides: report of five cases with ultrastructural observations. Br J Dermatol 1982; 106:643–649.
31. Goldberg DJ, Schinella RS, Kechijian P. Hypopigmented mycosis fungoides. Speculations about the mechanism of hypopigmentation. Am J Dermatopathol 1986; 8:326–330.
32. Chapman RS, Paul CJ. Poikiloderma atrophicans vasculare as a pointer to reticulosis of the skin. Postgrad Med J 1975; 51:463–467.
33. Lindae ML, Abel EA, Hoppe RT, Wood GS. Poikilodermatous mycosis fungoides and atrophic large-plaque parapsoriasis exhibit similar abnormalities of T-cell antigen expression. Arch Dermatol 1988; 124:366–372.
34. Wakelin SH, Stewart EJ, Emmerson RW. Poikilodermatous and verrucous mycosis fungoides. Clin Exp Dermatol 1996; 21:205–208.
35. Dougherty J. Poikiloderma atrophicans vasculare. Arch Dermatol 1971; 103:550–552.
36. Raznatovskii IM. Brocq's parapsoriases, their relationship to pokiloderma, mycosis fungoides and skin reticulosis Vestn. Dermatol Venerol 1976;42–46.
37. David M, Shanon A, Hazaz B, Sandbank M. Diffuse, progressive hyperpigmentation: an unusual skin manifestation of mycosis fungoides. J Am Acad Dermatol 1987; 16: 257–260.
38. Dummer R, Kamarashev J, Kempf W, Haffner AC, Hess-Schmid M, Burg G. Junctional CD8+ cutaneous lymphomas with nonaggressive clinical behavior: a CD8 variant of mycosis fungoides? Arch Dermatol 2002; 138:199–203.
39. Barnhill RL, Braverman IM. Progression of pigmented purpura-like eruptions to mycosis fungoides: report of three cases. J Am Acad Dermatol 1988; 19:25–31.
40. Cather JC, Farmer A, Jackow C, Manning JT, Shin DM, Duvic M. Unusual presentation of mycosis fungoides as pigmented purpura with malignant thymoma. J Am Acad Dermatol 1998; 39:858–863.
41. Toro JR, Sander CA, LeBoit PE. Persistent pigmented purpuric dermatitis and mycosis fungoides: simulant, precursor, or both? A study by light microscopy and molecular methods. Am J Dermatopathol 1997; 19:108–118.
42. Crowson AN, Magro CM, Zahorchak R. Atypical pigmentary purpura: a clinical, histopathologic, and genotypic study. Hum Pathol 1999; 30:1004–1012.
43. Georgala S, Katoulis AC, Symeonidou S, Georgala C, Vayopoulos G. Persistent pigmented purpuric eruption associated with mycosis fungoides: a case report and review of the literature. J Eur Acad Dermatol Venereol 2001; 15:62–64.

44. Heald PW, Glusac EJ. Unilesional cutaneous T-cell lymphoma: clinical features, therapy, and follow-up of 10 patients with a treatment-responsive mycosis fungoides variant. J Am Acad Dermatol 2000; 42:283–285.

45. Oliver GF, Winkelmann RK. Unilesional mycosis fungoides: a distinct entity. J Am Acad Dermatol 1989; 20:63–70.

46. Oliver GF, Winkelmann RK, Banks PM. Unilesional mycosis fungoides: clinical, microscopic and immunophenotypic features. Australas J Dermatol 1989; 30:65–71.

47. Resnik KS, Kantor GR, Lessin SR, Kadin ME, Chooback L, Cooper HS, Vonderheid EC. Mycosis fungoides palmaris et plantaris. Arch Dermatol 1995; 131:1052–1056.

48. McNiff JM, Schechner JS, Crotty PL, Glusac EJ. Mycosis fungoides et plantaris or acral pagetoid reticulosis? Am J Dermatopathol. 1998; 20:271–275.

49. Stasko T, Vander Ploeg DE, De Villez RL. Hyperkeratotic mycosis fungoides restricted to the palms. J Am Acad Dermatol 1982; 7:792–796.

50. Goldberg DJ, Stampien TM, Schwartz RA. Mycosis fungoides palmaris et plantaris: successful treatment with the carbon dioxide laser. Br J Dermatol 1997; 136:617–619.

51. Tomsick RS. Hyperkeratosis in mycosis fungoides. Cutis 1982; 29:621–623.

52. Tagami H, Aiba S, Ohkouchi K. Palmoplantar pustular lesions in mycosis fungoides. J Am Acad Dermatol 1991; 25:733–734.

53. Camisa C, Aulisio A. Pustular mycosis fungoides. Cutis 1994; 54:202–204.

54. Moreno JC, Ortega M, Conejo-Mir JS, Sanchez-Pedreno P. Palmoplantar pustulosis as a manifestation of cutaneous T cell lymphoma (mycosis fungoides). J Am Acad Dermatol 1990; 23:758–759.

55. Caputo R, Berti E, Monti M, Cavicchini S. A verrucoid epidermotropic OKT8-positive lymphoma. Am J Dermatopathol 1983; 5:159–164.

56. Sheehan-Dare RA, Goodfield MJ, Williamson DM, Cotterill JA. Ulceration of the palms and soles. An unusual feature of cutaneous T-cell lymphoma. Acta Derm Venereol 1990; 70:523–525.

57. Price NM, Fuks ZY, Hoffman TE. Hyperkeratotic and verrucous features of mycosis fungoides. Arch Dermatol 1977; 113:57–60.

58. Nicolis GD, Stratigos JD, Tosca AD, Capetanakis JA. Mycosis fungoides with verrucous lesions. Acta Derm Venereol 1979; 59:80–82.

59. Puig L, Musulen E, Fernandez-Figueras MT, Miralles J, Sitjas D, De Moragas JM. Mycosis fungoides associated with unusual epidermal hyperplasia. Clin Exp Dermatol 1996; 21:61–64.

60. Kanitakis C, Tsoitis G. Mycosis fungoides and follicular mucinosis with very prominent papillomatous and verrucous lesions (author's transl). Dermatologica 1977; 155:268–274.

61. Willemze R, Scheffer E, Van Vloten WA. Mycosis fungoides simulating acanthosis nigricans. Am J Dermatopathol 1985; 7:367–371.

62. Marzano AV, Borghi A, Facchetti M, Alessi E. Ichthyosiform mycosis fungoides. Dermatology 2002; 204:124–129.

63. Kutting B, Metze D, Luger TA, Bonsmann G. Mycosis fungoides presenting as an acquired ichthyosis. J Am Acad Dermatol 1996; 34:887–889.

64. Schmutz JL, Bisson J, Gillet-Terver. Pilotropic cutaneous lymphoma without mucinosis and ichthyosis. Nouv Dermatol 1977; 16:143–144.

65. Isaacson PG, Norton AJ. Cutaneous lymphomas. In: Isaacson PG, Norton AJ Extranodal Lymphomas. London: Churchill Livingstone, 1994:131–191.

66. Kazakov DV, Burg G, Kempf W. Clinicopathological spectrum of mycosis fungoides. J Eur Acad Dermatol Venereol 2004; 18:397–415.

67. Kuhn JJ, Wenig BM, Clark DA. Mycosis fungoides of the larynx. Report of two cases and review of the literature. Arch Otolaryngol Head Neck Surg 1992; 118:853–858.

68. Sirois DA, Miller AS, Harwick RD, Vonderheid EC. Oral manifestations of cutaneous T-cell lymphoma. A report of eight cases. Oral Surg Oral Med Oral Pathol 1993; 75:700–705.

23

Granulomatous Cutaneous T-cell Lymphomas

Werner Kempf, Dmitry V. Kazakov, and Günter Burg
Department of Dermatology, University Hospital, Zürich, Switzerland

Among lymphomas, non-necrotizing epithelioid granulomas are most commonly seen in association with Hodgkin lymphoma (1) where they can occur both in affected tissue (nodal and extranodal) as well as in otherwise unaffected organs. In contrast, granulomatous features are rarely found in primary cutaneous lymphomas (CL) (2,3). Distinct nosologic subtypes of CL with granulomatous features include granulomatous slack skin and granulomatous MF (Table 1). Granulomatous CTCL usually run a slowly progressive course. The impact of early therapeutic intervention on disease progression in this forms of CTCL is still unclear. Up to 50% of the cases develop nodal lymphomas which then have a potentially fatal outcome.

GRANULOMATOUS VARIANTS OF CTCL

Granulomatous variants of MF and SS are rarely seen (see also Chapter 22.3). In a study of 220 biopsies of MF and SS, granulomatous features were not detected (3). In another series, granulomas were found in biopsies from 4 of 39 (10%) patients with SS (4).

HISTOLOGY

Often granuloma formation is confined to limited areas in an otherwise classic histalogic manifestation of CTCL. In addition, not all biopsies display granulomatous features. Although granulomatous features may hide the underlying CTCL, typical clinical and histologic findings such as epidermotropism of tumor cells allow one to diagnose CTCL.

IMMUNOHISTOCHEMISTY

Tumor cells in granulomatous variants of CTCL display the same phenotypic pattern found in classic forms of the disease. Detection of clonal T-cell population is often the most useful diagnostic marker.

Table 1 Granulomatous Cutaneous T-cell Lymphomas

Granulomatous slack skin (GSS) (see Chapter 23.1)
Juvenile granulomatous cutaneous T-cell lymphoma (JG-CTCL) (see Chapter 23.2)
Granulomatous variants of CTCL
   Granulomatous mycosis fungoides (see Chapter 22)
   Granulomatous Sézary syndrome
   Granulomatous adult-T-cell leukemia/lymphoma

TREATMENT

The treatment is identical to that for MF.

CLINICAL COURSE AND PROGNOSIS

Whereas the occurrence of granulomas in MF has been considered to be a favorable prognostic sign by some authors (5), others have not confirmed this observation (6). It remains controversial whether the presence of granulomas has any prognostic significance in CTCL (7).

DIFFERENTIAL DIAGNOSIS

Sarcoidosis might be the most difficult and important differential diagnosis due to morphological similarities. Sarcoidosis has been reported to occur concurrently with lymphomas, in particular, in Hodgkin's disease, but also other forms of lymphomas (8). However, sarcoidosis is an inflammatory process and no clonal rearrangement of TCR genes can be observed, whereas own studies revealed a clonal T-cell population within granulomatous infiltrates of CTCL (unpublished data).

COMMENTS

The mechanism and significance of granuloma formation in lymphoid neoplasms are unknown. Various pathways for granuloma formation have been proposed. Immunologically, persistent antigens that are not totally eliminated by the host immune system can lead to granuloma formation. Alternatively, the granulomatous process may represent a local tissue response to the infiltrating malignant cells, but this hypothesis has been criticized because of the occurrence of granulomas in sites where no lymphoma is found. In addition, long-term treatment with interferon-alfa is able to induce granulomatous reactions and may be responsible for the skin changes in some patients.

REFERENCES

1. Sacks EL, Donaldson SS, Gordon J, Dorfman RF. Epithelioid granulomas associated with Hodgkin's disease: clinical correlations in 55 previously untreated patients. Cancer 1978; 41:562–567.
2. Randle HW, Banks PM, Winkelmann RK. Cutaneous granulomas in malignant lymphoma. Arch Dermatol 1980; 116:441–443.

3. Shapiro PE, Pinto FJ. The histologic spectrum of mycosis fungoides/Sezary syndrome (cutaneous T-cell lymphoma). A review of 222 biopsies, including newly described patterns and the earliest pathologic changes. Am J Surg Pathol 1994; 18:645–667.
4. Buechner SA, Winkelmann RK. Sezary syndrome. A clinicopathologic study of 39 cases. Arch Dermatol 1983; 119:979–986.
5. Ackerman AB, Flaxman BA. Granulomatous mycosis fungoides. Br J Dermatol 1970; 82:397–401.
6. Dabski K, Stoll HJ. Granulomatous reactions in mycosis fungoides. J Surg Oncol 1987; 34:217–229.
7. LeBoit PE, Zackheim HS, White CJ. Granulomatous variants of cutaneous T-cell lymphoma. The histopathology of granulomatous mycosis fungoides and granulomatous slack skin. Am J Surg Pathol 1988; 12:83–95.
8. Atwood W, Miller R, Nelson C. Sarcoidosis and the malignant lymphoreticular diseases. Arch Dermatol 1966; 94:144–151.

23.1. Granulomatous Slack Skin

Werner Kempf, Dmitry V. Kazakov, and Günter Burg
Department of Dermatology, University Hospital, Zürich, Switzerland

CLASSIFICATION

> WHO/ EORTC Classification (2005): Granulomatous slack skin (Variants and
>   subtypes of mycosis fungoides)
> WHO Classification (2001): Not listed
> REAL Classification (1997): Not listed
> EORTC Classification (1997): Granulomatous slack skin

DEFINITION

Granulomatous slack skin (GSS) is a rare granulomatous subtype of mycosis fungoides (see Chapter 21) with pathognomonic clinical features. The clinical condition was first described in 1968 by Bazex et al.(1) as "chalazodermie granulomateuse" and then by Convit et al.(2) as "progressive atrophying chronic granulomatous dermohypodermitis." Ackerman (3) introduced the term "granulomatous slack skin" in 1978.

CLINICAL FEATURES

GSS manifests usually in the third or fourth decade, but occurs also in childhood (4). Men seem to be more often affected than women (male:female ratio = 2:1). GSS is seen almost exclusively in whites. The disease starts with slightly infiltrated, poikilodermatous plaques. Predilection sites are the intertriginous body areas, especially the axillary and inguinal folds (Fig. 1). Progressive destruction of elastic fibers results in bulky pendulous skin folds (Fig. 2). Occasionally ulceration develops. The same changes may develop in patients with pre-existing MF (5).

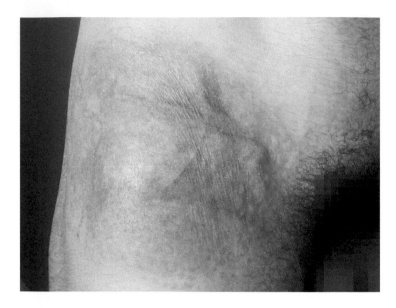

Figure 1   Large slightly infiltrated plaque in the groin as initial manifestation of GSS.

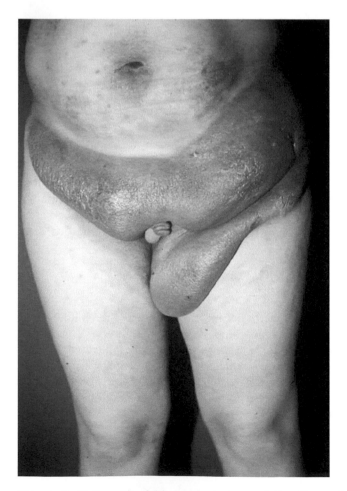

Figure 2   Bulky skin folds as final stage of the disease in a boy. (Courtesy of F.M. Camachoh M.D., Spain.)

Figure 3 Dense dermal lymphocytic infiltrate with scattered multinucleated giant cells.

HISTOLOGY

Early lesions of GSS show a bandlike infiltrate of small lymphocytes without significant nuclear atypia (6). In addition, there are characteristic syncytial giant cells with numerous nuclei at their periphery. More advanced lesions exhibit a dense lymphocytic infiltrate throughout the entire dermis (Fig. 3). While some lymphoid cells may have cerebriform nuclei, nuclear atypia is usually less pronounced than in classic MF. Numerous scattered multinucleated giant cells containing up to 40 nuclei are a hallmark (Fig. 4). Elastophagocytosis and emperipolesis, i.e., phagocytosis of lymphoid cells by giant cells, are present (Fig. 4). Elastic stains demonstrate the loss of elastic fibers within the infiltrates.

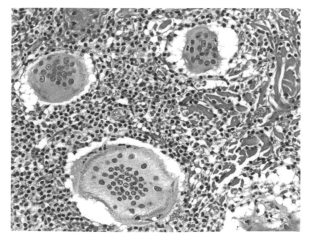

Figure 4 Characteristic multinucleated giant cells with numerous nuclei.

IMMUNOHISTOCHEMISTRY

Lymphoid tumor cells express CD4, CD45RO. Other T-cell markers like CD3, CD5, or CD7 may be absent. Rarely expression of CD30 is found. The giant cells are of histiocytic origin and thus are positive for histiocytic markers such as CD68 and Mac387.

MOLECULAR BIOLOGY

Clonal rearrangement of TCR genes can be detected in most cases and is a useful diagnostic tool in early stages of the disease (7). Trisomy 8 has been reported in two cases (8,9).

TREATMENT

Therapeutic approaches include surgical excision, photochemotherapy (PUVA), or intralesional or systemic interferon alpha in combination with retinoids. Finally, monoagent (methotrexate) or multiagent chemotherapy may be considered, especially in cases with extracutaneous involvement. No therapeutic regime has been able to induce complete remission. Recurrences are common.

CLINICAL COURSE AND PROGNOSIS

The disease runs an indolent, slowly progressive course over decades. Extracutaneous spread is rare. Occasionally granulomatous lymphoadenopathy occurs.

Granulomatous slack skin

Clinical features
   Onset in childhood or third to fourth decade, men > women, flexural areas, especially axillary and inguinal folds, initially infiltrated poikilodermatous plaques becoming bulky lax skin folds
Histology
   Dense lymphocytic infiltrate throughout the entire dermis with intermingled giant cells containing numerous peripherally located nuclei (up to 30 per giant cell)
Phenotype
   Lymphoid cells: T helper phenotype with loss of some antigens; giant cells: histiocytic markers
Genotype
   Clonal TCR gene rearrangement detected in most cases
Course
   Slowly progressive; risk of other cutaneous or nodal lymphomas (Hodgkin's disease) in 20% of the patients
Therapy
   Excision, photochemotherapy, or immunomodulators (IFN) in combination with retinoids, polychemotherapy in advanced stages with extracutaneous spread

---

Although the disease by itself does not reduce life expectancy, other cutaneous and nodal lymphomas such as MF, Hodgkin lymphoma, and peripheral T-cell lymphomas, NOS occur in approximately 20% of the patients (10).

DIFFERENTIAL DIAGNOSIS

Various granulomatous infiltrates of infectious or noninfectious origin have to be considered. The characteristic histologic features with the typical giant cells in the background of a dense lymphocytic infiltrate and elastophagocytosis allow the correct diagnosis in most cases. Generalized cutis laxa usually does not primarily affect flexural areas and often also involves the face. Mid-dermal elastolysis shows no proclivity for the development of pendulous skin folds. Neither cutis laxa nor mid-dermal elastolysis features dense lymphocytic infiltrates. Pseudoxanthoma elasticum may clinically appear similar involving flexural areas but has striking alterations in elastic fibers with calcium deposition.

COMMENTS

Some authors consider GSS as a distinct entity different from MF. In contrast to classical MF, GSS is in almost all cases confined to intertriginous areas, displays characteristic clinical features and runs a more benign course than classic MF. Nevertheless, we regard GSS as a granulomatous subtype within the group of MF (see also variants of MF Chapter 22.3).

REFERENCES

1. Bazex A, Dupre A, Christol B. Chalazodermic Besnier–Boeck–Schaumann disease? Bull Soc Fr Dermatol Syphiligr 1968; 75:448–449.
2. Convit J, Kerdel F, Goihman M, et al. Progressive, atrophing, chronic granulomatous dermohypodermitis. Autoimmune disease? Arch Dermatol 1973; 107:271.
3. Ackerman AB. Granulomatous slack skin. In: Ackerman AB, ed. Histologic Diagnosis of Inflammatory Skin Diseases. Philadelphia: Lea and Febiger, 1978:483–485.
4. Camacho FM, Burg G, Moreno JC, Campora RG, Villar JL. Granulomatous slack skin in childhood. Pediatr Dermatol 1997; 14:204–208.
5. van Haselen CW, Toonstra J, van der Putte SJ, van Dongen JJ, van Hees CL, van Vloten WA. Granulomatous slack skin. Report of three patients with an updated review of the literature. Dermatology 1998; 196:382–391.
6. LeBoit PE. Granulomatous slack skin. Dermatol Clin 1994; 12:375–389.
7. LeBoit PE, Beckstead JH, Bond B, Epstein WL, Frieden IJ, Parslow TG. Granulomatous slack skin: clonal rearrangement of the T-cell receptor beta gene is evidence for the lymphoproliferative nature of a cutaneous elastolytic disorder. J Invest Dermatol 1987; 89:183–186.
8. von den Driesch P, Mielke V, Simon MJ, Staib G, Tacke J, Sterry W. "Granulomatous slack skin"—kutanes elastolytisches Lymphom. Hautarzt 1994;45:861–865.
9. Balus L, Manente L, Remotti D, Grammatico P, Bellocci M. Granulomatous slack skin. Report of a case and review of the literature. Am J Dermatopathol 1996; 18:199–206.
10. Noto G, Pravata G, Miceli S, Arico M. Granulomatous slack skin: report of a case associated with Hodgkin's disease and a review of the literature. Br J Dermatol 1994; 131:275–279.

23.2. Juvenile Granulomatous Cutaneous T-cell Lymphoma

Werner Kempf and Günter Burg
Department of Dermatology, University Hospital, Zürich, Switzerland

CLASSIFICATION

WHO/EORTC Classification (2005): Not listed
WHO Classification (2001): Not listed
REAL Classification (1997): Not listed
EORTC Classification (1997): Not listed

DEFINITION

Rare variant of granulomatous mycosis fungoides (see Chapter 22) characterized by early onset, granulomatous clinical and histologic features in the absence of bulky skin folds, and risk for development of nodal lymphomas.

CLINICAL FEATURES

JG-CTCL manifests with poikilodermatous patchy or nodular, localized or disseminated skin lesions (Fig. 1), with onset in childhood or early adulthood (median age of six reported patients is 13 years, ranging from 4 to 23 years)(1). The course of the disease is slowly progressive. Several years to decades after disease onset, half of the patients develop nodal Hodgkin lymphoma or systemic large cell anaplastic CD30+ lymphoma.

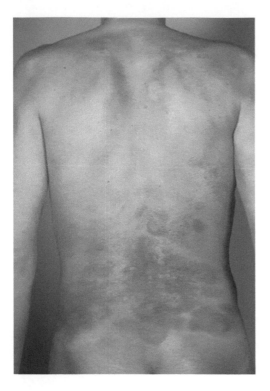

Figure 1 Infiltrated, hyperpigmented areas on the back.

HISTOLOGY

There is a patchy or nodular granulomatous infiltrate consisting of histiocytes, epithelioid cells, and a few multinucleated giant cells with a variable admixture of small well-differentiated lymphocytes (Fig. 2). Epidermotropism of T-cells is not found.

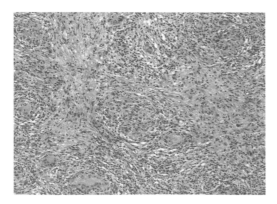

Figure 2 Dermal infiltrate with well-circumscribed granulomas containing giant cells and lymphocytes. Clinicopathologic correlation and molecular biologic studies are necessary to diagnose lymphoma.

IMMUNOHISTOCHEMISTRY

Lymphocytes express a CD3+ CD4+ T helper phenotype. CD30 expression is absent. Clonal rearrangement for TCR genes is found in all cases and represents an important diagnostic marker.

TREATMENT

The therapeutic approach is identical as in granulomatous MF.

CLINICAL COURSE AND PROGNOSIS

The disease is slowly progressive, but is associated with a high risk for the development of nodal lymphomas such as HD and ALCL which may be fatal.

DIFFERENTIAL DIAGNOSIS

Other granulomatous infiltrates of infectious and noninfectious cause must be excluded. Special stains and molecular studies help to exclude infectious processes and to demonstrate clonal T-cell population as a hint for JG-CTCL. In contrast to GSS, JG-CTCL does not display numerous characteristic giant cells or elastophagocytosis.

COMMENTS

Although JG-CTCL shows distinct nosologic features, we regard JG-CTCL as a variant of MF.

REFERENCE

1. Kempf W, Dummer R, Haeffner A, Panizzon R, Mueller B, Burg G. Juvenile granulomatous cutaneous T-cell lymphoma: a new entity in cutaneous lymphomas? (abstract). Am J Dermatopathol 1997; 19:497.

24

Sézary Syndrome (SS)

Werner Kempf, Dmitry V. Kazakov, and Günter Burg
Department of Dermatology, University Hospital, Zürich, Switzerland

CLASSIFICATION

WHO/EORTC Classification (2005): Sézary syndrome
WHO Classification (2001): Sézary syndrome
REAL Classification (1997): Sézary syndrome
EORTC Classification (1997): Sézary syndrome

DEFINITION

Sézary syndrome (SS) is a cutaneous T-cell lymphoma (CTCL) with distinct clinical features (erythroderma, palmoplantar hyperkeratosis, lymphadenopathy) and leukemic spread of neoplastic T-cells in peripheral blood (1). The term "Sézary syndrome" was proposed in 1961 by Taswell and Winkelmann (2). In 1938, Sézary and Bouvrain had described for the first time mononuclear cells with hyperconvoluted atypical nuclei in the skin and peripheral blood, for which they used the term "monster cells" (3).

Sézary syndrome

Clinical features
  Adult/elderly patients
  Erythroderma, palmoplantar hyperkeratosis, alopecia
  Pruritus
  Marked lymphoadenopathy
Histological features
  Often unspecific with perivascular or band-like lymphocytic infiltrate
  Variable epidermotropism of atypical lymphocytes
  Admixture of eosinophils and plasma cells
Immunophenotype
  CD2+, CD3+, CD5+, CD4+, CD8–, CD30–, CD45RO+
Molecular biology
  Clonal TCR rearrangement in majority of cases

(Continued)

Sézary syndrome (*Continued*)

Laboratory evaluation
  Detection of circulating atypical lymphocytes (> 1000 cells per microliter)
Treatment
  Extracorporeal photopheresis, PUVA, retinoids
Clinical course and prognosis
  10–70% 5-year-survival rate
  Aggressive after transformation

CLINICAL FEATURES

Sézary syndrome is an uncommon CTCL which accounts for less than 5% of CTCL (4,5). Sézary syndrome is characterized by distinct clinical features with erythroderma accompanied by intense and generalized pruritus, diffuse alopecia, palmoplantar hyperkeratosis and onychodystrophy as well as lymphadenopathy (Figs. 1–3). In the peripheral blood, lymphoid cells with hyperconvoluted nuclei (so-called Sézary or Lutzner cells) of varying size (8 to > 12 micrometer in diameter) and number are found (6). Interestingly, clinicopathologic manifestations of SS

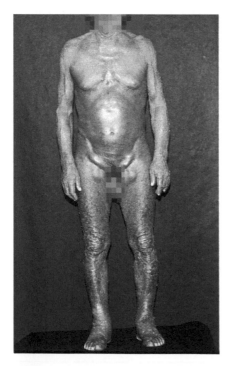

Figure 1 Erythroderma with striking lymphoadenopathy and edema of the lower extremities.

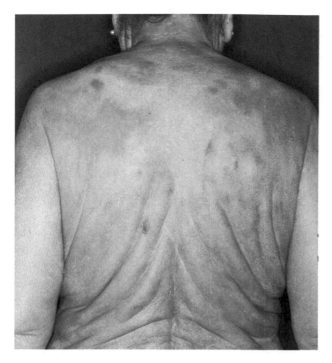

Figure 2   Massive edema (anasarca) creating thick skin folds on the back.

other than the classic one seem to be very rare or not yet identified. Granulomatous lesions harboring clonal T-cells in a patient with long-standing SS were recently described (7).

HISTOLOGY

A superficial perivascular infiltrate of small lymphoid cells is the most prevalent finding in skin biopsies of SS patients. Larger studies of SS biopsies demonstrated that a subepidermal perivascular or band-like infiltrate composed of predominantly small lymphocytes with or without nuclear atypia is the most common finding in SS,

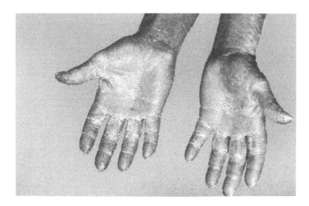

Figure 3   Palmar hyperkeratosis and erythema.

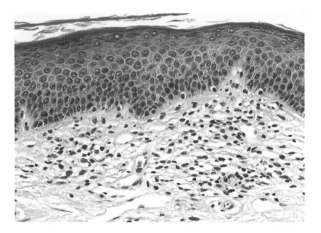

Figure 4 Sparse lymphocytic infiltrate in the upper dermis with few lymphocytes in the junctional zone.

present in about 40% of cases (8,9). The epidermis often shows psoriasiform acanthosis. Nonspecific findings are present in one-third of the biopsies (10) (Fig. 4). A band-like, variably intense, monomorphous infiltrate of small lymphocytes with or without nuclear atypia was found in approximately 30% of specimens (Fig. 5), whereas epidermotropism and lining-up of lymphocytes with cerebriform nuclei (MF-like pattern) was found in approximately 20–40%, half of which exhibited Pautrier collections (8,10) (Figs. 6 and 7). Pautrier collections are regarded as a specific, but relatively rare, finding in epidermotropic CTCL such as MF and SS (11). Edema is often present in initial stages of epidermotropic CTCL but may be replaced over time by fibrosis of papillary dermis. Occasionally, granulomatous features can be seen in SS lesions (8,12). Both intra-rater as well as inter-rater variability is high in the diagnosis of SS (13). Although Pautrier collections and acanthosis are more frequently present in SS than in MF, histological features do generally not allow differentiation between the two disorders (14,15). Pretreatment of skin lesions with PUVA or steroids may eliminate epidermotropic T-cells and render the

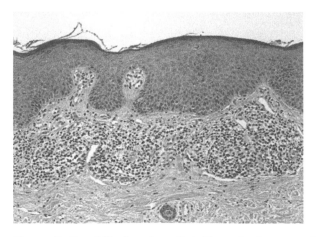

Figure 5 Band-like lymphocytic infiltrate in the upper dermis without epidermotropism.

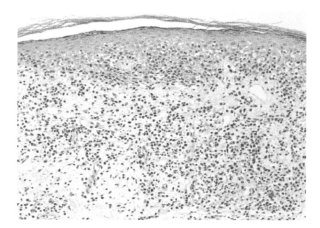

Figure 6 Perivascular lymphocytic infiltrate with lining up and epidermotropism of atypical lymphocytes as well as initial Pautrier microabscesses.

histologic findings nonspecific. Single apoptotic keratinocytes may indicate previous therapeutic intervention in such biopsies.

Lymph nodes show dermatopathic changes in early stages of the disease, whereas effacement of normal architecture by a dense, diffuse, and monotonous infiltration of small lymphoid cells is found in later specific involvement.

IMMUNOHISTOCHEMISTRY

Tumor cells in SS express a T helper phenotype (CD3+, CD4+, CD8–, CDW29+, CD30–, CD45RO+) and cutaneous lymphocyte antigen (CLA). Loss of T-cell antigens occurs in 66% of the cases with CD2 the one most commonly lost (16). Lymphocytosis with detection of an aberrant T-cell phenotype (e.g., loss of CD2, 3 or CD5, or coexpression of CD4 and CD8) can also be found by FACS analysis in some cases of SS. More than 40% of CD4+ CD7– cells are found in peripheral

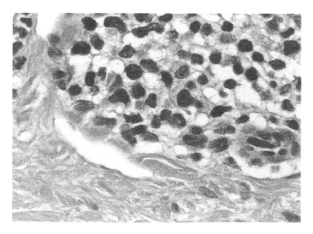

Figure 7 Atypical lymphocytes with convoluted nuclei.

blood of approximately half of SS patients, but not in patients with benign dermatoses (17). The percentage of CD4+CD7–cells correlates with Sézary cell count (18),
but the CD4+CD7–cells may not necessarily represent tumor cells. No differences in
expression of cellular interaction molecules such as ICAM-1, LFA-1, CD40 and
CD40 ligand, exist between MF and SS (15).

MOLECULAR BIOLOGY

T-cell clones in the skin or peripheral blood have been detected by Southern blot in
40 up to 87% and by PCR in 90% of cases. These clones can also be present in
peripheral blood of healthy elderly people. Peripheral blood T-cell clones not related
to the tumor cell clone have been found in patients with nonerythrodermic CTCL.
Allelotyping studies revealed allelic loss in 67% of patients with SS. High rates of loss
of heterozygosity were detected on 9p (46%) and 17p (42%) with lower rates on 2p
(12%), 6q (7%), and 10q (12%) (19).

DIAGNOSIS

Diagnosis of SS is based— as in most CL—on the combination of distinct clinical
features and detection of tumor cells in peripheral blood. Histological examination
not uncommonly shows nonspecific findings and is only of diagnostic value in cases
where the typical features of epidermotropic CTCL are present. Although a variety
of hematologic criteria have been developed for the diagnosis of SS (1), there is still
no widely accepted standard for SS. An absolute Sézary cell count of 1000 cells/mm^3
or more has often been used as cut-off for the diagnosis of SS (Fig. 8). However more
than 1000 cells/mm^3 can also be found in 5% of patients with benign dermatoses. A
Sézary cell percentage of 20% or more seems to be the best way to separate SS and
benign erythrodermic dermatoses. In addition, a CD4/8 ratios of 10 or more is a
further useful as criterion for SS, but this ratio approach also has its limitations
(20). In summary, both the ISCL and EORTC groups recommend demonstration
of clonal T-cells by molecular genetic studies and a significantly increased CD4/8
ratio (> 10) in the peripheral blood as useful additional diagnostic criteria (1,4).

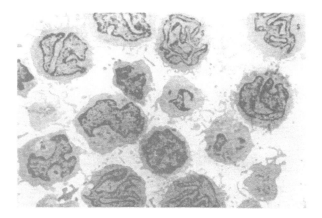

Figure 8   Sézary cells in peripheral blood (electron microscopy).

TREATMENT

In regard to the lack of widely accepted diagnostic criteria and controlled data for therapeutic interventions in SS, comparison of efficacy of various treatment schemes in SS is very difficult. Extracorporeal photopheresis, introduced by Edelson in 1987 (21) is considered as first line therapy of SS with response rates up to 87% (20). Alternatively, chemotherapy with methotrexate as low-dose single agent therapy may be effective with CR in about 40% of patients (22). Multiagent schemes including chlorambucil and prednisone such as CHOP may result in higher responses, which are usually short-lived (23). Also, PUVA, interferon-alpha and total skin electron beam and bexarotene have been employed. The impact of therapy on survival in SS has yet to be defined.

CLINICAL COURSE AND PROGNOSIS

Survival in SS is usually considered to be worse than in other epidermotropic forms of CTCL such as MF. One group reported a 5-year-survival of only 11% in 12 patients with SS (4). Recent studies indicate 5-year-survival rates of 33% (5). Increasing tumor burden in blood and lymph nodes is associated with worse prognosis (24). The presence of very large Sézary cells (> 14 micrometer in diameter) may indicate a worse prognosis (17,25). In addition, lack of expression of CD7 has been identified as negative prognostic factor (5-year-survival rate 20% vs. 67% in CD7– vs. CD7+ cases) (17). Transformation of SS to large-cell lymphoma, CD30–positive or negative, occurs in about 20% of patients. In our experience, transformation is usually first seen in lymph nodes, not in the skin (26). Expression of CD25 may be a marker for impending transformation (27).

DIFFERENTIAL DIAGNOSIS

Sézary syndrome has to be differentiated from erythrodermic phase of MF or other T-cell lymphomas, in which no tumor cells are found in peripheral blood, and erythroderma in the context of benign reactive conditions such as drug eruptions. The latter ones have also been referred to as drug-induced "pseudo-Sézary." The term "red man syndrome" describes patients with erythroderma, but lack of findings sufficient for the diagnosis of SS. Since nonspecific features and lack of epidermotropism of T-cells are found in a significant number of SS biopsies, repetitive biopsies and correlation of histologic findings with clinical features are crucial for differential diagnostic evaluation.

COMMENTS

The lack of widely accepted diagnostic criteria for SS renders comparison of studies in SS almost impossible, especially since benign erythrodermas of different etiology may have been included in previous studies. Moreover, prognostic data may dramatically vary due to differences in diagnostic criteria. Thus international multicenter studies applying defined diagnostic criteria for SS are urgently needed and ongoing to assess the value of therapeutic approaches and outcome in SS.

REFERENCES

1. Vonderheid EC, Bernengo MG, Burg G, Duvic M, Heald P, Laroche L, Olsen E, Pittelkow M, Russell-Jones R, Takigawa M, Willemze R. Update on erythrodermic cutaneous T-cell lymphoma: report of the international society for cutaneous lymphomas. J Am Acad Dermatol 2002; 46:95 106.
2. Taswell HF, Winkelmann RK. Sézary syndrome—a malignant reticulemic erythroderma. JAMA 1981; 177:465–472.
3. Sézary A, Bouvrain Y. Erythrodermie avec presence des cellules monstrueuses dans le derme et le sang circulant. Bull Soc Fr Dermatol Syphiligr 1938; 45:254–260.
4. Willemze R, Kerl H, Sterry W, Berti E, Cerroni L, Chimenti S, Diaz Perez JL, Geerts ML, Goos M, Knobler R, Ralfkiaer E, Santucci M, Smith N, Wechsler J, van Vloten WA, Meijer CJ. EORTC classification for primary cutaneous lymphomas: a proposal from the cutaneous lymphoma study group of the european organization for research and treatment of cancer. Blood 1997; 90:354–371.
5. Fink-Puches R, Zenahlik P, Back B, Smolle J, Kerl H, Cerroni L. Primary cutaneous lymphomas: applicability of current classification schemes (european organization for research and treatment of cancer, world health organization) based on clinicopathologic features observed in a large group of patients. Blood 2002; 99:800–805.
6. Lutzner MA, Jordan HW. The ultrastructure of an abnormal cell in Sézary's syndrome. Blood 1968; 31:719–726.
7. Carrozza PM, Kempf W, Kazakov DV, Dummer R, Burg G. A case of Sézary's syndrome associated with granulomatous lesions, myelodysplastic syndrome and transformation into CD30–positive large-cell pleomorphic lymphoma. Br J Dermatol 2002; 147:582–586.
8. Buechner SA, Winkelmann RK. Sézary syndrome. A clinicopathologic study of 39 cases. Arch Dermatol 1983; 119:979–986.
9. Shapiro PE, Pinto FJ. The histologic spectrum of mycosis fungoides/Sézary syndrome (cutaneous T-cell lymphoma). A review of 222 biopsies, including newly described patterns and the earliest pathologic changes. Am J Surg Pathol 1994; 18:645–667.
10. Trotter MJ, Whittaker SJ, Orchard GE, Smith NP. Cutaneous histopathology of Sézary syndrome: a study of 41 cases with a proven circulating T-cell clone. J Cutan Pathol 1997; 24:286–291.
11. Sentis HJ, Willemze R, Scheffer E. Histopathologic studies in Sézary syndrome and erythrodermic mycosis fungoides: a comparison with benign forms of erythroderma. J Am Acad Dermatol 1986; 15:1217–1226.
12. Haneke E. Granulomatöses Sézary-Syndrom mit Epithelinseln. Z Hautkr 1984; 59: 951–961.
13. Walsh NM, Prokopetz R, Tron VA, Sawyer DM, Watters AK, Murray S, Zip C. Histopathology in erythroderma: review of a series of cases by multiple observers. J Cutan Pathol 1994; 21:419–423.
14. Imai S, Burg G, Braun-Falco O. Mycosis fungoides and Sézary's syndrome show distinct histomorphological features. Dermatologica 1986; 173:131–135.
15. Kamarashev J, Burg G, Kempf W, Hess Schmid M, Dummer R. Comparative analysis of histological and immunohistological features in mycosis fungoides and Sézary syndrome. J Cutan Pathol 1998; 25:407–412.
16. Harmon CB, Witzig TE, Katzmann JA, Pittelkow MR. Detection of circulating T cells with CD4+CD7- immunophenotype in patients with benign and malignant lymphoproliferative dermatoses J Am Acad Dermatol 1996; 35:404–410.
17. Bernengo MG, Quaglino P, Novelli M, Cappello N, Doveil GC, Lisa F, De Matteis A, Fierro MT, Appino A. Prognostic factors in Sézary syndrome: a multivariate analysis of clinical, haematological and immunological features. Ann Oncol 1998; 9:857–863.

18. Dummer R, Nestle FO, Niederer E, Ludwig E, Laine E, Grundmann H, Grob P, Burg G. Genotypic, phenotypic and functional analysis of CD4+CD7+ and CD4+CD7− T lymphocyte subsets in Sézary syndrome. Arch Dermatol Res 1999; 291:307–311.
19. Scarisbrick JJ, Woolford AJ, Russell-Jones R, Whittaker SJ. Allelotyping in mycosis fungoides and Sézary syndrome: common regions of allelic loss identified on 9p, 10q, and 17p. J Invest Dermatol 2001; 117:663–670.
20. Russell-Jones R, Whittaker S. Sézary syndrome: diagnostic criteria and therapeutic options. Semin Cutan Med Surg 2000; 19:100–108.
21. Edelson R, Berger C, Gasparro F, Jegasothy B, Heald P, Wintroub B, Vonderheid E, Knobler R, Wolff K, Plewig G. Treatment of cutaneous T-cell lymphoma by extracorporeal photochemotherapy. Preliminary results. N Engl J Med 1987; 316:297–303.
22. Zackheim HS, Epstein EJ. Low-dose methotrexate for the Sézary syndrome. J Am Acad Dermatol 1989; 21:757–762.
23. Rosen ST, Foss FM. Chemotherapy for mycosis fungoides and the Sézary syndrome. Hematol Oncol Clin North Am 1995; 9:1109–1116.
24. Scarisbrick JJ, Whittaker S, Evans AV, Fraser-Andrews EA, Child FJ, Dean A, Russell-Jones R. Prognostic significance of tumor burden in the blood of patients with erythrodermic primary cutaneous T-cell lymphoma. Blood 2001; 97:624–630.
25. Vonderheid EC, Sobel EL, Nowell PC, Finan JB, Helfrich MK, Whipple DS. Diagnostic and prognostic significance of Sézary cells in peripheral blood smears from patients with cutaneous T cell lymphoma. Blood 1985; 66:358–366.
26. Midiaelis S, Kazakov DV, Brug G, Dummer R, Kempf W. Extracutaneous transformation into a high-grade lymphoma: a potential pitfall in managment of patients with Sézary's Syndrome. Int Am J Dermatopathol, In press .
27. Stefanato CM, Tallini G, Crotty PL. Histologic and immunophenotypic features prior to transformation in patients with transformed cutaneous T-cell lymphoma: is CD25 expression in skin biopsy samples predictive of large cell transformation in cutaneous T-cell lymphoma? Am J Dermatopathol 1998; 20:1–6.

25

CD30+ T-cell Lymphoproliferative Disorders of the Skin

Werner Kempf and Günter Burg
Department of Dermatology, University Hospital, Zürich, Switzerland

The CD30-positive T-cell lymphoproliferative disorders of the skin (CD30+LPD) represent a distinctive group of primary cutaneous T-cell lymphoma (CTCL) which have been recognized as nosologic entities in recent lymphoma classifications. The CD30+ LPD of the skin comprise a clinical and morphologic spectrum of diseases including lymphomatoid papulosis (LyP), primary cutaneous anaplastic large T-cell lymphoma (CD30+ ALCL) as well as so called borderline cases (1,2). The hallmark of the tumor cells is the expression of CD30, a cytokine receptor belonging to the tumor necrosis factor receptor (TNFR) superfamily. Although they share CD30 expression as a common immunophenotypic feature, the diseases within the group of CD30+LPD differ in their clinical and histological presentations (3–5).

REFERENCES

1. Kadin ME. The spectrum of Ki-1+ custaneous lymphomas. Curr Probl Dermatol 1990; 19:132–143.
2. Kaudewitz P, Burg G. Lymphomatoid papulosis and Ki-1 (CD30)-positive cutaneous large cell lymphomas. Semin Diagn Pathol 1991; 8:117–124.
3. Willemze R, Beljaards RC. Spectrum of primary cutaneous CD30 (Ki-1)-positive lymphoproliferative disorders. A proposal for classification and guidelines for management and treatment. J Am Acad Dermatol 1993; 28:973–980.
4. Paulli M, Berti E, Rosso R, Boveri E, Kindl S, Klersy C, Lazzarino M, Borroni G, Menestrina F, Santucci M. CD30/Ki-1-positive lymphoproliferative disorders of the skin—clinicopathologic correlation and statistical analysis of 86 cases: a multicentric study from the european organization for research and treatment of cancer cutaneous lymphoma project group. J Clin Oncol 1995; 13:1343–1354.
5. Drews R, Samel A, Kadin ME. Lymphomatoid papulosis and anaplastic large cell lymphomas of the skin. Semin Cutan Med Surg 2000; 19:109–117.

25.1. Lymphomatoid Papulosis

Werner Kempf, Günter Burg, and Dmitry V. Kazakov
Department of Dermatology, University Hospital, Zürich, Switzerland

CLASSIFICATION

WHO/EORTC Classification (2005): Primary cutaneous CD30+ lymphoproliferative disorders of the skin–lymphomatoid papulosis

WHO Classification (2001): Primary cutaneous CD30 lymphoproliferative disorders of the skin–lymphomatoid papulosis

REAL Classification (1997): Not listed

EORTC Classification (1997): Lymphomatoid papulosis

DEFINITION

Lymphomatoid papulosis (LyP), described in 1968 by Macaulay (1), is a chronic recurrent, self-healing papulo-nodular skin eruption with histologic features of a malignant lymphoma.

CLINICAL FEATURES

The overall estimated prevalence is 1–2 cases per 1,000,000 population with a male: female ratio of 1.5:1 (2). Usually, LyP affects people in their third or fourth decade (median age:45 years), but it can be seen in patients of all ages.

LyP is characterized by disseminated papules or nodules, which evolve and regress over a few weeks sometimes leaving behind scars. Often several papules are clustered (Fig. 1). The number of lesions in LyP can vary from few to hundreds (3). Although no definite predilection site has been identified, LyP lesions more often arise on the trunk, especially the buttocks, and extremities. In contrast to CD30+ LTCL, the face is less frequently involved in LyP. The individual LyP lesion starts as an erythematous, usually asymptomatic papule (initial stage). Within days or

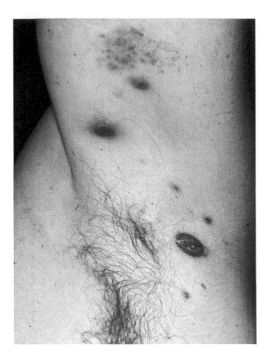

Figure 1 Lymphomatoid papulosis: grouped papules with a larger superficially ulcerated nodule on the arm.

few weeks, the papules become red brown, hemorrhagic, or pustular. Some lesions undergo ulceration (ulcerative stage). This stage is followed by complete spontaneous regression of the lesion, often leaving behind hyper- or hypopigmented scars with varioliform aspect (Fig. 2). The individual lesions usually last for several weeks (2–8 weeks) (4,5). The duration of the disorder is highly variable ranging from several weeks to years, even decades.

Clinicopathologic variants of LyP include regional LyP (6), follicular, pustular, and rare mucosal involvement with oral lesions (7).

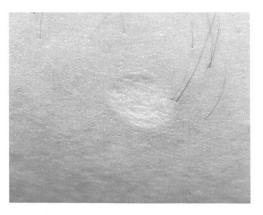

Figure 2 Lymphomatoid papulosis: varioliform scar after spontaneous regression of a nodule.

Table 1 Definition Criteria for the Different Histologic Types of LyP According to EORTC Classification for Cutaneous Lymphomas

Histologic type	Morphologic criteria
LyP type A	Scattered CD30+ blast cells in an extensive inflammatory infiltrate
LyP type B	Mycosis fungoides-like histology with atypical CD30-negative T-cells with cerebriform nuclei
LyP type C	Large clusters of CD30+ cells with few inflammatory cells, histologically suggesting a CD30+ (anaplastic) large-cell lymphoma

HISTOLOGY

The histological features of LyP are variable and considerably depend on the stage of the lesions and disease. Three histologic subtypes (types A, B and C) have been delineated (8) which represent a spectrum with overlapping features (Table 1). In fully developed LyP lesions, a wedge-shaped diffuse dermal infiltrate with or without overlying ulceration is found (Fig. 3). The infiltrate contains medium-sized to large pleomorphic or anaplastic lymphoid cells with irregular nuclei, sparse chromatin, and mitotic activity (Fig. 4). These atypical lymphoid cells are scattered or grouped in small clusters. Epidermotropism can be present. In addition, there are numerous inflammatory cells such as neutrophils, eosinophils and histiocytes as well as few plasma cells and a prominent edema in the upper dermis. Cases with scattered tumor cells intermingled with numerous inflammatory cells are designated LyP type A, whereas LyP type C features cohesive sheets of large atypical lymphoid cells with only a few intermingled reactive inflammatory cells (Fig. 5). A third histologic presentation, often referred to as type B, is characterized by an epidermotropic infiltrate resembling histologic features of MF or SS and harbors atypical lymphoid cells with cerebriform nuclei. Differentiation between MF, SS, and LyP type B cannot be accomplished with routine light microscopy alone. Although distinction of different histologic subtypes may be of interest, often various histologic manifestations of LyP lesions can be seen at the same time in the same patient.

IMMUNOHISTOCHEMISTRY

The tumor cells in LyP are of T-cell origin with a CD3+, CD4+, CD8−, CD30+, CD56+ (10%) phenotype and additional expression of activation markers such as HLA-DR and CD25 (interleukin 2-receptor) thus representing a proliferation of activated T helper cells (9–12) (Figs. 6 and 7). Usually one or more T-cell antigens such as CD2 and CD5 are expressed, whereas CD7 expression is often absent. The CD15, which is a characteristic marker for Reed–Sternberg cells in HD, is usually not expressed by tumor cells in LyP. In contrast to tumor cells expressing CD30 as a hallmark of LyP type A and type C, the small tumor cells with cerebriform nuclei in LyP type B are usually negative for CD30. Recent studies indicated that almost all tumor cells in LyP and CD30+ LTCL express cytotoxic molecules such as TIA-1 and granzyme B (13).

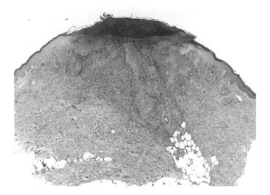

Figure 3 Lymphomatoid papulosis: wedge-shaped lymphocytic infiltrate with crusted superficial ulceration.

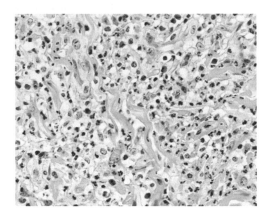

Figure 4 Lymphomatoid papulosis: mixed infiltrate consisting of large atypical lymphocytes,
eosinophils, and neutrophils (LyP, type A).

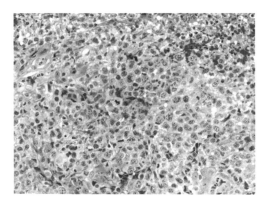

Figure 5 Lymphomatoid papulosis: cohesive sheets of large atypical lymphocytes with only
few neutrophils (LyP, type C).

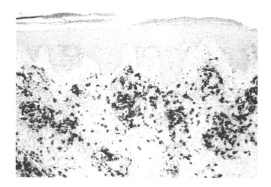

Figure 6 Lymphomatoid papulosis: grouped and scattered CD30+ lymphocytes of varying size (immunohistochemistry).

MOLECULAR BIOLOGY

Clonal rearrangement of TCR-genes has been detected in 40–100% of LyP lesions by Southern blot technique or PCR. In archival formalin-fixed and paraffin-embedded skin biopsies, the rate of detection of clonal T-cell population is lower and may be restricted to certain histologic subforms of LyP (own unpublished data). Cytogenetic studies have demonstrated chromosomal deletions and rearrangements of chromosomes 1, 7, 9, and 10 (14). The t(2;5) (p23;q35) translocation characteristic of systemic anaplastic large cell lymphomas is not detected in LyP (15,16).

The etiology of LyP is still unknown. A virus as causative factor has been suggested. Various studies have demonstrated absence of HTLV-1 and 2, EBV and human herpesviruses 6, 7, and 8 in LyP (17). Recently, endogenous retroviral elements have been identified in LyP, but their role has still to be defined (18). Interaction of CD30 and CD30L as well as TGF-beta with its receptor are essential for growth regulation (19,20).

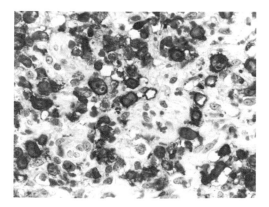

Figure 7 Lymphomatoid papulosis: large CD30+ tumor cells with characteristic staining of cell membranes and the Golgi apparatus (perinuclear dot).

TREATMENT

Various therapeutic approaches in LyP have been employed. However, LyP can usually not be cured. Moreover, there are no data indicating that any kind of therapeutic intervention in LyP alters the natural history of the disease or prevents progression to other malignant lymphomas (21). Methotrexate (10–20 mg weekly) is the most effective therapy resulting in rapid clearance of the skin lesions in 90% of patients (22). Relapses occur in most patients after withdrawal of MTX. Alternative therapies include photochemotherapy (PUVA, bath PUVA), retinoids, and interferon-alpha. Oral or topical steroids are effective in some cases, but their efficacy has not been proven by larger studies. In children, antibiotic therapy may sometimes be useful (Eric vondemeid, MD, personal communication).

CLINICAL COURSE AND PROGNOSIS

In general, primary cutaneous CD30+ LPD exhibit a favorable prognosis with 5-year-survival rates 100% in LyP (23,24). In 5–20% of patients with LyP, development of other cutaneous and nodal lymphomas is observed (5,24). Such lymphomas can develop prior to, concurrent with, or after the manifestation of LyP and other CD30+ LPD and are usually referred to as LyP-associated malignant lymphomas (25) and include mycosis fungoides (MF), Hodgkin's disease (HD), and systemic or cutaneous CD30+ ALCL with a fatal outcome in 2% of affected patients (24). No risk factors have been identified which definitely indicate likely progression to associated lymphomas in LyP patients. Since fascin expression occurs at a significantly higher rate in LyP cases associated with systemic lymphomas, its expression might serve as a putative prognostic marker (20).

Lymphomatoid papulosis

Clinical features
    Recurrent grouped papules and nodules. Spontaneous regression after weeks with
        or without ulceration and scars
Histological features
    Wedge-shaped mixed-cellular infiltrate with large atypical lymphocytes,
        granulocytes, and eosinophils
    Mitotic activity of large atypical lymphocytes. Ulceration may be found
Immunophenotype
    CD3+, CD4+, CD30+, TIA-1+
Molecular biology
    Clonal TCR gene rearrangement variably detected
Treatment
    Observation, heliotherapy, PUVA, chemotherapy (methotrexate)
Clinical course
    Benign, but recurrent. In 5–15% of patients development of a second lymphoid
        neoplasm

DIFFERENTIAL DIAGNOSIS

Diagnostic criteria for LyP include (i) the occurrence of recurrent, self-healing papulo-nodular skin lesions, often arranged in crops, (ii) spontaneous regression—with or without transient ulceration—of the individual skin lesions, often concurrently with the development of new lesions in the same or another body region, (iii) and histologic features of CD30+ T-cell lymphoma ranging from few scattered CD30+ tumor cells with numerous admixed inflammatory reactive cells to cohesive sheets of anaplastic tumor cells. Because of overlapping histologic and immunophenotypical features in CD30+ LPD and to avoid misinterpretation of histologic findings in LyP as high-malignant lymphoma, the final diagnosis has to include careful correlation with clinical manifestations of the disease when evaluating infiltrates with CD30+ tumor cells.

A variety of inflammatory and neoplastic disorders can mimic clinically and/or histologically LyP. Moreover, during the last years, several disorders with expression of CD30 by reactive or neoplastic cells have been described. Those "LyP simulators" include pityriasis lichenoides, arthropod bite reactions, parasitic infestations (e.g., scabies), viral infections, and pseudolymphomatous drug eruptions containing CD30-positive cells. These experiences emphasize that expression of CD30 by itself is not a sufficient diagnostic tool for CD30+ LPD.

COMMENTS

The distinction of three different histologic LyP types has so far not proven to be of clinical or prognostic significance and is thus not supported by all experts in the field.

Sometimes, the development of large nodules up to several centimeters in diameter is observed in LyP patients; they may last for months until spontaneous regression occurs (8). It is still a matter of debate whether such lesions should be considered as part of the spectrum of clinical manifestation of LyP, or whether those large nodular lesions rather represent concurrent CD30+ ALCL.

REFERENCES

1. Macaulay WL. Lymphomatoid papulosis. A continuing self-healing eruption, clinically benign–histologically malignant. Arch Dermatol 1968; 97:23–30.
2. Wang HH, Lach L, Kadin ME. Epidemiology of lymphomatoid papulosis. Cancer 1992; 70:2951–2957.
3. Sanchez NP, Pittelkow MR, Muller SA, Banks PM, Winkelmann RK. The clinicopathologic spectrum of lymphomatoid papulosis: study of 31 cases. J Am Acad Dermatol 1983; 8:81–94.
4. Braun Falco O, Nikolowski J, Burg G, Schmoeckel C. Lymphomatoide Papulose. Ubersicht und eigene Beobachtungen an vier Patienten. Hautarzt 1983; 34:59–65.
5. Kadin ME. The spectrum of Ki-1+ cutaneous lymphomas. Curr Probl Dermatol 1990; 19:132–143.
6. Scarisbrick JJ, Evans AV, Woolford AJ, Black MM, Russell Jones R. Regional lymphomatoid papulosis: a report of four cases. Br J Dermatol 1999; 141:1125–1128.
7. Kato N, Tomita Y, Yoshida K, Hisai H. Involvement of the tongue by lymphomatoid papulosis. Am J Dermatopathol 1998; 20:522–526.
8. Willemze R, Meyer CJ, Van Vloten WA, Scheffer E. The clinical and histological spectrum of lymphomatoid papulosis. Br J Dermatol 1982; 107:131–144.

9. Burg G, Hoffmann Fezer G, Nikolowski J, Schmoeckel C, Braun Falco O, Stunkel K. Lymphomatoid papulosis: a cutaneous T-cell pseudolymphoma. Acta Derm Venereol 1981; 61:491–496.

10. Kaudewitz P, Stein H, Burg G, Mason M, Braun-Falco O. Detection of Sternberg–Reed and Hodgkin cell specific antigen on atypical cells in lymphomatoid papulosis (poster). 2nd International Conference on Malignant Lymphoma, Lugano, June 13–16, 1984.

11. Kadin ME. Common activated helper-T-cell origin for lymphomatoid papulosis, mycosis fungoides, and some types of Hodgkin's disease. Lancet 1985; 2:864–865.

12. Kaudewitz P, Burg G, Stein H, Klepzig K, Mason DY, Braun Falco O. Monoclonal antibody patterns in lymphomatoid papulosis. Dermatol Clin 1985; 3:749–757.

13. Kummer JA, Vermeer MH, Dukers D, Meijer CJ, Willemze R. Most primary cutaneous CD30-positive lymphoproliferative disorders have a CD4-positive cytotoxic T-cell phenotype. J Invest Dermatol 1997; 109:636–640.

14. Peters K, Knoll JH, Kadin ME. Cytogenetic findings in regressing skin lesions of lymphomatoid papulosis. Cancer Genet Cytogenet 1995; 80:13–16.

15. DeCoteau JF, Butmarc JR, Kinney MC, Kadin ME. The t(2;5) chromosomal transloca- tion is not a common feature of primary cutaneous CD30+ lymphoproliferative disor- ders: comparison with anaplastic large-cell lymphoma of nodal origin. Blood 1996; 87:3437–3441.

16. Ott G, Katzenberger T, Siebert R, DeCoteau JF, Fletcher JA, Knoll JH, Kalla J, Rosenwald A, Ott MM, Weber Matthiesen K, Kadin ME, Muller Hermelink HK. Chromosomal abnormalities in nodal and extranodal CD30+ anaplastic large cell lymphomas: infrequent detection of the t(2;5) in extranodal lymphomas. Genes Chromosomes Cancer 1998; 22:114–121.

17. Kempf W, Kadin ME, Kutzner H, Lord CL, Burg G, Letvin NL, Koralnik IJ. Lympho- matoid papulosis and human herpesviruses—A PCR-based evaluation for the presence of human herpesvirus 6, 7 and 8 related herpesviruses. J Cutan Pathol 2001; 28:29–33.

18. Kempf W, Kadin ME, Dvorak AM, Lord CC, Burg G, Letvin NL, Koralnik IJ. Endo- genous retroviral elements, but not exogenous retroviruses, are detected in CD30- positive lymphoproliferative disorders of the skin. Carcinogenesis 2003; 24:301–306.

19. Mori M, Manuelli C, Pimpinelli N, Mavilia C, Maggi E, Santucci M, Bianchi B, Cappugi P, Giannotti B, Kadin ME. CD30-CD30 ligand interaction in primary cutaneous CD30(+) T-cell lymphomas: a clue to the pathophysiology of clinical regression. Blood 1999; 94:3077–3083.

20. Kadin ME, Levi E, Kempf W. Progression of lymphomatoid papulosis to systemic lymphoma is associated with escape from growth inhibition by TGF-beta and CD30 ligand. Ann N Y Acad Sci 2001; 941:59–68.

21. Drews R, Samel A, Kadin ME. Lymphomatoid papulosis and anaplastic large cell lymphomas of the skin. Semin Cutan Med Surg 2000; 19:109–117.

22. Vonderheid EC, Sajjadian A, Kadin ME. Methotrexate is effective therapy for lympho- matoid papulosis and other primary cutaneous CD30-positive lymphoproliferative disor- ders. J Am Acad Dermatol 1996; 34:470–481.

23. Paulli M, Berti E, Rosso R, Boveri E, Kindl S, Klersy C, Lazzarino M, Borroni G, Menestrina F, Santucci M. CD30/Ki-1-positive lymphoproliferative disorders of the skin—clinicopathologic correlation and statistical analysis of 86 cases: a multicentric study from the European organization for research and treatment of cancer cutaneous lymphoma project Group. J Clin Oncol 1995; 13:1343–1354.

24. Bekkenk MW, Geelen FA, van Voorst Vader PC, Heule F, Geerts ML, van Vloten WA, Meijer CJ, Willemze R. Primary and secondary cutaneous CD30(+) lymphoproliferative disorders: a report from the Dutch cutaneous lymphoma group on the long-term follow- up data of 219 patients and guidelines for diagnosis and treatment. Blood 2000; 95: 3653–3661.

25. Kadin ME. Lymphomatoid papulosis and associated lymphomas. How are they related?. Arch Dermatol 1993; 129:351–353.

**Primary Cutaneous Anaplastic Large
Cell Lymphoma**

Werner Kempf, Dmitry V. Kazakov, and Günter Burg
Department of Dermatology, University Hospital, Zürich, Switzerland

CLASSIFICATION AND TERMINOLOGY

WHO/EORTC Classification(2005): Primary cutaneous anaplastic large cell
   lymphoma.
WHO Classification(2001): Primary cutaneous anaplastic large cell lymphoma
REAL Classification(1997): Anaplastic large cell lymphoma, CD30+
EORTC Classification(1997): Primary cutaneous large cell T-cell lymphoma,
   CD30+

DEFINITION

Primary cutaneous anaplastic large cell lymphoma (CD30+ ALCL) is a neoplasm
composed of large atypical lymphocytes of either pleomorphic, anaplastic, or immunoblastic cytomorphology expressing CD30 antigen. Clinically, CD30+ ALCL is
divided into a primary (de novo) form and a secondary form originating from
another lymphoma by transformation. Primary cutaneous and primary nodal
CD30+ ALCL are distinct clinical entities that have identical morphologic features,
but differ in age of onset, immunophenotype, and prognosis (1). In this book,
primary cutaneous large cell pleomorphic CD30+ CTCL and primary cutaneous
CD30+ ALCL are used as synonyms. According to the EORTC classification
(2), CD30+ large cell lymphomas are defined by CD30 expression of at least 75%
of the large pleomorphic or anaplastic lymphoid cells.

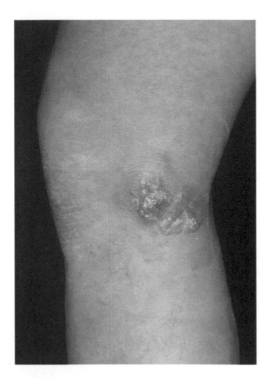

Figure 1   Solitary, large, ulcerated nodule on the leg.

CLINICAL FEATURES

Anaplastic large cell lymphoma represents the second most common form of CL, with a prevalence of 1–2 per million, occurring mainly in people in their sixth decade, with a male preponderance (male:female ratio = 2–3:1) (3,4). Children can also have ALCL. The vast majority of primary cutaneous ALCL in HIV-infected individuals are also CD30+ (5). The clinicopathologic features are otherwise identical to those of ALCL occurring in immunocompetent patients.

ALCL usually manifests as an asymptomatic, solitary, firm, and often ulcerated nodule (Fig. 1) (3,6). The extremities and head are sites of predilection (3,7,8). Approximately 20% of the patients have multifocal disease, i.e., two or more lesions at multiple anatomic sites (4). Most patients experience a history of rapidly growing tumors over a time span of 4–6 weeks without preceding longstanding patches or plaques. If there is no therapeutic intervention, spontaneous regression has been reported to occur in 10–42% of the tumor lesions (3,4), which led to the original description of regressing atypical histiocytosis (RAH) (9).

HISTOLOGY

There is a dense nodular infiltrate of atypical lymphoid cells, extending through all levels of the dermis into the subcutis. Epidermotropism is an inconsistent feature. The morphologic hallmarks are large, bizarre cells with irregularly shaped nuclei and one or more nucleoli and an abundant clear or eosinophilic cytoplasm

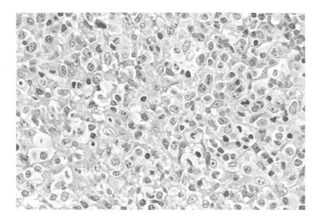

Figure 2 Cohesive sheets of large, atypical tumor cells with mitoses.

(Fig. 2). Tumor cells usually grow in dense cohesive sheets, reminiscent of nodular malignant melanoma or undifferentiated carcinoma, and may be multinucleated (Fig. 2). Mitoses are frequent.M Clusters of small reactive lymphocytes are found within and around the tumor. Eosinophils, plasma cells, and dendritic cells are usually few in ALCL. The lymphoma can also present with an extensive infiltrate of neutrophils and is then described as *neutrophil-rich or pyogenic CD30+ ALCL* (N-ALCL) (10,11). Clinically, N-ALCL is characterized by ulceration and purulent secretion due to formation of small abscesses within the tumor tissue. Remarkably, these lymphomas are almost exclusively limited to the face. Small aggregations or scattered CD30+ medium to large pleomorphic lymphoid cells are found within a diffuse mixed-cellular infiltrate with numerous neutrophilic abscesses.

IMMUNOHISTOCHEMISTRY

Primary cutaneous CD30+ ALCLs have an activated T-cell phenotype with expression of T-cell associated antigens CD2, CD3, CD4, and CD45RO, and activation markers such as CD25 (IL-2R), CD30, CD71, and HLA-DR. According to the

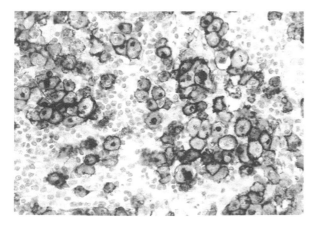

Figure 3 Expression of CD30 by almost all tumor cells.

Table 1 Expression of Differentiation and Activation Markers in Various CD30+ LPD

Disorder	CD30	CD15	CD45RO	ALK	EMA	HOXC5
LyP	+	∓ (50%?)	+	−	−	n.a.
1°cut ALCL	+	−	+	− (rarely +)		∣∣
2°cut ALCL (syst. ALCL)	+	∓ (HD-like ALCL +!)	−	+ (65%)	+	∓
HL	+	+	−	−	−	n.a.

Abbreviations: LyP, lymphomatoid papulosis; ALCL, anaplastic large-cell lymphoma; HL, Hodgkin lymphoma; EMA, epithelial membrane antigen.

EORTC classification, CD30+ large cell lymphomas are defined by CD30 expression of at least 75% of the large pleomorphic or anaplastic lymphoid cells (2) (Fig. 3). Variable loss of T-cell antigens (CD2, CD3, CD5) can be found (7). Expression of T-cell markers on tumor cells is usually weaker than that on reactive lymphocytes (3). In contrast to nodal ALCL, primary cutaneous forms do not express EMA, but may express the cutaneous lymphocyte antigen (CLA, HECA-452). Table 1 shows other markers that are variably expressed in nodal and cutaneous ALCL along with ALK and EMA.

MOLECULAR BIOLOGY

Most cases (over 90%) of primary cutaneous ALCL display clonal rearrangement of TCR genes in Southern blot and PCR (12). A high percentage of nodal CD30+ ALCL have a t(2;5) (p23;q35) translocation, resulting in expression of NPM–ALK protein (p80); this translocation is not or only in a small percentage of primary cutaneous CD30+ ALCL found. This is of particular importance, since lack of ALK expression in cutaneous lymphomas is not a prognostic factor, whereas ALK-negative nodal lymphomas show a significantly worse prognosis compared to their ALK-positive counterparts (79% vs. 46% 5-year survival rate) (13).

TREATMENT

For solitary CD30+ ALCL arising de novo, surgical excision or radiation therapy (total dose 4000 cGy) is the first-line treatment. In addition, radiation therapy is usually considered for recurrences of ALCL after surgical excision. In cases with cutaneous or extracutaneous spread, where surgical excision and radiation therapy is not practical, single or multiagent chemotherapy is indicated. Unfortunately, it seems not be very effective (8).

CLINICAL COURSE AND PROGNOSIS

Primary cutaneous CD30+ ALCL has a favorable prognosis, with 5-year survival rates of 90% (4,14). Spontaneous regression and age less than 60 years are associated with a better prognosis, while extracutaneous disease and age greater than 60 years have a worse outlook. Cytomorphology (anaplastic or pleomorphic and immunoblastic) seems not to be a prognostic factor (14). Recurrences are observed

---

Primary cutaneous anaplastic large cell lymphoma

Clinical features
  Solitary, rapidly growing, ulcerated nodule
Histological features
  Cohesive sheets of anaplastic tumor cells
  Sparse reactive inflammatory infiltrate
Immunophenotype
  CD2+, CD3+, CD5+, CD4+, CD45RO+, CD30+, ALK–
Molecular biology
  Clonal TCR rearrangement in majority of cases
Treatment
  Excision, ionizing radiation, methotrexate, chemotherapy in disseminated forms
Clinical course and prognosis
  Favorable (> 90% 5-year survival rate)

---

in up to 40% of the cases (4) and do not require different treatment than initial lesions (15). Extracutaneous spread occurs in 10% of the patients, in particular in those with multiple grouped or multifocal tumor lesions. Regional lymph nodes may be involved, but the survival rate is similar to that of patients with skin lesions only (4). Fatal outcome is observed in up to 12% of the patients. Up to 40% of CD30+ ALCLs show spontaneous regression (16). If complete tumor regression occurs, no further treatment is necessary; usually the rapid tumor growth in the first weeks makes therapeutic intervention necessary.

DIFFERENTIAL DIAGNOSIS

Undifferentiated epithelial, mesenchymal, and melanocytic tumors with anaplastic morphology have to be distinguished by immunohistochemistry. Differentiation of LyP type C and CD30+ ALCL requires correlation with clinical features. Staging is mandatory to exclude secondary cutaneous forms of ALCL, which require aggressive treatment with multiagent polychemotherapy. No single marker is specific enough to distinguish between primary and secondary cutaneous forms of ALCL.

COMMENTS

There is a considerable debate about the terminology of tumor cell morphology in large cell lymphomas, which is mainly due to contradictory opinions as to whether the terms "pleomorphic" and "anaplastic" can and should be used as synonyms. In this book, primary cutaneous large cell pleomorphic CD30+ CTCL and primary cutaneous CD30+ ALCL are used as synonyms. In the EORTC classification, ALCL is not regarded as a separate entity, but as a subform of large T-cell lymphoma. On the other hand, pleomorphic lymphomas of whatever tumor cell size are not listed in the REAL and WHO classifications, but are part of the large group of "peripheral T-cell lymphomas, not otherwise specified (NOS)." Some (including the authors) feel that the cytomorphologic differences between tumor cells in ALCL do not have any prognostic implications and, moreover, that there are no reliable criteria to distinguish between large pleomorphic and large anaplastic cells (2).

REFERENCES

1. Stein H, Foss HD, Durkop H, Marafioti T, Delsol G, Pulford K, Pileri S, Falini B. CD30(+) anaplastic large cell lymphoma: a review of its histopathologic, genetic, and clinical features. Blood 2000; 96:3681–3695.

2. Willemze R, Kerl H, Sterry W, Berti E, Cerroni L, Chimenti S, Diaz Perez JL, Geerts ML, Goos M, Knobler R, Ralfkiaer E, Santucci M, Smith N, Wechsler J, van Vloten WA, Meijer CJ. EORTC classification for primary cutaneous lymphomas: a proposal from the Cutaneous Lymphoma Study Group of the European Organization for Research and Treatment of ancer. Blood 1997; 90:354–371.

3. Kaudewitz P, Burg G, Stein H. Ki-1 (CD30) positive cutaneous anaplastic large cell lymphomas. Curr Probl Dermatol 1990; 19:150–156.

4. Bekkenk MW, Geelen FA, van Voorst Vader PC, Heule F, Geerts ML, van Vloten WA, Meijer CJ, Willemze R. Primary and secondary cutaneous CD30(+) lymphoproliferative disorders: a report from the Dutch Cutaneous Lymphoma Group on the long-term follow-up data of 219 patients and guidelines for diagnosis and treatment. Blood 2000; 95:3653–3661.

5. Kerschmann RL, Berger TG, Weiss LM, Herndier BG, Abrahms KM, Heon V, Schulze K, Kaplan LD, Resnik SD, LeBoit PE. Cutaneous presentations of lymphoma in human immunodeficiency virus disease. Predominance of T cell lineage. Arch Dermatol 1995; 131:1281–1288.

6. Kadin ME. The spectrum of Ki-1+ cutaneous lymphomas. Curr Probl Dermatol 1990; 19:132–143.

7. Kaudewitz P, Stein H, Dallenbach F, Eckert F, Bieber K, Burg G, Braun Falco O. Primary and secondary cutaneous Ki-1+ (CD30+) anaplastic large cell lymphomas. Morphologic, immunohistologic, and clinical-characteristics.. Am J Pathol 1989; 135: 359–367.

8. Beljaards RC, Kaudewitz P, Berti E, Gianotti R, Neumann C, Rosso R, Paulli M, Meijer CJ, Willemze R. Primary cutaneous CD30-positive large cell lymphoma: definition of a new type of cutaneous lymphoma with a favorable prognosis. A European Multicenter Study of 47 patients. Cancer 1993; 71:2097–2104.

9. Flynn KJ, Dehner LP, Gajl Peczalska KJ, Dahl MV, Ramsay N, Wang N. Regressing atypical histiocytosis: a cutaneous proliferation of atypical neoplastic histiocytes with unexpectedly indolent biologic behavior. Cancer 1982; 49:959–970.

10. McCluggage WG, Walsh MY, Bharucha H. Anaplastic large cell malignant lymphoma with extensive eosinophilic or neutrophilic infiltration. Histopathology 1998; 32:110–115.

11. Burg G, Kempf W, Kazakov DV, Dummer R, Frosch PJ, Lange-Ionescu S, Nishikawa T, Kadin ME. Pyogenic lymphoma of the skin: a peculiar variant of primary cutaneous neutrophil-rich CD30+ anaplastic large-cell lymphoma. Clinicopathological study of four cases and review of the literature. Br J Dermatol 2003; 148:580–586.

12. Macgrogan G, Vergier B, Dubus P, Beylot Barry M, Belleannee G, Delaunay MM, Eghbali H, Beylot C, Rivel J, Trojani M, Vital C, De Mascarel A, Bloch B, Merlio JP. CD30-positive cutaneous large cell lymphomas. A comparative study of clinico-pathologic and molecular features of 16 cases. Am J Clin Pathol 1996; 105:440–450.

13. Gascoyne RD, Aoun P, Wu D, Chhanabhai M, Skinnider BF, Greiner TC, Morris SW, Connors JM, Vose JM, Viswanatha DS, Coldman A, Weisenburger DD. Prognostic significance of anaplastic lymphoma kinase (ALK) protein expression in adults with anaplastic large cell lymphoma. Blood 1999; 93:3913–3921.

14. Paulli M, Berti E, Rosso R, Boveri E, Kindl S, Klersy C, Lazzarino M, Borroni G, Menestrina F, Santucci M, et al. CD30/Ki-1-positive lymphoproliferative disorders of the skin—clinicopathologic correlation and statistical analysis of 86 cases: a multicentric study from the European Organization for Research and Treatment of Cancer Cutaneous Lymphoma Project Group. J Clin Oncol 1995; 13:1343–1354.

15. Drews R, Samel A, Kadin ME. Lymphomatoid papulosis and anaplastic large cell lymphomas of the skin. Semin Cutan Med Surg 2000; 19:109–117.
16. Beljaards RC, Willemze R. The prognosis of patients with lymphomatoid papulosis associated with malignant lymphomas. Br J Dermatol 1992; 126:596–602.

26

Subcutaneous Panniculitis-like T-cell Lymphoma

Werner Kempf, Dmitry V. Kazakov, and Günter Burg
Department of Dermatology, University Hospital, Zürich, Switzerland

CLASSIFICATION

WHO/EORTC Classification (2005): Subcutaneous panniculitis-like T-cell lymphoma

WHO Classification (2001): Subcutaneous panniculitis-like T-cell lymphoma

REAL Classification (1997): Subcutaneous panniculitis-like T-cell lymphoma

EORTC Classification (1997): Subcutaneous panniculitis-like T-cell lymphoma

DEFINITION

Subcutaneous panniculitis-like T-cell lymphoma (SPTCL) is a lymphoproliferative disease originating and presenting primarily in the subcutaneous fat tissue, displaying various phenotypic variants.

CLINICAL FEATURES

The disease presents with multiple indurated plaques or tumors predominantly located on the lower legs and to a lesser extent the trunk (1–3). The neoplastic infiltrates simulate panniculitis. The skin lesions may ulcerate (Fig. 1). Systemic features such as fever, malaise, fatigue, myalgias, chills and weight loss are not uncommon. Some patients develop a hemophagocytic syndrome with resultant cytopenia which may be in part due to release of cytokines, particularly TNFalpha and IFNgamma (4). Mostly patients in their fifth decade are affected. There is no gender predilection.

HISTOLOGY

The histopathologic hallmark of this type of CTCL is the subcutaneous localization and growth pattern of usually nonepidermotropic, focal infiltrates simulating lobular

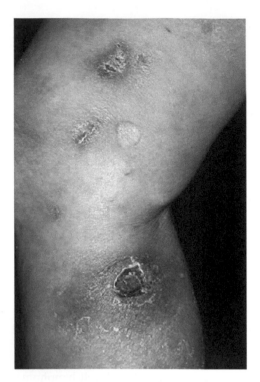

Figure 1 Subcutaneous panniculitis-like T-cell lymphoma: infiltrated subcutaneous nodules with ulceration on the leg.

panniculitis (2,3) (Fig. 2). Karyorrhexis and fat necrosis are prominent features. The tumor cells are lymphoid cells of varying size, often with chromatin-dense nuclei. Rimming of adipocytes by tumor cells is a common, but not specific, finding for SPCTL (Fig. 3). Many histiocytes are found and erythrophagocytosis can be present. Since the lymphoproliferative process is focal, large and deep biopsies are mandatory to establish diagnosis. During evolution, the dermis may become involved by tumoral infiltrates, especially in cases with $\gamma/\delta+$/CD56+ phenotype (5).

IMMUNOHISTOCHEMISTRY

Tumor cells express T-cell-associated antigens CD2+, CD3+, CD5+, CD4–, CD8+, CD43+ and expression of cytotoxic proteins such as TIA-1, granzyme B and per-forin (3). A TCR α/β (βF1+) phenotype is much more frequently found than a TCR γ/δ (TCRδ-1+) phenotype. Clonal rearrangement of TCR genes is present in the majority of the cases. Rarely, CD56+ (TCR $\alpha/\beta+$), CD4+ CD56+, and CD30+ forms of SPTCL have been described (6,7). TCR γ/δ (TCRδ-1+) positive cases preferentially express Vδ2 in contrast to γ/δ hepatosplenic T cell lymphomas expressing Vδ1 (8). The SPTCL are thought to arise from normal T lymphocytes, which reside in the subcutis and express the Vδ2 gene.

Some cases of SPTCL, in particular the ones in Asians, are associated with EBV. The EBV may play a role in the development of hemophagocytosis associated with SPTCL (9). Most cases of SPTCL in Western countries are EBV-negative (3,10,11).

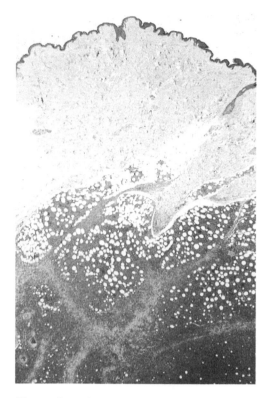

Figure 2 Subcutaneous panniculitis-like T-cell lymphoma: dense subcutaneous lymphocytic infiltrate extending into the deep dermis.

TREATMENT

For cases of SPTCL with a course expected to be aggressive (i.e., especially cases with expression of a TCR $\gamma/\delta+$/CD56+ phenotype), multiagent chemotherapy, possibly followed by allogeneic BMT may be useful.

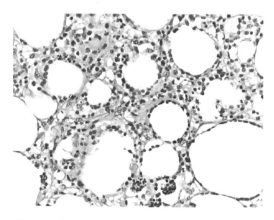

Figure 3 Subcutaneous panniculitis-like T-cell lymphoma: rimming of adipocytes by medium sized pleomorphic tumor cells and collections of nuclear fragments (bean bag cells).

Subcutaneous panniculitis-like T-Cell lymphoma

Clinical features
   Location on lower extremities and trunk
   Deep-seated plaques or nodules which may ulcerate
Histological features
   Subcutaneous lymphocytic infiltrate. Minimal dermal or epidermal involvement.
      Rimming of fat lobules by pleomorphic medium to large lymphocytes.
      Karyorrhexis with macrophages, erythrophagocytosis
Immunophenotype
   CD2+, CD3+, CD5+, CD4-/+, CD8+/−, CD43+, TIA-1+, Granzyme B+
      and perforin+
   TCR α/β (bF1+)≫TCR γ/δ (TCRδ-1+) > CD4+ CD56+≫CD30+
Molecular biology
   Clonal TCR rearrangement in most cases
Treatment
   Not standardized.
Clinical course and prognosis
   Indolent slowly progressive course more common in TCR α/β (βF1+) cases.
      Rapid and aggressive course with fatal outcome in TCR γ/δ (TCRδ-1+)
      cases. Hemophagocytic syndrome with systemic signs in some patients

CLINICAL COURSE AND PROGNOSIS

The disease usually runs an indolent, slowly progressive course (sometimes even with spontaneous remission). On occasion, rapid and aggressive course with dissemination of skin lesions, systemic spread to bone marrow, lung, and liver, sepsis, hemophagocytic syndrome, and fatal outcome occurs (1,12). A correlation exists between the course of the disease and the immunophenotype of tumor cells. A TCR $\alpha/\beta+$ phenotype may be indicative of a more indolent course, whereas expression of TCR $\gamma/\delta+$ phenotype appears to be associated with an aggressive course and worse prognosis (7,13).

DIFFERENTIAL DIAGNOSIS

On clinical grounds, erythema nodosum or other forms of panniculitis are the most common differential diagnostic considerations. Histologically, SPTCL can be misinterpreted as lupus panniculitis or histiocytic cytophagic panniculitis, which is a reactive process associated with variable systemic diseases, which usually presents with a hemorrhagic diathesis due to hemophagocytosis but without proliferation of lymphoid tumor cells.

COMMENTS

Since the phenotype of tumor cells has been linked to aggressiveness of the disease, immunophenotyping has both therapeutic and prognostic implications. Alpha/beta expressing forms can be distinguished from gamma/delta positive forms. Due to their aggressive course, SPTCL expressing a gamma/delta phenotype belong to the group of cutaneous gamma/delta lymphoma in the WHO–EORTC classification. Cases with dermal involvement on the first biopsy may give rise to difficulties in classification. In cases where dermal involvement is prominent, it has been recommended to classify such cases as peripheral T-cell lymphoma (pleomorphic or unspecified). Correlation with clinical features is essential for further differentiation. On rare occasion, primary subcutaneous B-cell lymphoma may be found, expanding the spectrum of primary subcutaneous lymphomas (14).

REFERENCES

1. Perniciaro C, Zalla MJ, White JJ, Menke DM. Subcutaneous T-cell lymphoma. Report of two additional cases and further observations. Arch Dermatol 1993; 129:1171–1176.
2. Mehregan, Su WP, Kurtin PJ. Subcutaneous T-cell lymphoma: a clinical, histopathologic, and immunohistochemical study of six cases. J Cutan Pathol 1994; 21:110–117.
3. Salhany KE, Macon WR, Choi JK, Elenitsas R, Lessin SR, Felgar RE, Wilson DM, Przyblski GK, Lister J, Wasik MA, Swerdlow SH. Subcutaneous panniculitis-like T-cell lymphoma: clinicopathologic, immunophenotypic, and genotypic analysis of alpha/beta and gamma/delta subtypes. Am J Surg Pathol 1998; 22:881–893.
4. Lay JD, Tsao CJ, Chen JY, Kadin ME, Su IJ. Upregulation of tumor necrosis factor-alpha gene by Epstein–Barr virus and activation of macrophages in Epstein–Barr virus-infected T cells in the pathogenesis of hemophagocytic syndrome. J Clin Invest 1997; 100:1969–1979.
5. Takimoto Y, Imanaka F, Sasaki N, Nanba K, Kimura N. Gamma/delta T cell lymphoma presenting in the subcutaneous tissue and small intestine in a patient with capillary leak syndrome. Int J Hematol 1998; 68:183–191.
6. Park SB, Cho KH, Kim CW. Subcutaneous tissue involvement of CD30-positive large cell lymphoma. J Dermatol 1998; 25:553–555.
7. Jang KA, Choi JH, Sung KJ, Moon KC, Koh JK, Kwon YM, Chi HS. Primary CD56+ nasal-type T/natural killer-cell subcutaneous panniculitic lymphoma: presentation as haemophagocytic syndrome. Br J Dermatol 1999; 141:706–709.
8. Przybylski GK, Wu H, Macon WR, Finan J, Leonard DG, Felgar RE, DiGiuseppe JA, Nowell PC, Swerdlow SH, Kadin ME, Wasik MA, Salhany KE. Hepatosplenic and subcutaneous panniculitis-like gamma/delta T cell lymphomas are derived from different Vdelta subsets of gamma/delta T lymphocytes. J Mol Diagn 2000; 2:11–19.
9. Craig AJ, Cualing H, Thomas G, Lamerson C, Smith R. Cytophagic histiocytic panniculitis—a syndrome associated with benign and malignant panniculitis: case comparison and review of the literature. J Am Acad Dermatol 1998; 39:721–736.
10. Burg G, Dummer R, Wilhelm M, Nestle F, Ott MM, Feller A, Hefner H, Lanz U, Schwinn A, Wiede J. A subcutaneous delta-positive T-cell lymphoma that produces interferon gamma. N Engl J Med 1991; 325:1078–1081.
11. Kumar S, Krenacs L, Medeiros J, Elenitoba-Johnson KS, Greiner TC, Sorbara L, Kingma DW, Raffeld M, Jaffe ES. Subcutaneous panniculitic T-cell lymphoma is a tumor of cytotoxic T lymphocytes. Hum Pathol 1998; 29:397–403.
12. Gonzalez CL, Medeiros LJ, Braziel RM, Jaffe ES. T-cell lymphoma involving subcutaneous tissue. A clinicopathologic entity commonly associated with hemophagocytic syndrome. Am J Surg Pathol 1991; 15:17–27.
13. Yamashita Y, Tsuzuki T, Nakayama A, Fujino M, Mori N. A case of natural killer/T cell lymphoma of the subcutis resembling subcutaneous panniculitis-like T cell lymphoma. Pathol Int 1999; 49:241–246.
14. Kazakov DV, Burg G, Dummer R, Palmedo G, Muller , Kempf W. Primary subcutaneous follicular centre cell lymphoma with involvement of the galea: a case report and short review of the literature. Br J Dermatol 2002; 146:663–666.

27

Primary Cutaneous Peripheral T-cell Lymphoma, Unspecified

27.1. Cytotoxic Lymphomas

Werner Kempf, Dmitry V. Kazakov, Reinhard Dummer, and Günter Burg
Department of Dermatology, University Hospital, Zürich, Switzerland

The spectrum of cytotoxic lymphomas of the skin is heterogeneous and includes CD8+ T-cell, T/NK-cell, and NK-cell lymphomas as well as neoplasms related to myelomonocytic leukemia. As a common hallmark, the tumor cells display cytotoxic proteins. There is no widely accepted classification (and or even nomenclature) of this group of lymphomas. Immunophenotyping plays a crucial role in diagnosing cytotoxic lymphomas. Future developments will clarify, which forms of cytotoxic lymphoma in fact represent cytotoxic variants of well-established CL such as MF and which ones are distinct nosologic entities. In accordance with the basic principle

Table 1 Cytotoxic Lymphomas with Primary or Secondary Cutaneous Involvement

---

Primary cutaneous CD8+ cytotoxic lymphoma
Epidermotropic forms
  MF-like hypo- or hyperpigmented types
  Aggressive type
  Sezary syndrome-like variant
Nonepidermotropic forms
  Nodular type
Extranodal NK/T-cell lymphoma
Nasal type
Subcutaneous panniculitis-like lymphoma
Gamma/delta lymphoma
Lymphoblastoid NK-cell lymphoma/leukemia
CD4+ CD56+ blastic lymphoma/leukemia
Aggressive T/NK cell lymphoma/leukemia

Note: CD30+ lymphoproliferative disorders of the skin such as lymphomatoid papulosis and CD30+ ALCL have usually a CD4+ T-helper cell phenotype, but often express cytotoxic molecules such as TIA-1.

of recent lymphoma classifications (WHO, REAL, and EORTC) to delineate nosologic entities, the aim of this chapter is to describe those forms of cytotoxic lymphomas with primary or secondary skin involvement which display distinct clinical,
pathologic, and immunophenotypic features (Table 1). It is essential to identify
lymphomas with a cytotoxic phenotype, since some forms exhibit an aggressive
course which has therapeutic implications (1–4).

CYTOTOXIC MOLECULES

Cytotoxic molecules are expressed by cytotoxic T cells and NK cells, but have also
been found in CD4+ T cells of primary cutaneous CD30+ LPD. These molecules
mediate cell lysis and include perforin (cytolysin), serine esterases (granzymes),
and the granule membrane-associated cytotoxic protein TIA-1. TIA-1 is expressed
by both activated and nonactivated NK cells and cytotoxic T cells (3,5), whereas
other proteins such as granzyme and perforin are primarily expressed only by activated cells. Thus, TIA-1 serves as a useful marker to identify cytotoxic lymphomas.
NK and T/NK cells (NK-like cytotoxic T lymphocytes) express CD56, also known
as N-CAM. In lymphoblastoid neoplasms, the CD56+ tumor cells probably represent precursor cells related to a myelomonocytic lineage or dendritic cells rather than
NK-cells. Differential expression of cytotoxic molecules and killer cell inhibitory
receptors have been observed in CD8+ and CD56+ cutaneous lymphomas (6).

REFERENCES

1. Jaffe ES, Chan JK, Su IJ, Frizzera G, Mori S, Feller AC, Ho FC. Report of the Workshop
    on Nasal and Related Extranodal Angiocentric T/Natural Killer Cell Lymphomas. Defi-
    nitions, differential diagnosis, and epidemiology. Am J Surg Pathol 1996; 20:103–111.
2. Chan JK, Sin VC, Wong KF, Ng CS, Tsang WY, Chan CH, Cheung MM, Lau WH.
    Nonnasal lymphoma expressing the natural killer cell marker CD56: a clinicopathologic
    study of 49 cases of an uncommon aggressive neoplasm. Blood 1997; 89:4501–4513.
3. Felgar RE, Macon WR, Kinney MC, Roberts S, Pasha T, Salhany KE. TIA-1 expression
    in lymphoid neoplasms. Identification of subsets with cytotoxic T lymphocyte or natural
    killer cell differentiation. Am J Pathol 1997; 150:1893–1900.
4. Santucci M, Pimpinelli N, Massi D, Kadin ME, Meijer CJ, Muller-Hermelink HK, Paulli M,
    Wechsler J, Willemze R, Audring H, Bernengo MG, Cerroni L, Chimenti S, Chott A,
    Diaz-Perez JL, Dippel E, Duncan LM, Feller AC, Geerts ML, Hallermann C, Kempf W,
    Russell-Jones R, Sander C, Berti E. Cytotoxic/natural killer cell cutaneous lymphomas.
    Report of EORTC Cutaneous Lymphoma Task Force Workshop. Cancer 2003; 97:
    610–627.
5. Boulland ML, Kanavaros P, Wechsler J, Casiraghi O, Gaulard P. Cytotoxic protein
    expression in natural killer cell lymphomas and in alpha beta and gamma delta peripheral
    T-cell lymphomas. J Pathol 1997; 183:432–439.
6. Kamarashev J, Burg G, Mingari MC, Kempf W, Hofbauer G, Dummer R. Differential
    expression of cytotoxic molecules and killer cell inhibitory receptors in CD8+ and
    CD56+ cutaneous lymphomas. Am J Pathol 2001; 158:1593–1598.

27.1.1. CD8+ Cytotoxic Cutaneous T-cell Lymphomas

Werner Kempf, Reinhard Dummer, Dmitry V. Kazakov, and Günter Burg
Department of Dermatology, University Hospital, Zürich, Switzerland

Among this group, which belongs to the peripheral T-cell lymphomas, unspecified in the WHO classification, at least four subforms can be distinguished (Table 1). Two forms are histologically characterized by epidermotropic CD8+ T-cells. Clinically, they differ in regard to their course with one form being slowly progressive like classic MF, whereas the other form shows an aggressive behavior. Two other less common variants are an erythrodermic Sézary syndrome (SS) -like form and a nodular, nonepidermotropic type (1). Only the primary cutaneous aggressive epidermotropic CD8+ T-cell lymphoma is considered as provisional entity in the WHO-EORTC consensus classification.

MF-LIKE HYPO- OR HYPERPIGMENTED FORM OF CYTOTOXIC CD8+ T-CELL LYMPHOMA

This variant manifests with hypo- or hyperpigmented patches or plaques mostly on the trunk, clinically resembling classic MF (Fig. 1) (2,3). The hypopigmented form seems to affect predominantly children and adolescents (3), whereas the hyperpigmented form has been reported in patients over 50 years of age (2). Histologically, lining-up along the junctional zone and epidermotropism of small T-cells is found

Table 1 Primary Cutaneous CD8+ Cytotoxic Lymphomas

Epidermotropic forms
MF-like hypo- or hyperpigmented types
Aggressive type
  Sézary syndrome-like variant
Non-epidermotropic forms
  Nodular type

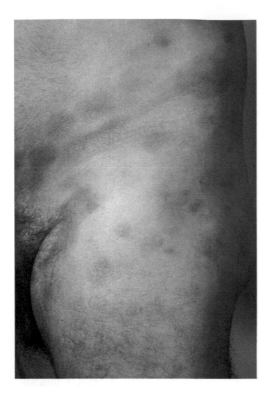

Figure 1 Hyperpigmented patches.

(Fig. 2); changes which are indistinguishable from classic MF or SS. Immunophenotyping is crucial and reveals that the epidermotropic T-cells express CD8 and CD3, but are negative for CD4 (Fig. 3 A–C). Clonal rearrangement of T-cell receptor genes can be detected in most of the cases (3). The therapeutic approach is identical

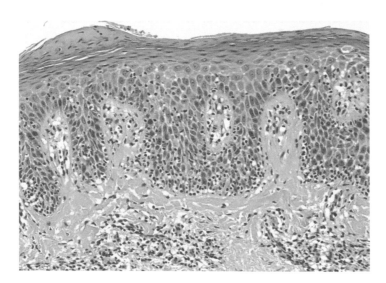

Figure 2 Epidermotropic infiltrate with prominent lining up of lymphocytes along the junctional zone.

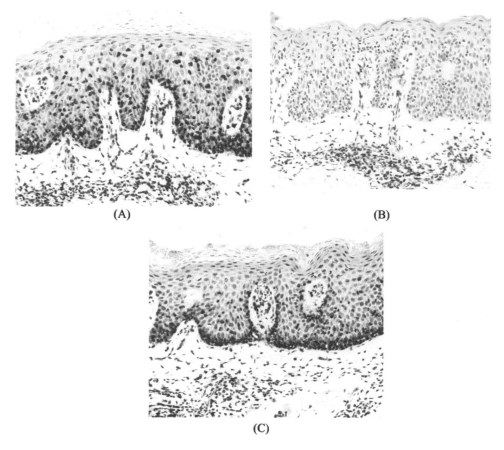

Figure 3 Neoplastic lymphocytes express CD3 as a pan T-cell marker(A), but are negative for CD4 (in contrast to classic MF) (B), and positive for CD8 (C).

to classic MF. Good response to PUVA was reported in a patient with hyperpigmented form (2). The course seems to be comparable to classic MF (4).

It remains to be clarified whether this form of lymphoma should perhaps be designated rather as hypo- or hyperpigmented MF with CD8+ cytotoxic phenotype, since this phenotype is the only distinguishing feature from classic MF, or whether this form reflects a distinct entity within the group of cytotoxic CD8+ CTCL.

PRIMARY CUTANEOUS AGGRESSIVE EPIDERMOTROPIC CD8+ T-CELL LYMPHOMA

Another epidermotropic form of CD8+ CTCL is often characterized by an aggressive course (5). Generalized patches, plaques, papulonodular lesions, and tumors have been described (Fig. 4); the clinical picture has been compared to disseminated pagetoid reticulosis or MF, respectively. Histologically, a band-like infiltrate of pleomorphic T-cells or immunoblasts with epidermotropism and epidermal changes with acanthosis, spongiosis, intraepidermal blistering, and necrosis are seen. The tumor cells express CD3, CD8, CD7, CD45RA, and beta F1 as well as TIA-1. A CD2– CD7+ phenotype seems to be associated with a more aggressive course (6).

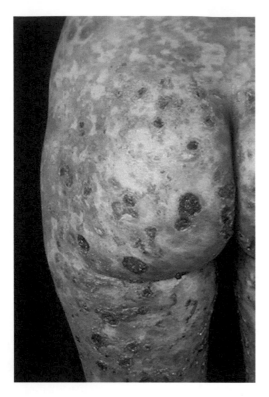

Figure 4 Aggressive type: disseminated partly eroded plaques.

An aggressive course with extracutaneous spread to CNS, visceral organs, and oral mucosa is common with a median survival of 32 months (5). Similar cases with an aggressive course have sometimes shown angiocentric and angiodestructive growth (7–9). Patients with erythroderma and peripheral blood involvement consistent with SS but also expressing CD8 have also been identified (1).

NODULAR FORM OF CYTOTOXIC CD8+ CTCL

Along with the epidermotropic variants of CD8+ CTCL, other patients present with nodular lesions of varying size and number, with a highly variable outcome ranging from complete remission after topical steroids, radiotherapy, or chemotherapy to death within 29 months (1).

REFERENCES

1. Lu D, Patel KA, Duvic M, Jones D. Clinical and pathological spectrum of CD8-positive cutaneous T-cell lymphomas. J Cutan Pathol 2002; 29:465–472.
2. Dummer R, Kamarashev J, Kempf W, Haffner AC, Hess-Schmid M, Burg G. Junctional CD8+ cutaneous lymphomas with nonaggressive clinical behavior: a CD8+ variant of mycosis fungoides? Arch Dermatol 2002; 138:199–203.
3. El Shabrawi-Caelen L, Cerroni L, Kerl H. The clinicopathologic spectrum of cytotoxic lymphomas of the skin. Semin Cutan Med Surg 2000; 19:118–123.

4. Santucci M, Pimpinelli N, Massi D, Kadin ME, Meijer CJ, Muller-Hermelink HK, Paulli M, Wechsler J, Willemze R, Audring H, Bernengo MG, Cerroni L, Chimenti S, Chott A, Diaz-Perez JL, Dippel E, Duncan LM, Feller AC, Geerts ML, Hallermann C, Kempf W, Russell-Jones R, Sander C, Berti E. Cytotoxic/natural killer cell cutaneous lymphomas. Report of EORTC Cutaneous Lymphoma Task Force Workshop. Cancer 2003; 97:610–627.

5. Berti E, Tomasini D, Vermeer MH, Meijer CJ, Alessi E, Willemze R. Primary cutaneous CD8-positive epidermotropic cytotoxic T cell lymphomas. A distinct clinicopathological entity with an aggressive clinical behavior. Am J Pathol 1999; 155:483–492.

6. Agnarsson BA, Vonderheid EC, Kadin ME. Cutaneous T cell lymphoma with suppressor/cytotoxic (CD8) phenotype: identification of rapidly progressive and chronic subtypes. J Am Acad Dermatol 1990; 22:569–577.

7. Jensen JR, Thestrup-Pedersen K. Subpopulations of T lymphocytes in a patient with fulminant mycosis fungoides. Acta Derm Venereol 1980; 60:159–161.

8. Fujiwara Y, Abe Y, Kuyama M, Arata J, Yoshino T, Akagi T, Miyoshi K. CD8+ cutaneous T-cell lymphoma with pagetoid epidermotropism and angiocentric and angio-destructive infiltration. Arch Dermatol 1990; 126:801–804.

9. Urrutia S, Piris MA, Orradre JL, Martinez B, Cruz MA, Garcia AD. Cytotoxic/suppressor (CD8+, CD4–) cutaneous T-cell lymphoma with aggressive course. Am J Dermatopathol 1990; 12:603–606.

27.1.2. Cutaneous Gamma/Delta T-cell Lymphoma

Werner Kempf, Dmitry V. Kazakov, and Günter Burg
Department of Dermatology, University Hospital, Zürich, Switzerland

CLASSIFICATION

WHO/EORTC Classification (2005): Primary cutaueous peripharal T-cell lymphoma, unspecified, Cutaneous γ/δ-positive T-cell lymphoma (provisional)
WHO Classification (2001): peripharal T-cell lymphoma, unspecified
REAL Classification (1997): peripharal T-cell lymphoma, unspecified
EORTC Classification (1997): Not listed

DEFINITION

Gamma/delta T-cell lymphomas are characterized by the expression of TCR delta and the absence of beta F1. They belong to the group of peripheral T-cell lymphomas, unspecified.

CLINICAL FEATURES

Nonhepatosplenic gamma/delta T-cell lymphomas have a proclivity for mucosal or cutaneous sites (1). Primary cutaneous lymphomas expressing gamma/delta TCR are very rare. Clinically, gamma/delta lymphoma of the skin manifests with multiple plaques, tumors, or subcutaneous nodules especially on the extremities (2).

HISTOLOGY

There are dense infiltrate mainly in the mid-dermis of small to intermediate-sized tumor cells with irregular nuclei. Epidermotropism of reactive CD4+ T-cells, ulceration, and periadnexal infiltration are present in one-third of the biopsies (3). Some cases belong to the group of subcutaneous panniculitis-like T-cell lymphoma (4).

195

IMMUNOHISTOCHEMISTRY

The immunophenotypic hallmark is expression of TCR delta and the absence of beta F1. Tumor cells may express CD3, CD4, or CD8, but are often double negative (CD4– and CD8–) (3,5) and positive for TIA-1, granzyme B, and perforin (2). Most of the so-called CD4– CD8– double negative cutaneous T-cell lymphoma belongs to this group of gamma/delta lymphoma (3,5). CD30, CD56, and TdT are not expressed.

MOLECULAR BIOLOGY

Clonal rearrangement of TCR genes can be detected in almost all cases. Cutaneous gamma/delta T-cell lymphomas are EBV-negative (2).

TREATMENT

Multiagent chemotherapy is indicated in most cases.

CLINICAL COURSE AND PROGNOSIS

The disease has an aggressive course with a proclivity for rapid multifocal cutaneous dissemination, spread to bone marrow or lymph nodes and fatal outcome (2,3).

DIFFERENTIAL DIAGNOSIS

Immunophenotyping and molecular studies are essential to identify and to differentiate this subtype from other forms of CTCL.

REFERENCES

1. Arnulf B, Copie-Bergman C, Delfau-Larue MH, Lavergne-Slove A, Bosq J, Wechsler J, Wassef M, Matuchansky C, Epardeau B, Stern M, Bagot M, Reyes F, Gaulard P. Nonhepatosplenic gammadelta T-cell lymphoma: a subset of cytotoxic lymphomas with mucosal or skin localization. Blood 1998; 91:1723–1731.
2. Toro JR, Beaty M, Sorbara L, Turner ML, White J, Kingma DW, Raffeld M, Jaffe ES. Gamma delta T-cell lymphoma of the skin: a clinical, microscopic, and molecular study. Arch Dermatol 2000; 136:1024–1032.
3. Jones D, Vega F, Sarris AH, Medeiros LJ. CD4– CD8– "Double-negative" cutaneous T-cell lymphomas share common histologic features and an aggressive clinical course. Am J Surg Pathol 2002; 26:225–231.
4. Burg G, Dummer R, Wilhelm M, Nestle F, Ott MM, Feller A, Hefner H, Lanz U, Schwinn A, Wiede J. A subcutaneous delta-positive T-cell lymphoma that produces interferon gamma. N Engl J Med 1991; 325:1078–1081.
5. Ralfkiaer E, Wollf-Sneedorff A, Thomsen K, Geisler C, Vejlsgaard GL. T-cell receptor gamma delta-positive peripheral T-cell lymphomas presenting in the skin: a clinical, histological and immunophenotypic study. Exp Dermatol 1992; 1:31–36.

27.2. Primary Cutaneous Peripheral T-cell Lymphoma, Unspecified Noncytotoxic Variants

27.2.1. Primary Cutaneous CD4-Positive Small- to Medium-Sized Pleomorphic T-cell Lymphoma

Werner Kempf, Dmitry V. Kazakov, and Günter Burg
Department of Dermatology, University Hospital, Zürich, Switzerland

CLASSIFICATION

WHO/EORTC Classification (2005): Primary cutaneous Peripheral T-cell-lymphoma, unspecified; Primary cutaneous CD4-positive small/medium-sized pleomorphic T-cell lymphoma(provisional)
WHO Classification (2001): Peripheral T-cell lymphoma, unspecified
REAL Classification (1997): Peripheral T-cell lymphoma, unspecified
EORTC Classification (1997): CTCL, pleomorphic small/medium-sized

DEFINITION

Primary cutaneous CD4-positive small to medium-sized pleomorphic T-cell lymphoma (SM-PTCL) is a noncytotoxic form of peripheral T-cell lymphoma, unspecified characterized by small to medium-sized tumor cells expressing CD4. While only a linked number of cases have been reported, SM-PTCL is a provisional entity in the EORTC classification and WHO–EORTC consensus classification (1).

CLINICAL FEATURES

The SM-PTCL presents with localized (in most cases) or widespread, mostly asymptomatic and indurated papules, nodules or violaceous plaques without any preceding history of patches (2,3) (Fig. 1). Ulceration may occur. The mean age at diagnosis is approximately 50–60 years with a wide range. There is no gender predilection.

197

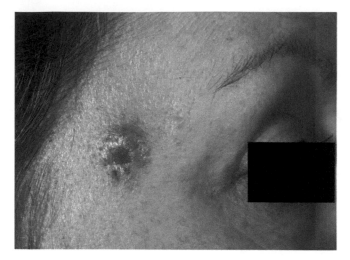

Figure 1 CD30-negative small to medium-sized pleomorphic lymphoma: solitary erythematous nodule on the temple (with biopsy site).

HISTOLOGY

The lymphoid infiltrate is monomorphous, predominantly perivascular and periadnexal or nodular and extends to the subcutaneous tissue. It consists of small to medium-sized pleomorphic lymphoid cells with irregular hyperchromatic nuclei and a pale scanty cytoplasm (2) (Fig. 2). Mitoses are found. Eosinophils and plasma cells may be admixed. Epidermotropism is absent in most cases, but granulomatous features are found in a subset of cases.

IMMUNOHISTOCHEMISTRY

The tumor cells have a CD3+ CD4+ T helper phenotype CD3+ CD8+ similar cases were reported (2). Loss of T-cell antigens has been observed. Tumor cells are nega-

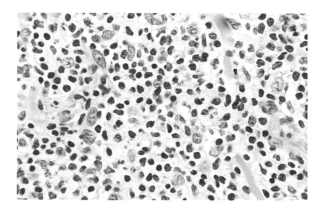

Figure 2 CD30-negative small to medium-sized pleomorphic lymphoma: diffuse infiltrate of small to medium-sized lymphocytes with convoluted nuclei and abundant cytoplasm. Prominent endothelial cells.

tive for CD30. The CD20+ B-cells may be admixed and account for up to 20% of the infiltrate (3).

MOLECULAR BIOLOGY

Clonal rearrangement of TCR genes has been detected in almost all cases, and may be useful in distinguishing SPTCL from pseudolymphoma.

TREATMENT

For solitary lesions, excision or radiotherapy is effective. Relapses have been reported (2). For disseminated lesions, PUVA, cyclophospamide, and interferon alpha have been reported to be effective (4,5).

CLINICAL COURSE AND PROGNOSIS

The prognosis of CD30-negative small to medium-sized pleomorphic lymphoma is favorable (1,2).

DIFFERENTIAL DIAGNOSIS

Small to medium sized pleomorphic T-cell infiltrates can be observed in MF, but a history of preceding patches points to the correct diagnosis. While T-cell pseudolymphoma may present with small pleomorphic T-cells, but they do not show monoclonal rearrangement of TCR genes. The cells in small cell variant of CD30+ large T-cell lymphoma or lymphomatoid papulosis express CD30.

REFERENCES

1. Willemze R, Kerl H, Sterry W, Berti E, Cerroni L, Chimenti S, Diaz Perez JL, Geerts ML, Goos M, Knobler R, Ralfkiaer E, Santucci M, Smith N, Wechsler J, van Vloten WA, Meijer CJ. EORTC classification for primary cutaneous lymphomas: a proposal from the cutaneous lymphoma study group of the European organization for research and treatment of cancer. Blood 1997; 90:354–371.
2. Friedmann D, Wechsler J, Delfau MH, Esteve E, Farcet JP, de Muret A, Parneix-Spake A, Vaillant L, Revuz J, Bagot M. Primary cutaneous pleomorphic small T-cell lymphoma. A review of 11 cases. The French study group on cutaneous lymphomas. Arch Dermatol 1995; 131:1009–1015.
3. Kim YC, Vandersteen DP. Primary cutaneous pleomorphic small/medium-sized T-cell lymphoma in a young man. Br J Dermatol 2001; 144:903–905.
4. Sterry W, Siebel A, Mielke V. HTLV-1-negative pleomorphic T-cell lymphoma of the skin: the clinicopathological correlations and natural history of 15 patients. Br J Dermatol 1992; 126:456–462.
5. Beljaards RC, Meijer CJ, Van der Putte SC, Hollema H, Geerts ML, Bezemer PD, Willemze R. Primary cutaneous T-cell lymphoma: clinicopathological features and prognostic parameters of 35 cases other than mycosis fungoides and CD30-positive large cell lymphoma. J Pathol 1994; 172:53–60.

27.2.2. Primary Cutaneous Peripheral T-cell Lymphomas, Unspecified, Other Forms

Werner Kempf, Dmitry V. Kazakov, and Günter Burg
Department of Dermatology, University Hospital, Zürich, Switzerland

CLASSIFICATION

WHO/EORTC Classification (2005): Primary cutaneous peripheral T-cell lymphoma, unspecified

WHO Classification (2001): Peripheral T-cell lymphoma, unspecified

REAL Classification (1997): Peripheral T-cell lymphoma, unspecified

EORTC Classification (1997): Large cell CTCL, CD30–

DEFINITION

Most cases within this group cytomorphologically represent large-cell pleomorphic lymphomas with large pleomorphic cells which—by definition—do not express CD30 (1,2). It belongs to the group of noncytotoxic peripheral T-cell lymphomas. Recent studies show that many cases included previously in this group in fact, belong to extranodal T/NK-cell lymphoma, blastic NK-cell lymphoma (synonym: agranular CD4+ CD56+ hematodermic neoplasm), and other distinct entities (3). CD30– PLTCL per se is a rare lymphoma whose clinicopathologic features have yet to be defined. It is listed as a separate entity only in the EORTC classification (2). In WHO classification, this lymphoma falls under the group of peripheral T-cell lymphomas, unspecified.

HISTOPATHOLOGY

The tumor cells are characterized by pleomorphic nuclei, which may be medium-sized or large (Fig. 1). In addition, small reactive lymphocytes, eosinophils, and plasma cells may be present.

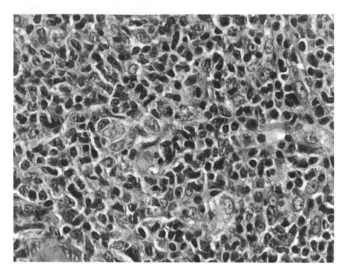

Figure 1 CD30– large pleomorphic lymphoma: diffuse infiltrate of large lymphocytes with pleomorphic nuclei and abundant cytoplasm.

IMMUNOHISTOCHEMISTRY

The tumor cells express T-cell associated antigens (CD2, CD3, CD5), but usually lack CD7; most cases are CD4+, but rare cases of CD8+ have been reported.

MOLECULAR BIOLOGY

Molecular studies reveal clonal rearrangement of TCR genes.

TREATMENT

Only a few cases of CD30– PTCL have been reported and no standard therapy has been established.

CLINICAL COURSE AND PROGNOSIS

The prognosis seems to be worse than in other CTCL with 5-year survival rates of approximately 60% or less with primary cutaneous immunoblastic lymphomas having the worst prognosis (2,4). Disseminated skin lesions and elevated serum lactate dehydrogenase (LDH) levels seem to be indicators of a poor prognosis (1). Other parameters including age, sex, and mode of initial treatment have no significant effect on the survival time (4).

DIFFERENTIAL DIAGNOSIS

CD30+ anaplastic large T-cell lymphoma must be ruled out, as it has a far better prognosis than CD30– PTCL. When PTCL arises in the context of transformation of pre-existing MF or SS, only the history provides the answer. Since many cytotoxic lymphomas and related disorders are composed of medium to large cells, immuno-phenotyping is crucial to identify extranodal NK and T/NK-cell lymphomas, nasal and nasal type, as well as blastic NK-cell lymphoma with expression of CD56+ as a common hallmark. In ATLL, significant epidermotropism with formation of intrae-pidermal microabscesses is seen and leukemic spread of tumor cells found. Merkel cell carcinoma is characterized by expression of CK 20 (perinuclear dot-like pattern).

COMMENTS

The distinction between small- and large-cell pleomorphic CTCL is made in the EORTC classification of cutaneous lymphomas (2). In the WHO classification, these cases are lumped together in the group of peripheral T-cell lymphomas, unspecified.

REFERENCES

1. Joly P, Vasseur E, Esteve E, Leibowitch M, Tilly H, Vaillant L, Wechsler J, Thomine E, De Muret A, Dreyfus F, et al. Primary cutaneous medium and large cell lymphomas other than mycosis fungoides. An immunohistological and follow-up study on 54 cases. French Study Group for Cutaneous Lymphomas. Br J Dermatol 1995; 132:506–512.
2. Willemze R, Kerl H, Sterry W, Berti E, Cerroni L, Chimenti S, Diaz Perez JL, Geerts ML, Goos M, Knobler R, Ralfkiaer E, Santucci M, Smith N, Wechsler J, van Vloten WA, Meijer CJ. EORTC classification for primary cutaneous lymphomas: a proposal from the Cutaneous Lymphoma Study Group of the European Organization for Research and Treatment of Cancer. Blood 1997; 90:354–371.
3. Petrella T, Dalac S, Maynadie M, Mugneret F, Thomine E, Courville P, Joly P, Lenormand B, Arnould L, Wechsler J, Bagot M, Rieux C, Bosq J, Avril MF, Bernheim A, Molina T, Devidas A, Delfau-Larue MH, Gaulard P, Lambert D. CD4+ CD56+ cuta-neous neoplasms: a distinct hematological entity? Groupe Francais d'Etude des Lymphomes Cutanes (GFELC). Am J Surg Pathol 1999; 23:137–146.
4. Beljaards RC, Meijer CJ, Van der Putte SC, Hollema H, Geerts ML, Bezemer PD, Willemze R. Primary cutaneous T-cell lymphoma: clinicopathological features and prognostic parameters of 35 cases other than mycosis fungoides and CD30-positive large cell lymphoma. J Pathol 1994; 172:53–60.

28

Extranodal NK/T-cell Lymphoma, Nasal Type

Werner Kempf, Reinhard Dummer, Dmitry V. Kazakov, and Günter Burg
Department of Dermatology, University Hospital, Zürich, Switzerland

CLASSIFICATION

WHO/EORTC Classification (2005): Extranodal NK/T-cell lymphoma,
   nasal type
WHO Classification (2001): Extranodal NK/T-cell lymphoma, nasal type
REAL Classification (1997): Extranodal NK/T-cell lymphoma, nasal type
EORTC Classification (1997): Not listed

DEFINITION

While the clinicopathologic and phenotypic features of nasal/nasal type NK/T-cell
lymphomas and aggressive NK cell leukemia/lymphoma are well characterized (1,2)
there is a considerable heterogeneity—clinical as well as histological and immunophenotypic—among other extranodal NK/T-cell lymphomas (3). In addition, the
nomenclature shows overlaps and contradictions, making comparison of cases and
delineation of characteristic features difficult. The unifying feature is expression of
CD56 by tumor cells. The majority of cases also express cytotoxic proteins and some
are EBV-positive.

CLINICAL FEATURES

The classic *nasal extranodal NK/T-cell lymphoma* occurs more frequently in Asia and
Latin America and is associated with EBV. It involves the skin (mostly secondarily),
upper respiratory tract and gastrointestinal tract. Large ulcerations in the area of the
nose are the hallmark of the disease and led to the old term "lethal midline granuloma". Specific skin lesions include maculopapular rashes, plaques and ulcerated
nodules (4).

   In general, *extranodal NK/T-cell lymphoma of nasal type* affect predominantly
young and middle-aged men (4). Papulonodular lesions are the most common clin-

ical manifestation (5,6). Systemic symptoms including fever, malaise and weight loss are common in cutaneous (forms of extranodal NK/T-cell lymphoma).

HISTOLOGY

Histologically, there is often an angiocentric and angiodestructive growth pattern (in up to 75% of the cases) and pleomorphic lymphocytes of varying size are present. Azurophilic granules containing cytotoxic molecules are a characteristic finding in NK cell lymphomas; they can be best identified with Giemsa stain (5). Necrotic areas are also common.

IMMUNOHISTOCHEMISTRY

Tumor cells express CD56 and cytotoxic molecules in NK/T-cell lymphomas. In addition, in NK/T-cell lymphomas CD3 (cytoplasmic CD3e) and CD45RO+ may be expressed, but not CD4 and CD45RA.

MOLECULAR BIOLOGY

Clonal rearrangement is rarely found and only in NK/T-cell lymphoma, whereas germline configuration of TCR genes is found in pure NK-cell lymphomas. EBV is found in most cases of secondary cutaneous NK/T and NK-cell lymphomas, but rarely in primary cutaneous forms (3,7,8).

TREATMENT

Polychemotherapy is first-line treatment possibly followed by autologous or hetero-logous bone marrow transplantation (3).

CLINICAL COURSE AND PROGNOSIS

Both NK and NK/T-cell lymphomas presenting in the skin have an aggressive course in most cases with median survival of 15 months (8). Involvement or spread to extracutaneous sites is common; organs affected include the liver, spleen, salivary glands, lungs and gastrointestinal tract. The presence of extracutaneous disease at presentation portends a poor prognosis, while expression of CD30 seems to indicate a more favorable prognosis (8).

REFERENCES

1. Jaffe ES, Chan JK, Su IJ, Frizzera G, Mori S, Feller AC, Ho FC. Report of the workshop on nasal and related extranodal angiocentric t/natural killer cell lymphomas. Definitions, differential diagnosis, and epidemiology. Am J Surg Pathol 1996; 20:103–111.

2. Chan JK, Sin VC, Wong KF, Ng CS, Tsang WY, Chan CH, Cheung MM, Lau WH. Nonnasal lymphoma expressing the natural killer cell marker CD56: a clinicopathologic study of 49 cases of an uncommon aggressive neoplasm. Blood 1997; 89:4501–4513.
3. Santucci M, Pimpinelli N, Massi D, Kadin ME, Meijer CJ, Muller-Hermelink HK, Paulli M, Wechsler J, Willemze R, Audring H, Bernengo MG, Cerroni L, Chimenti S, Chott A, Diaz-Perez JL, Dippel E, Duncan LM, Feller AC, Geerts ML, Hallermann C, Kempf W, Russell-Jones R, Sander C, Berti E. Cytotoxic/natural killer cell cutaneous lymphomas. Report of EORTC cutaneous lymphoma task force workshop. Cancer 2003; 97:610–627.
4. Wong KF, Chan JK, Ng CS. CD56 (NCAM)-positive malignant lymphoma. Leuk Lymphoma 1994; 14:29–36.
5. Savoia P, Fierro MT, Novelli M, Quaglino P, Verrone A, Geuna M, Bernengo MG. CD56-positive cutaneous lymphoma: a poorly recognized entity in the spectrum of primary cutaneous disease. Br J Dermatol 1997; 137:966–971.
6. Kato N, Yasukawa K, Onozuka T, Kikuta H. Nasal and nasal-type T/NK-cell lymphoma with cutaneous involvement. J Am Acad Dermatol 1999; 40:850–856.
7. Takeshita M, Yoshida K, Suzumiya J, Kikuchi M, Kimura N, Uike N, Okamura T, Nakayama J, Komiyama S. Cases of cutaneous and nasal CD56 (NCAM)-positive lymphoma in Japan have differences in immunohistology, genotype, and etiology. Hum Pathol 1999; 30:1024–1034.
8. Mraz-Gernhard S, Natkunam Y, Hoppe RT, LeBoit P, Kohler S, Kim YH. Natural killer/natural killer-like T-cell lymphoma, CD56+, presenting in the skin: an increasingly recognized entity with an aggressive course. J Clin Oncol 2001; 19:2179–2188.

Hydroa-like Lymphoma

Dmitry V. Kazakov, Günter Burg, and Werner Kempf
Department of Dermatology, University Hospital, Zürich, Switzerland

CLASSIFICATION

WHO/EORTC Classification (2005): Not listed
WHO Classification (2001): Not listed
REAL Classification (1997): Not listed
EORTC Classification (1997): Not listed

DEFINITION

Hydroa-like lymphoma (HLL) encompasses a group of rare lymphoproliferative disorders associated with chronic EBV infection. While the clinical features are similar to severe hydroa vacciniforme (HV), the patients with HLL have the potential to progress to overt hematological neoplasms.

CLINICAL FEATURES

Most affected patients are children or young adults of Asian (Japan, Korea, Taiwan) and Latin American origin (Mexico) (1–5). Edema, vesiculopapular eruptions, small blisters, crusts, necrotic areas, and scars occur mainly on the face and limbs (Figs. 1 and 2). The oral mucosae may be involved. The lesions are not induced or exacerbated by UV radiation. The history may reveal previous similar recurrent eruptions. There is often high fever, malaise, weight loss, failure to thrive, lymphadenopathy, and hepatosplenomegaly. Some patients report hypersensitivity to insect bites, which may be a trigger factor (6). Laboratory tests often show leukopenia, anemia, thrombocytopenia, and signs of impaired liver function. In addition, antibodies to EBV can be detected in the serum.

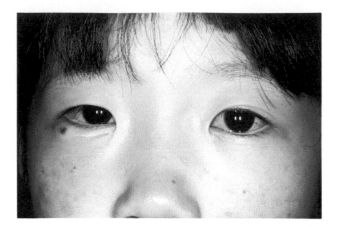

Figure 1   Vesiculopapules on the eyelid and cheeks. Note presence of conjunctivitis. (Courtesy of K. Iwatsuki. From Burg G, LeBoit Ph, eds. Unusual Lymphomas. Steinkopff-Verlag, 2001.)

HISTOLOGY

The epidermis shows reticular degeneration and necrosis. There is a dense perivascular/periadnexal nodular infiltrate in the dermis containing medium-sized lymphocytes with irregular, hyperchromatic nuclei. In some cases, the infiltrate displays a prominent angiocentric/angiodestructive pattern (7). In other patients,

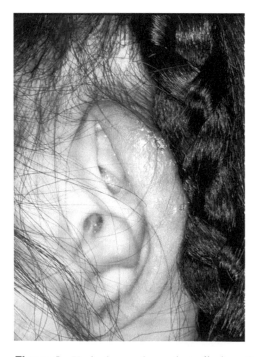

Figure 2   Vesiculopapules and small ulceration on the ear. (Courtesy of K. Iwatsuki. From Burg G, LeBoit Ph, eds. Unusual Lymphomas. Steinkopff-Verlag, 2001.)

there is septal or lobular panniculitis in company with vasculitis affecting small and medium-sized vessels in the mid- and/or deep dermis or involving large veins in the subcutis (9).

IMMUNOHISTOCHEMISTRY

The atypical cells express T-cell markers (CD3, CD45RO). B-cell-associated antigens, BCL-2 protein, and CD56 are negative. In cases with angiocentric infiltrates, CD30 antigen is expressed on 10–40% of the atypical cells (7). Only very few cells ($< 1\%$) show positive reaction for latent membrane protein 1 (LMP-1—a substance expressed by cells latently infected by EBV).

MOLECULAR BIOLOGY

EBV DNA sequences are detected by PCR in the great majority of cases. In situ hybridization studies demonstrate that 3–10% of the cells are positive for EBV-encoded small nuclear RNA (EBER) in early stages of the disease. Clonal TRC-γ gene rearrangements have been detected only in patients with accompanying large granular cell lymphocytes (LGL) in the peripheral blood (5).

TREATMENT

Antibiotics, antiseptics, and corticosteroids (both topical and systemic) or thalidomide are useful in some cases. Carotenoids and chloroquine are not usually helpful. Various chemotherapy regimes have been tried but it is not clear whether they are beneficial in the absence of malignant transformation and whether they can influence the survival.

CLINICAL COURSE AND PROGNOSIS

A subset of patients deteriorate very rapidly and die of severe infectious complications, septicemia, and/or multiorgan failure. In other cases, the disease can be controlled but the patients are apt to progress after years to various lymphomas or LGL leukemia. There are no clear-cut markers to predict which patients will die early in the course of the disease. The mortality rate (37.5–50%) is somewhat higher in the patients with angiocentric/angiodestructive features and panniculitis.

DIFFERENTIAL DIAGNOSIS

The lesions in HLL are similar to those seen in HV but tend to be larger and deeper causing extensive loss of tissue and sometimes resulting in severe disfigurement. In addition, HLL differs from typical HV by the presence of lesions both in sun-exposed and non-exposed areas, systemic involvement, normal response to minimal doses of UVA and UVB, and presence of atypical lymphocytes histologically. Other entities that should be differentiated clinically from HLL are pityriasis lichenoides et varioliformis acuta, papulonecrotic tuberculid, and polymorphous light eruption. At a histological level, HLL with prominent angiocentric/angiodestructive features should be differentiated from nasal T/NK lymphoma. Absence of expression of NK-associated antigens is a clue to HLL.

Hydroa-like lymphoma

Clinical features
  Children and young adults
  Asian or Latin American origin
  Papular, vesicular, necrotic lesions, and scars
  Sun-exposed and covered areas
  Fever, malaise, failure to thrive, weight loss
  Lymphadenopathy, hepatosplenomegaly
Histological features
  Epidermal necrosis
  Atypical lymphocytes
  Angiodestruction or panniculitis
Immunophenotype
  CD3+, CD45RO+, CD56−, CD30 ±
Molecular biology
  EBV DNA in majority of cases
Laboratory evaluation
  Leukopenia (rarely lymphocytosis)
  Anemia
  Thrombocytopenia
  Elevated transaminases, low protein
  Antibodies to EBV
Treatment
  Antibiotics, corticosteroids (both topical and systemic), thalidomide,
    chemotherapy
Clinical course and prognosis
  Early death or progression to lymphoma or leukemia often

COMMENTS

HLL has been described in the literature under various designations, namely atypical HV, angiocentric cutaneous T-cell lymphoma of childhood (ACTCLC), edematous scarring vasculitic panniculitis, and EBV-associated lymphoproliferative eruption. All these disorders may be not separate entities but represent a spectrum of EBV-associated lymphoproliferative disease which affect mainly children from certain world regions where EBV infections are common. On one end of the spectrum is atypical HV—a smoldering stage of the disease. The malignant end of the spectrum corresponds probably to ACTCLC, edematous vasculiticpanniculitis, and papulonecrotic skin eruptions in patients who over time develop LGL leukemia. Progression of atypical HV to lymphoma or LGL leukemia is accompanied by an increase of the viral load, with up to 60% EBER-positive cells found in the infiltrate.

REFERENCES

1. Barrionuevo C, Anderson VM, Zevallos-Giampietri E, Zaharia M, Misad O, Bravo F, Caceres H, Taxa L, Martinez MT, Wachtel A, Piris MA. Hydroa-like cutaneous T-cell lymphoma: a clinicopathologic and molecular genetic study of 16 pediatric cases from Peru. Appl Immunohistochem Mol Morphol 2002; 10:7–14.
2. Cho KH, Kim CW, Heo DS, Lee DS, Choi WW, Rim JH, Han WS. Epstein–Barr virus-associated peripheral T-cell lymphoma in adults with hydroa vacciniforme-like lesions. Clin Exp Dermatol 2001; 26:242–247.
3. Iwatsuki K, Ohtsuka M, Akiba H, Kaneko F. Atypical hydroa vacciniforme in child-hood: from a smoldering stage to Epstein–Barr virus-associated lymphoid malignancy. J Am Acad Dermatol 1999; 40:283–284.
4. Iwatsuki K, Ohtsuka M, Harada H, Han G, Kaneko F. Clinicopathologic manifesta-tions of Epstein–Barr virus-associated cutaneous lymphoproliferative disorders. Arch Dermatol 1997; 133:1081–1086.
5. Asada H, Okada N, Tei H, Yamamura T, Hashimoto K, Kondo K, Yamanishi K, Yoshikawa K. Epstein–Barr virus-associated large granular lymphocyte leukemia with cutaneous infiltration. J Am Acad Dermatol 1994; 31:251–255.
6. Iwatsuki K, Xu Z, Takata M, Iguchi M, Ohtsuka M, Akiba H, Mitsuhashi Y, Take-noshita H, Sugiuchi R, Tagami H, Kaneko F. The association of latent Epstein–Barr virus infection with hydroa vacciniforme. Br J Dermatol 1999; 140:715–721.
7. Magana M, Sangueza P, Gil-Beristain J, Sanchez-Sosa S, Salgado A, Ramon G, Sangueza OP. Angiocentric cutaneous T-cell lymphoma of childhood (hydroa-like lymphoma): a distinctive type of cutaneous T-cell lymphoma. J Am Acad Dermatol 1998; 38:574–579.
8. Ruiz-Maldonado R, Parrilla FM, Orozco-Covarrubias ML, Ridaura C, Tamayo Sanchez L, Duran McKinster C. Edematous, scarring vasculitic panniculitis: a new multisystemic disease with malignant potential. J Am Acad Dermatol 1995; 32:37–44.
9. Oono T, Arata J, Masuda T, Ohtsuki Y. Coexistence of hydroa vacciniforme and malignant lymphoma. Arch Dermatol 1986; 122:1306–1309.
10. Yoon TY, Yang TH, Hahn YS, Huh JR, Soo Y. Epstein–Barr virus-associated recurrent necrotic papulovesicles with repeated bacterial infections ending in sepsis and death: consideration of the relationship between Epstein–Barr virus infection and immune defect. J Dermatol 2001; 28:442–447.

29

Adult T-cell Leukemia/Lymphoma

Werner Kempf, Dmitry V. Kazakov, and Günter Burg
Department of Dermatology, University Hospital, Zürich, Switzerland

CLASSIFICATION

> WHO/EORTC Classification (2005): Adult T-cell leukemia/lymphoma
> WHO Classification (2001): adult T-cell leukemia/lymphoma
> REAL Classification (1997): adult T-cell leukemia/lymphoma
> EORTC Classification (1997): not included

DEFINITION

Adult T-cell leukemia/lymphoma (ATLL) is a peripheral T-cell lymphoma, etiologically associated with human T-cell leukemia virus I (HTLV-1) (1,2). HTLV-1 infection and ATLL is endemic in southwestern Japan and the Caribbean (3). The disease is rare in Europe and U.S.A. (4). There is a considerable spectrum of clinical manifestations and histologic features in ATLL (4,5).

CLINICAL FEATURES

An acute, a chronic, a lymphomatous and a smoldering subtype can be differentiated. Skin involvement occurs in about 50% of the cases during the course of the disease, presenting as purpuric papules, nodules or tumors, or as erythroderma. ATLL may simulate MF in nonendemic areas (6) (Fig. 1). Peripheral blood smears show atypical lymphoid cells with convoluted nuclei (so called flower cells) (Fig. 2) and leukocytosis, sometimes in conjunction with anemia. Additional findings are hypoalbuminemia, hypergammaglobulinemia, and hypercalcemia. Bone marrow involvement, lymphadenopathy, hepatosplenomegaly, and pulmonary infiltrates are frequently found only in patients with acute ATLL.

HISTOLOGY

Histologically, ATLL shows features of MF. A perivascular or diffuse infiltrate of medium to large pleomorphic cells is found in the upper dermis. Tumor cells show

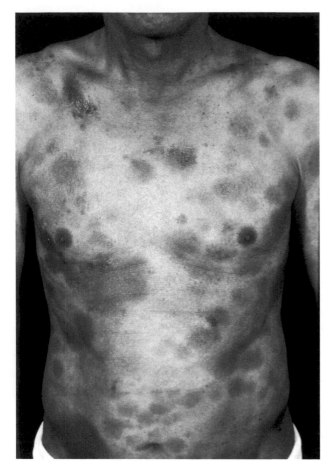

Figure 1 Multiple patches and plaques, which can easily be mistaken for mycosis fungoides. (Kindly provided by Prof. Ueki, Japan.)

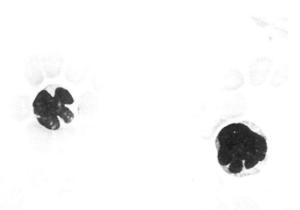

Figure 2 A typical lymphocytes with multilobular convoluted nuclei (flower cells).

pronounced nuclear pleomorphism. Epidermotropism of lymphoid cells with formation of Pautrier microabscesses (or collections), which can contain nuclear dust, may
be present. Plasma cells and eosinophils are less frequent than in MF. In chronic and
smoldering variants of ATLL, small neoplastic lymphocytes with only minimal
cytologic atypia are found. Granulomatous and angiodestructive features have
been reported (7). Some cases of ATLL manifest as CD30+ anaplastic large cell
lymphoma (8,9).

IMMUNOHISTOCHEMISTRY

There is a pronounced heterogeneity of the phenotype of neoplastic cells in patients
with ATLL. Usually, they show a helper/inducer T-cell phenotype (CD4+, CD8−);
however, other phenotypic profiles may be seen in some of the cases (CD4−, CD8+
or CD4−, CD8−). In addition, tumor cells express activation markers CD25 (IL2
receptor) and large cells may express CD30. ALK-1, TIA-1, and granzyme B are
negative. T-cell antigens such as CD7 may be lost on tumor cells.

MOLECULAR BIOLOGY

Clonal rearrangement of TCR genes is found in the majority of ATLL cases. HTLV-
1 can be found in lesional skin biopsies of patients with ATLL (10). The HTLV-1I
tax gene can always be detected in the ATLL tissues, whereas segments of the pol
gene were not detected in half the cases (11). The p40 tax protein of HTLV-1 results
in transcriptional activation and is, besides additional genetic factors, one of the
main pathogenetic factors in ATLL (12).

TREATMENT

Multiagent chemotherapy is therapy of choice for acute and lymphomatous cases.
However, the combination of zidovudine (AZT) and interferon alfa (IFN) showed
tumoricid activity, even in patients in whom prior cytotoxic therapy has failed
(13). Major responses were achieved in almost 60% of the patients, including
complete remission in 26% (13). In conclusion, IFN and AZT improves the
outcome of ATLL patients and helps to maintain clinical responses (14).

COURSE AND PROGNOSIS

The prognosis of ATLL is generally poor. Clinical subtype, age, increased serum calcium and LDH levels have been identified as major prognostic factors, whereas the
size of tumor cells does not have prognostic implications (15). Patients with acute or
lymphomatous forms of ATLL have poor prognosis (weeks to one year) and often
die due to concurrent infections (4). Chronic and smoldering forms are mostly slowly
progressive, but may undergo transformation into acute form of ATLL. Rarely,
Hodgkin lymphoma associated with EBV may develop in patients with HTLV-1
associated ATLL (16).

Adult T-cell leukemia/lymphoma

Clinical features
Most common in Japan, Caribbean, rare in Europe and U.S.A.
Purpuric papules, nodules or tumors, or erythroderma
Histological features
Perivascular or diffuse infiltrate of medium to large pleomorphic cells. Epidermotropism.
Immunophenotype
CD2+, CD3+, CD4+, CD25+, CD30+/−, some cases CD8+
Molecular biology
Clonal TCR rearrangement in the majority of cases
Laboratory evaluation
Leukocytosis with circulating atypical lymphocytes (flower cells).
Hypoalbuminemia, hypergammaglobulinemia, and hypercalcemia
Treatment
Multiagent chemotherapy. Zidovudine (AZT) and interferon alfa (IFN)
Clinical course and prognosis
Course dependent on subtype. Poor prognosis.

DIFFERENTIAL DIAGNOSIS

Differential diagnoses include MF, SS, and pleomorphic medium to large-cell T-cell lymphomas. Correlation of clinical and histologic features is essential to establish correct diagnosis. Moreover, detection of HTLV-1 by serology or molecular techniques is crucial for the diagnosis of ATLL.

REFERENCES

1. Yamaguchi K, Takatsuki K. Adult T cell leukaemia–lymphoma. Baillieres Clin Haematol 1993; 6:899–915.
2. Siegel R, Gartenhaus R, Kuzel T. HTLV-I associated leukemia/lymphoma: epidemiology, biology, and treatment. Cancer Treat Res 2001; 104:75–88.
3. Levine PH, Jaffe ES, Manns A, Murphy EL, Clark J, Blattner WA. Human T-cell lymphotropic virus type I and adult T-cell leukemia/lymphoma outside Japan and the Caribbean Basin. Yale J Biol Med 1988; 61:215–222.
4. Pawson R, Richardson DS, Pagliuca A, Kelsey SM, Hoque S, Breuer J, Newland AC, Mufti GJ. Adult T-cell leukemia/lymphoma in London: clinical experience of 21 cases. Leuk Lymphoma 1998; 31:177–185.
5. Plumelle Y, Pascaline N, Nguyen D, Panelatti G, Jouannelle A, Jouault H, Imbert M. Adult T-cell leukemia-lymphoma: a clinico-pathologic study of twenty-six patients from Martinique. Hematol Pathol 1993; 7:251–262.
6. D'Incan M, Antoniotti O, Gasmi M, Fonck Y, Chassagne J, Desgranges C, Souteyrand P. HTLV-I-associated lymphoma presenting as mycosis fungoides in an HTLV-I non-endemic area: a viro-molecular study. Br J Dermatol 1995; 132:983–988.
7. Ohtake N, Setoyama M, Fukumaru S, Kanzaki T. A case of adult T-cell leukemia/lymphoma (ATLL) with angiocentric and angiodestructive features. J Dermatol 1997; 24:165–169.
8. Takahara T, Masutani K, Kajiwara E, Sadoshima S, Misago M, Sasaguri Y, Onoyama K. Adult T-cell leukemia/lymphoma in which the pathohistological diagnosis was identical to that of Ki-1 positive anaplastic large cell lymphoma. Intern Med 1999; 38:824–828.

9. Kumura T, Hino M, Yamane T, Ohta K, Nakao T, Wakasa K, Tatsumi N. Triple-negative (CD3−/CD4−/CD8−) adult T cell leukemia/lymphoma, histologically presenting as CD30 (Ki-1)-positive anaplastic large cell lymphoma with clonal Epstein–Barr virus genome. Leukemia 2001; 15:994–995.

10. Setoyama M, Katahira Y, Hamada T, Tashiro M, Yashiki S, Tanaka Y, Tozawa H, Sonoda S. Expression of human T-cell lymphotropic virus type-1 gene products in the short-term cultured skin tissues of an adult T-cell leukemia/lymphoma patient with cutaneous manifestations. J Dermatol 1992; 19:133–139.

11. Shibata D, Tokunaga M, Sasaki N, Nanba K. Detection of human T-cell leukemia virus type I proviral sequences from fixed tissues of seropositive patients. Am J Clin Pathol 1991; 95:536–539.

12. Franchini G. Molecular mechanisms of human T-cell leukemia/lymphotropic virus type I infection. Blood 1995; 86:3619–3639.

13. Gill PS, Harrington W Jr, Kaplan MH, Ribeiro RC, Bennett JM, Liebman HA, Bernstein-Singer M, Espina BM, Cabral L, Allen S, et al. Treatment of adult T-cell leukemia–lymphoma with a combination of interferon alfa and zidovudine. N Engl J Med 1995; 332:1744–1748.

14. Matutes E, Taylor GP, Cavenagh J, Pagliuca A, Bareford D, Domingo A, Hamblin M, Kelsey S, Mir N, Reilly JT. Interferon alpha and zidovudine therapy in adult T-cell leukaemia lymphoma: response and outcome in 15 patients. Br J Haematol 2001; 113:779–784.

15. Yamamura M, Yamada Y, Momita S, Kamihira S, Tomonaga M. Circulating interleukin-6 levels are elevated in adult T-cell leukaemia/lymphoma patients and correlate with adverse clinical features and survival. Br J Haematol 1998; 100:129–134.

16. Hayashi T, Yamabe H, Haga H, Akasaka T, Kadowaki N, Ohno H, Okuma M, Fukuhara S. Synchronous presentation of Epstein–Barr virus-associated Hodgkin's disease and adult T-cell leukemia/lymphoma (ATLL) in a patient from an endemic area of ATLL. Int J Hematol 1995; 61:215–222.

30

Cutaneous Manifestations in Other Mature T-cell Neoplasms

30.1. Angioimmunoblastic T-cell Lymphoma

Dmitry V. Kazakov, Günter Burg, and Werner Kempf
Department of Dermatology, University Hospital, Zürich, Switzerland

CLASSIFICATION

> WHO/EORTC Classification (2005): Angioimmunoblastic T-cell lymphoma
> WHO Classification (2001): Angioimmunoblastic T-cell lymphoma
> REAL Classification (1997): Angioimmunoblastic T-cell lymphoma
> EORTC Classification (1997): Not listed

DEFINITION

Angioimmunoblastic T-cell lymphoma (AITL) is a systemic malignant lymphopro-liferative disorder characterized by a clonal growth of atypical lymphoid cells accompanied by the proliferation of high endothelial venules and follicular dendritic cells. This entity was identified in the early 1970s by Frizzera and colleagues (1), who used the term angioimmunoblastic lymphadenopathy with dysproteinemia or immu-noblastic lymphadenopathy, which they considered an abnormal immune reaction.

CLINICAL FEATURES

Most patients are middle-aged or elderly people. There is no gender predilection. Presenting complaints include fever, weight loss, night sweats, lymphadenopathy, hepato and splenomegaly. Examination of peripheral blood may reveal anemia, an elevated sedimentation rate, leukocytosis, neutropenia, or thrombocytopenia, as well as polyclonal hypergammaglobulinemia, positive rheumatoid factors, and anti-smooth muscle antibodies. Skin involvement occurs in up to 50% of cases, usually in the form of a generalized maculopapular eruption with a predilection for the trunk

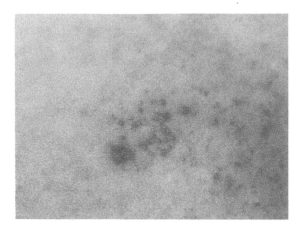

Figure 1   Angioimmunoblastic T-cell lymphoma: grouped papules on the trunk.

mimicking a viral exanthem or drug eruption (Fig. 1). In some cases, the eruption is triggered by a drug or infection (2). Other reported skin manifestations include urticaria, purpura, erythemato-squamous plaques, prurigo-like lesions, erythroderma, erosions, and necrotic lesions (3).

HISTOLOGY

The skin involvement can be subdivided into four histologic types (3). (1) A nonspecific pattern with scant superficial perivascular infiltrates composed of eosinophils and lymphocytes without atypia accompanied by hyperplasia of the capillaries (Fig. 2a). (2) A distinct pattern suggesting AITL, characterized by prominent vascular hyperplasia accompanied by sparse perivascular infiltrates composed of pleomorphic lymphocytes with medium-sized to large reniform nuclei. Reed–Sternberg-like cells can be seen. (3) The third pattern reveals dense infiltrates of pleomorphic cells involving superficial and deep dermis in combination with vascular hyperplasia (4). The fourth pattern has small vessel vasculitis without nuclear atypia of the infiltrating lymphoid cells (Fig. 2b).

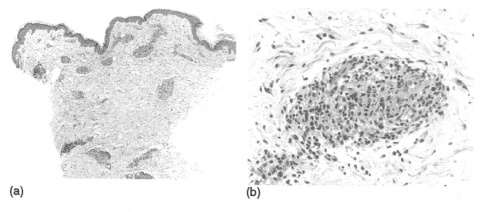

(a)   (b)

Figure 2   (a) Angioimmunoblastic T-cell lymphoma: perivascular sharply demarcated infiltrates filling the entire dermis. (b) Vasculitic changes.

IMMUNOHISTOCHEMISTRY

The neoplastic lymphocytes express the phenotype of mature T-helper cells (CD3+, CD4+, CD8+/−). Aberrant loss of some T-associated antigens can be seen. Staining for factor XIIIa reveals increased numbers of dermal dendritic cells in the infiltrate. The reactive infiltrate is composed of mature B cells, plasma cells, and histiocytes.

MOLECULAR BIOLOGY

The study of TCRγ gene with PCR-based techniques allows the identification of the same clone in the skin, lymph nodes, and peripheral blood. In most cases, a clonal population is present even in "non-specific" lesions. There are rare reports on the identification of Epstein–Barr virus by in situ hybridization in skin lesions of AITL (2) Trisomy 3 has been found (4).

TREATMENT

Aggressive treatment modalities are usually required.

CLINICAL COURSE AND PROGNOSIS

The disease runs an aggressive course with a mortality rate ranging from 50% to 70% and a median survival ranging from 11 to 30 months. Patients often succumb to infectious complications; some of them develop secondary EBV-positive B-cell nodal lymphomas.

Angioimmunoblastic T-cell lymphoma

Clinical features
    Middle-aged or elderly patients, B symptoms, lymphadenopathy, hepato- and
       splenomegaly, arthritis, pleural effusion, ascites. Maculopapular rash
       resembling viral exanthem or drug eruption
Histological features
    Non-specific superficial perivascular dermatitis, vasculitis or infiltrates with
       atypical cells. Eosinophils and vascular hyperplasia
Immunophenotype
    Mature T-helper cells (CD3+, CD4+, CD8+/−. Increased numbers of dermal
       dendritic cells (factor XIIIa +)
Laboratory evaluation
    Anemia, elevated sedimentation rate, leukocytosis, neutropenia,
       thrombocytopenia, polyclonal hypergammaglobulinemia.
Treatment
    Chemotherapy
Prognosis
    Poor: median survival 11–30 months

DIFFERENTIAL DIAGNOSIS

The differential diagnosis of AITL can be difficult both clinically and histologically. The abnormal laboratory findings can be helpful in distinguishing AITL from viral exanthems or drug eruptions. Histologically, the presence of vascular hyperplasia, eosinophils, and increased numbers of dermal dendritic cells can be a clue to the diagnosis of AITL.

COMMENTS

The diagnosis of specific cutaneous involvement of AITL should be made only when the lymphoma has been found in the lymph nodes.

REFERENCES

1. Frizzera G, Moran EM, Rappaport H. Angio-immunoblastic lymphadenopathy. Diagnosis and clinical course. Am J Med 1975; 59:803–818.
2. Brown HA, Macon WR, Kurtin PJ, Gibson LE. Cutaneous involvement by angioimmunoblastic T-cell lymphoma with remarkable heterogeneous Epstein–Barr virus expression. J Cutan Pathol 2001; 28:432–438.
3. Martel P, Laroche L, Courville P, Larroche C, Wechsler J, Lenormand B, Delfau MH, Bodemer C, Bagot M, Joly P. Cutaneous involvement in patients with angioimmunoblastic lymphadenopathy with dysproteinemia: a clinical, immunohistological, and molecular analysis. Arch Dermatol 2000; 136:881–886.
4. Schlegelberger B, Himmler A, Godde E, Grote W, Feller AC, Lennert K. Cytogenetic findings in peripheral T-cell lymphomas as a basis for distinguishing low-grade and high-grade lymphomas. Blood 1994; 83:505–511.

30.2. T-Zone Lymphoma

Dmitry V. Kazakov, Günter Burg, and Werner Kempf
Department of Dermatology, University Hospital, Zürich, Switzerland

CLASSIFICATION

WHO/EORTC Classification (2005): Not listed
WHO Classification (2001): Peripheral T-cell lymphoma, T-zone variant
REAL Classification (1997): Peripheral T-cell lymphoma, unspecified
EORTC Classification (1997): Not listed

DEFINITION

T-zone lymphoma (TZL) belongs to the group of (nodal) peripheral T-cell lymphoma, unspecified, characterized by a clonal expansion of T-zone lymphocytes accompanied by the proliferation of other normal T-zone constituents. It was first described by Lennert and Mohri in 1978 (1). Nonspecific cutaneous changes such as maculopapular or erythematous exanthems or pruritus are seen in approximately one-third of cases. Specific cutaneous involvement is exceedingly rare.

CLINICAL FEATURES

TZL affects primarily patients in the fifth and sixth decades (range between 15 and 82 years of age) with a slight male predominance (male:female ratio approximately 1.5:1) (2,3). Patients most often present with lymph node enlargement and hepatosplenomegaly. Specific skin lesions in the early stages are papules and nodules (Fig. 1). As the disease progresses, large dermal and/or deep-seated subcutaneous tumors can develop (2–4).

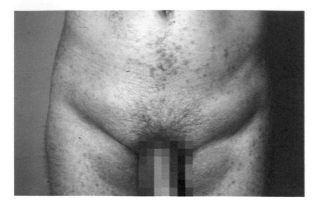

Figure 1 Scattered papules along with plaques overlying inguinal lymphadenopathy.

HISTOLOGY

The papular and nodular lesions contain perivascular and periadnexal infiltrates in the upper and mid-dermis composed predominantly of small lymphocytes admixed with a few medium-sized cells with clear cytoplasm and immunoblasts. In more advanced lesions, the infiltrate is diffuse and can extend into the subcutis. Small to medium-sized lymphocytes with minimal nuclear pleomorphism and clear halo cytoplasm are the predominant cell type (Fig. 2). Eosinophils are found in substantial numbers. There is an increase in the number of small blood vessels with prominent endothelial cells (2–6).

IMMUNOHISTOCHEMISTRY

The tumor cells express T-cell associated antigens CD3, CD4, CD43, CD45RO. Cyto-toxic molecules are not expressed. There are high numbers of tumor-associated macro-

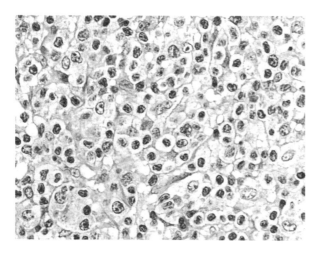

Figure 2 Medium-sized lympocytes with pleomorphic nuclei and abundant pale cytoplasm.

phages (S-100, CD68, Mac387) and dermal dendritic cells (factor XIIIa). Irregular networks of follicular dendritic cells (CD21) corresponding to the remnants of follicles are present (2–6). Clusters of reactive B cells (CD79a+, CD20+) expressing bcl-2 protein may be seen (7).

MOLECULAR BIOLOGY

TCR genes are clonally rearranged both in lymph nodes and skin. The most frequently observed cytogenetic abnormality is trisomy 3 (8,9).

TREATMENT

TZL is notably resistant to treatment. Various aggressive chemotherapy regimes (CHOP, ChlVPP, UKALLXA, F-MACHOP) alone or combined with radiation therapy or bone marrow transplantation have been used with rather unsatisfying results (2–4).

CLINICAL COURSE AND PROGNOSIS

TZL lymphoma has an aggressive clinical course with a tendency to early dissemination. The reported median survival is 23 months (2,3). Lung involvement is seen in 40% of cases. Less frequently, the bone marrow can be involved and in some cases leukemic conversion may occur. Widespread visceral involvement is usually associated with an unfavorable course. Rare patients may follow a prolonged, indolent course over many years (7).

T-zone lymphoma

Clinical features
   Skin rarely involved
   Papulo-nodular lesions
   Lymphadenopathy, hepatosplenomegaly
Histological features
   Perivascular or diffuse infiltrates of uniform medium-sized lymphocytes with
      clear, halo cytoplasm, immunoblasts, and eosinophils
   Proliferation of postcapillary venules
Immunophenotype
   CD3+, CD4+, CD45RO+, CD43+, CD8–
   Increased numbers of macrophages (CD68)
   Increased numbers of dendritic cells (FXIIIa)
   Remnants of follicles (CD21)
Molecular biology
   Clonal rearrangement of TCR genes
Treatment
   Multiagent chemotherapy
   Clinical course and prognosis
   Aggressive course

DIFFERENTIAL DIAGNOSIS

Cutaneous involvement in TZL should be differentiated from pleomorphic T-cell lymphomas with predominant proliferation of medium-sized cells and skin involvement by angioimmunoblastic T-cell lymphoma (AILT)(10). Pleomorphic T-cell lymphoma cells display prominent nuclear pleomorphism in contrast to uniform cells with limited nuclear pleomorphism of TZL. Clinicopathological clues to AILT are polyclonal hypergammaglobulinemia, frequent pronounced systemic symptoms (arthritis, pleural effusion, ascites), hemolytic anemia, positive rheumatoid factors, and antismooth muscle antibodies. Since a diffuse involvement of the subcutis is a typical finding in the advanced stages of TZL, it must be distinguished from subcutaneous panniculitis-like T-cell lymphoma. The latter starts primarily in the subcutis and is characterized by the rimming of the tumor cells around lipocytes, macrophages engulfing neoplastic cells, and erythrophagocytosis.

COMMENTS

In some cases, the skin lesions appear simultaneously with or even precede systemic symptoms and lymph node enlargement (4,7). Therefore, clinical investigation of the patients with skin eruptions suggesting TZL is mandatory. The diagnosis of specific cutaneous involvement of TZL should be based on the evidence of the lymphoma in the lymph nodes.

REFERENCES

1. Lennert K Mohri N. Malignant lymphoma, lymphocytic, T-zone type (T-zone lymphoma). In: Lennert K, ed. Malignant Lymphomas Other Than Hodgkin's disease. Berlin: Springer, 1978:196–209.
2. Krajewski AS, Myskow MW, Cachia PG, Salter DM, Sheehan T, Dewar AE. T-cell lymphoma: morphology, immunophenotype and clinical features. Histopathology 1988; 13:19–41.
3. Helborn D, Brittinger G, Lennert K. T-zonen-lymphom. Klinisches bild, therapie and prognose. Blut 1979; 39:117–131.
4. Bernengo MG, Massobrio R. Cutaneous manifestations in T-zone lymphoma. Curr Probl Dermatol 1990; 19:161–166.
5. Siegert W, Nerl C, Engelhard M, Brittinger G, Tiemann M, Parwaresch R, Heinz R, Huhn D. Peripheral T-cell non-Hodgkin's lymphomas of low malignancy: prospective study of 25 patients with pleomorphic small cell lymphoma, lymphoepitheloid cell (Lennert's) lymphoma and T-zone lymphoma. Br J Haematol; 1994; 87:529–534.
6. Liang R, Todd D, Chan TK, Wong KL, Ho F, Loke SL. Peripheral T cell lymphoma. J Clin Oncol 1987; 5:750–755.
7. Kazakov DV, Kempf W, Michaelis S, Schmid U, Cogliatti S, Dummer R, Burg G. T-zone lymphoma with cutaneous involvement: a case report and review of the literature. Br J Dermatol 2002; 146:1096–1100.
8. Godde-Salz E, Schwarze EW, Stein H, Lennert K, Grote W. Cytogenetic findings in T-zone lymphoma. J Cancer Res Clin Oncol 1981; 101:81–89.
9. Schlegelberger B, Feller AC. Classification of peripheral T-cell lymphomas: cytogenetic findings support the updated Kiel classification. Leuk Lymphoma 1996; 20:411–416.

10. Takagi N, Nakamura S, Ueda R, Osada H, Obata Y, Kitoh K, Suchi T, Takahashi T. A phenotypic and genotypic study of three node-based, low-grade peripheral T-cell lymphomas: angioimmunoblastic lymphoma, T-zone lymphoma, and lymphoepithelioid lymphoma. Cancer 1992; 69:2571–2582.

31

Primary Cutaneous Marginal Zone B-cell Lymphoma

Werner Kempf, Dmitry V. Kazakov, and Günter Burg
Department of Dermatology, University Hospital, Zürich, Switzerland

CLASSIFICATION

WHO/EORTC Classification (2005): Primary cutaneous marginal zone B-cell lymphoma

WHO Classification (2001): Extranodal marginal zone lymphoma of MALT type

EORTC Classification (1997): Primary cutaneous immunocytoma/marginal zone B-cell lymphoma

REAL Classification (1997): Extranodal marginal zone B-cell lymphoma

DEFINITION

Primary cutaneous marginal zone lymphoma (MZL) represents a low-grade cutaneous B-cell lymphoma.

CLINICAL FEATURES

Because of considerable controversies in the classification of cutaneous B-cell lymphoma (CBCL), the incidence and clinicopathologic features of primary cutaneous MZL are still insufficiently delineated. Some authors consider MZL the most prevalent form of CBCL, whereas others regard it as a relatively rare type (1,2).

Marginal zone lymphoma affects most commonly adults aged over 40 years. Conflicting data on gender preponderance have been reported (3,4). In contrast to follicle center lymphoma (FCL), which is often located on the head and neck, the sites of predilection of MZL are the trunk and arms. Disseminated MZL or tumors on the

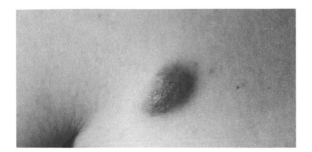

Figure 1   Solitary nodule on the left shoulder.

lower aspects of the legs are rare (4,5). Most often cutaneous MZL presents with red to violaceous infiltrated plaques or nodules with an erythematous periphery (Fig. 1) (2,4).

HISTOLOGY

There is a nodular or diffuse infiltrate composed of small- to medium-sized lymphocytes possessing slightly irregular nuclei with moderately dispersed chromatin and inconspicuous nucleoli and an abundant, pale cytoplasm (marginal zone cells) (6,7). Some cells have a monocytoid appearance (reniform nuclei) or show prominent plasma cell differentiation (8) (Fig. 3). The characteristic "inverse pattern" may been seen on scanning magnification, typified by darker centers surrounded by brighter zones of pale-staining cells (Fig. 2). Reactive follicles are also present in the majority of cases. The tumor cells proliferate mainly around the follicles and are apt to colonize them. The colonized follicles lack a distinct germinal center/mantle zone demarcation and have a more variable cellular composition, including marginal zone cells, centrocytes, and centroblasts. The cellular population in the interfollicular areas is represented by small lymphocytes, lymphoplasmacytoid cells, and aggregations of plasma cells. Occasionally, the infiltrate is arranged around adnexal structures analogous to lymphoepithelioid lesions of MALT-lymphoma of the gastrointestinal tract (4).

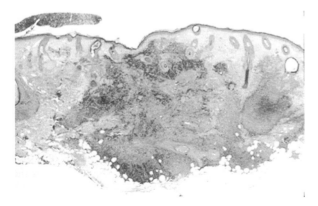

Figure 2   Large, partly confluent nodular lymphocytic infiltrates involving the subcutis. The centers of the nodules are darker than the periphery (inverse pattern).

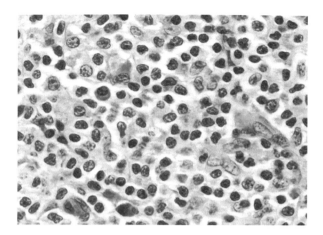

Figure 3 Monocytoid B lymphocytes with admixture of plasma cells.

IMMUNOHISTOCHEMISTRY

The neoplastic cells have the following immunophenotype: CD19+, CD20+, CD22+, CD79a+, CD5−, CD10−, CD23−, bcl-6−, bcl-2+. Monotypic expression of immunoglobulin light chains is seen in the majority of cases. Anti-CD21 staining often reveals regular and irregular networks of follicular dendritic cells (FDC) corresponding to the follicles (Fig. 4). In some cases large, expanded, diffuse FDC networks may be seen. Germinal center cells in the colonized and reactive follicles as well as in the expanded FDC networks are usually bcl-6+, bcl-2−. CD30+ blasts can often be found.

MOLECULAR BIOLOGY

IgH genes are monoclonally rearranged in the majority (>70%) of the cases (9). The t(14;18) translocation resulting in overexpression of bcl-2 is usually not present,

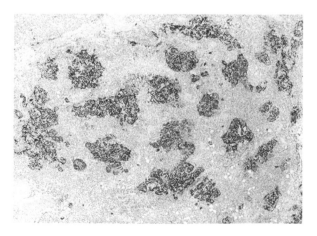

Figure 4 CD21 staining for follicular dendritic cells demonstrating both regular and irregular networks.

found only in a minority of primary cutaneous MZL (10). *Borrelia burgdorferi* infection has been identified in a subset of MZL (11).

TREATMENT

Surgical excision and/or local radiotherapy is the treatment of choice for solitary or grouped MZL lesions. Complete response rates up to 100% after radiotherapy have been reported (4). Antibiotic therapy (doxycycline 100 mg t.i.d. for 3–6 weeks) may be effective especially in cases associated with Borrelia infection (12), but also in some of the Borrelia-negative cases.

CLINICAL COURSE AND PROGNOSIS

In general, MZL exhibits a favorable prognosis with 5-year-survival rates between 90% and 100%. Just as is the case with other low-grade CBCL, MZL shows a marked tendency for recurrences which occur in 33–66% of patients. The prognosis is not worse in patients with recurrent tumors. In one study, 23% of patients developed extracutaneous spread, some of them with large-cell transformation (4). Rarely, MZL runs a fatal course.

DIFFERENTIAL DIAGNOSIS

The most relevant differential diagnoses are primary cutaneous follicle center lymphoma (FCL), immunocytoma and cutaneous B-cell pseudolymphoma (B-

---

Primary cutaneous marginal zone B-cell lymphoma

Clinical features
  Adults aged over 40 years
  Red to violaceous infiltrated plaques or nodules with an erythematous
    periphery on trunk and arms
Histological features
  Nodular or diffuse infiltrate of small- to medium-sized lymphocytes with
    pale cytoplasm
Immunophenotype
  CD19+, CD20+, CD22+, CD79a+, CD5–, CD10–, CD23–, bcl-6–, bcl-2+.
    Regular and irregular networks of CD21+ follicular dendritic cells
Molecular biology
  IgH genes are monoclonally rearranged in the majority (>70%).
    t(14;18) translocation usually not present
Laboratory evaluation
  Search for Borrelia infection
Treatment
  Antibiotics, excision, ionizing radiation, rituximab
Clinical course and prognosis
  Excellent prognosis, tendency to recur

PSL). All three diseases also have a good outlook. By definition, B-cell PSL does not spread to extracutaneous sites and never runs a fatal course. In contrast to MZL, only reactive germinal centers with distinct mantle zones, regular networks of CD21+ FDC and tingible body macrophages are found. Clonality of IgH genes or restricted expression of Ig light chains is not found in the vast majority in B-PSL. Clonal cases of B-PSL may even represent MZL or FCL. Marginal zone lymphoma and FCL share many clinical as well as histologic features. The inverse pattern with darker centers of the nodular infiltrates of MZL, sheets or collections of plasma cells, and the presence of numerous cells with lymphoplasmacytoid or monocytoid morphology argue for MZL. Immunohistochemistry may be helpful for differentiating between these two forms. FCL expresses bcl-6 uniformly and usually expresses CD10 and bcl-6, while MZL is negative for bcl-6 and CD10, but bcl-2 positive (13). Colonized follicles in MZL contain numerous bcl-6– and bcl-2+ cells. Coexpression of CD20 and CD43 is seen in many cases of FCL, but not found in MZL (3). The issue of the nosologic relationship of MZL and immunocytoma (lymphoplasmacytic lymphoma) has not yet been clarified (14). In immunocytoma diffuse infiltrates of lymphoplasmacytoid cells and Dutcher bodies (intranuclear PAS-positive inclusions) are typically found. However, Dutcher bodies are not completely specific for immunocytoma. A further differential diagnostic consideration is cutaneous follicular hyperplasia with monotypic plasma cells which may be closely related or even identical to MZL.

REFERENCES

1. Slater D. Primary cutaneous B-cell lymphomas. Arch Dermatol 1997; 133:1604–1605.
2. Willemze R, Kerl H, Sterry W, Berti E, Cerroni L, Chimenti S, Diaz Perez JL, Geerts ML, Goos M, Knobler R, Ralfkiaer E, Santucci M, Smith N, Wechsler J, van Vloten WA, Meijer CJ. EORTC classification for primary cutaneous lymphomas: a proposal from the Cutaneous Lymphoma Study Group of the European Organization for Research and Treatment of Cancer. Blood 1997; 90:354–371.
3. Baldassano MF, Bailey EM, Ferry JA, Harris NL, Duncan LM. Cutaneous lymphoid hyperplasia and cutaneous marginal zone lymphoma: comparison of morphologic and immunophenotypic features. Am J Surg Pathol 1999; 23:88–96.
4. Servitje O, Estrach T, Pujol RM, Blanco A, Fernandez-Sevilla A, Petriz L, Peyri J. Primary cutaneous marginal zone B-cell lymphoma: a clinical, histopathological, immunophenotypic and molecular genetic study of 22 cases. Br J Dermatol 2002; 147:1147–1158.
5. Cerroni L, Signoretti S, Hofler G, Annessi G, Putz B, Lackinger E, Metze D, Giannetti A, Kerl H. Primary cutaneous marginal zone B-cell lymphoma: a recently described entity of low-grade malignant cutaneous B-cell lymphoma. Am J Surg Pathol 1997; 21:1307–1315.
6. Spencer J, Perry ME, Dunn Walters DK. Human marginal-zone B cells. Immunol Today 1998; 19:421–426.
7. Tomaszewski MM, Abbondanzo SL, Lupton GP. Extranodal marginal zone B-cell lymphoma of the skin: a morphologic and immunophenotypic study of 11 cases. Am J Dermatopathol 2000; 22:205–211.
8. de la Fouchardiere A, Balme B, Chouvet B, Sebban C, Perrot H, Claudy A, Bryon PA, Coiffier B, Berger F. Primary cutaneous marginal zone B-cell lymphoma: a report of 9 cases. J Am Acad Dermatol 1999; 41:181–188.
9. Child FJ, Woolford AJ, Calonje E, Russell Jones R, Whittaker SJ. Molecular analysis of the immunoglobulin heavy chain gene in the diagnosis of primary cutaneous B cell lymphoma. J Invest Dermatol 2001; 117:984–989.

10. Child FJ, Russell Jones R, Woolford AJ, Calonje E, Photiou A, Orchard G, Whittaker SJ. Absence of the t(14;18) chromosomal translocation in primary cutaneous B-cell lymphoma. Br J Dermatol 2001; 144:735–744.

11. Cerroni L, Zochling N, Putz B, Kerl H. Infection by *Borrelia burgdorferi* and cutaneous B-cell lymphoma. J Cutan Pathol 1997; 24:457–461.

12. Roggero E, Zucca E, Mainetti C, Bertoni F, Valsangiacomo C, Pedrinis E, Borisch B, Piffaretti JC, Cavalli F, Isaacson PG. Eradication of *Borrelia burgdorferi* infection in primary marginal zone B-cell lymphoma of the skin. Hum Pathol 2000; 31:263–268.

13. de Leval L, Harris NL, Longtine J, Ferry JA, Duncan LM. Cutaneous B-cell lymphomas of follicular and marginal zone types: use of Bcl-6, CD10, Bcl-2, and CD21 in differential diagnosis and classification. Am J Surg Pathol 2001; 25:732–741.

14. Duncan LM, LeBoit PE. Are primary cutaneous immunocytoma and marginal zone lymphoma the same disease? Am J Surg Pathol 1997; 21:1368–1372</title

15. Schmid U, Eckert F, Griesser H, Steinke C, Cogliatti SB, Kaudewitz P, Lennert K. Cutaneous follicular lymphoid hyperplasia with monotypic plasma cells. A clinicopathologic study of 18 patients. Am J Surg Pathol 1995; 19:12–20.

31.1. Immunocytoma

Günter Burg and Werner Kempf
Department of Dermatology, University Hospital, Zürich, Switzerland

CLASSIFICATION

WHO/EORTC Classification (2005): Primary cutaneous marginal zone B-cell lymphomas (MALT type), variant: immunocytoma

WHO Classification (2001): Extranodal marginal zone lymphoma of mucosa-associated lymphoid tissue (MALT lymphoma)

REAL Classification (1997): Immunocytoma/lymphoplasmacytic lymphoma

EORTC Classification (1997): Immunocytoma (marginal zone B-cell lymphoma)

DEFINITION

Immunocytoma is a variant of primary cutaneous marginal zone B-cell lymphoma with high numbers of monotypic plasma cells and lymphoplasmacytoid cells.

CLINICAL FEATURES

Marginal zone lymphomas including immunocytoma represent 50–80% of cutaneous B-cell lymphomas, which in turn compose 20–25% of all cutaneous lymphomas.

Primary cutaneous immunocytoma presents as red brown nodules or plaques with smooth surface (Fig. 1), sometimes arising on the background of acrodermatitis chronica atrophicans (Fig. 2) (1–3).

HISTOLOGY

The infiltrates present a typical B-cell pattern with well-circumscribed nodules in the dermis extending in some instances into the subcutaneous tissue (Fig. 3). The epidermis is not involved. The predominant cells are small well-differentiated lymphocytes,

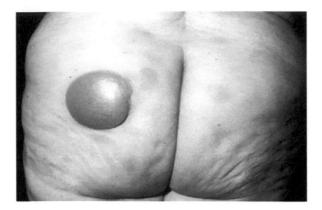

Figure 1   Large nodule with smooth surface on the buttock. (Kindly provided by H. Kerl.)

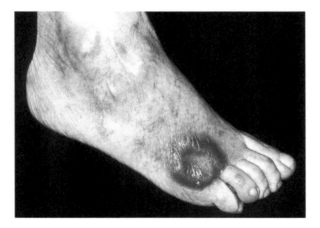

Figure 2   Similar lesion on the background of acrodermatitis chronica atrophicans.

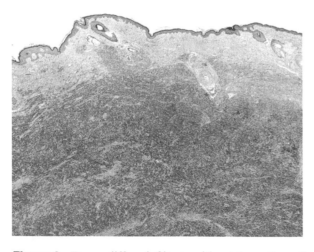

Figure 3   Dense diffuse infiltrate without formation of germinal centers.

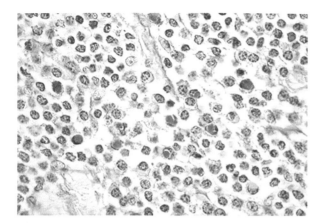

Figure 4 Plasmacytoid differentiated cells, some of which exhibit intranuclear inclusions (Dutcher bodies) (PAS staining). (Kindly provided by H. Kerl.)

lymphoplasmocytoid cells, and mature plasma cells. Intranuclear (Dutcher bodies) and intracytoplasmatic PAS-positive globular inclusions, representing immunoglobulin deposits, are common (Fig. 4). These features can also be found in other B-cell lymphomas, particularly B-cell chronic lymphocytic leukemia, marginal zone and follicle center cell lymphomas, and therefore cannot be regarded as specific for immunocytoma even though they are very typical.

IMMUNOHISTOCHEMISTRY

Phenotypically, the cells have surface and monotypic cytoplasmic Ig, usually of IgM type (4), express B-cell associated antigens (CD20, CD79a) and lack CD5, CD10, CD23 bcl-6 allowing discrimination from follicle center lymphoma and marginal zone lymphoma. In contrast to infiltrates in chronic lymphocytic leukemia, infiltrating cells in immunocytoma are CD5–.

MOLECULAR BIOLOGY

Immunoglobulin heavy and light chain genes are clonally rearranged. Translocation of t(9;14) gene has been reported in nodal immunocytomas (5). The Bcl-2 oncogene, normally involved in nodal follicular or follicle center lymphomas, is in germ-line configuration in cutaneous immunocytoma. In MALT lymphomas, the etiologic role of *Helicobacter pylori* is well established: induction of reactive lymphoid hyperplasia may be followed by transformation into malignant B-cell lymphoma. *Borrelia burgdorferi* has been pathogenetically implicated in cutaneous B-cell pseudolymphomas and B-cell lymphomas (6–8), including immunocytoma (1).

TREATMENT

Treatment of immunocytoma follows the rules for treatment of other low-grade malignant B-cell lymphomas. Solitary lesions can be removed surgically or treated with ionizing radiation. In Borrelia-associated cases, antibiotic treatment (doxycy-

---

Immunocytoma

Clinical features
    Nodules with smooth surface, occasionally in Borrelia infection
Histological features
    Nodular infiltrates of lymphoplasmacytoid cells and plasma cells
Immunophenotype
    Monotypic cytoplasmic Ig, usually of IgM type CD20+, CD79a+,
        CD5–, CD10–, CD23–
Molecular biology
    Clonal IgH rearrangement in majority of cases
Laboratory evaluation
    Search for Borrelia infection
Treatment
    Antibiotics, excision, radiotherapy, rituximab
Clinical course and prognosis
    Excellent prognosis

---

cline 100 mg bid for 6–8 weeks) is the therapy of choice. Multiple disseminated lesions have to be treated systemically by low dose chlorambucil (4 mg/day) with steroids or methotrexate (15–25 mg/once a week). Anti-CD20 antibodies (Rituximab) may be effective even though plasma cells are CD20–.

CLINICAL COURSE AND PROGNOSIS

The prognosis is exceptionally good with 5-year-survival rates approaching 100% (9,10).

DIFFERENTIAL DIAGNOSIS

From a clinical point of view, all the types of cutaneous B-cell lymphomas and B-cell pseudolymphomas (11) have to be considered. Histologically, there are overlapping features with marginal zone B-cell lymphoma (12) which resulted in the classification of immunocytoma as a morphological variant of marginal zone B-cell lymphoma. Plasmacytoma and cutaneous follicular lymphoid hyperplasia with monotypic plasma cells, which most probably also represents marginal zone B-cell lymphoma, are the most important differential diagnoses.

REFERENCES

1. Braun-Falco O, Guggenberger K, Burg G, Fateh-Moghadam A. Immunozytom unter dem Bild einer Acrodermatitis chronica atrophicans. Hautarzt 1978; 29:644–647.
2. Kerl H, Burg G. Immunocytomas and immunoblastic lymphomas of the skin. Hautarzt 1979; 30:666–672.
3. Rijlaarsdam JU, van der Putte SC, Berti E, Kerl H, Rieger E, Toonstra J, Geerts ML, Meijer CJ, Willemze R. Cutaneous immunocytomas: a clinicopathologic study of 26 cases. Histopathology 1993; 23:117–125.

4. Burg G, Braun-Falco O. Cutaneous Lymphomas, Pseudolymphomas and Related Disorders. Berlin, Heidelberg, New York, Tokyo: Springer-Verlag, 1983.

5. Iida S, Rao PH, Nallasivam P, Hibshoosh H, Butler M, Louie DC, Dyomin V, Ohno H, Chaganti RS, Dalla-Favera R. The t(9;14)(p13;q32) chromosomal translocation associated with lymphoplasmacytoid lymphoma involves the PAX-5 gene. Blood 1996; 88:4110–4117.

6. Cerroni L, Zochling N, Putz B, Kerl H. Infection by *Borrelia burgdorferi* and cutaneous B-cell lymphoma. J Cutan Pathol 1997; 24:457–461.

7. Garbe C, Stein H, Dienemann D, Orfanos CE. *Borrelia burgdorferi*-associated cutaneous B cell lymphoma: clinical and immunohistologic characterization of four cases. J Am Acad Dermatol 1991; 24:584–590.

8. Kutting B, Bonsmann G, Metze D, Luger TA, Cerroni L. *Borrelia burgdorferi*-associated primary cutaneous B cell lymphoma: complete clearing of skin lesions after antibiotic pulse therapy or intralesional injection of interferon alfa-2a. J Am Acad Dermatol 1997; 36:311–314.

9. Willemze R, Kerl H, Sterry W, Berti E, Cerroni L, Chimenti S, Diaz Perez JL, Geerts ML, Goos M, Knobler R, Ralfkiaer E, Santucci M, Smith N, Wechsler J, van Vloten WA, Meijer CJ. EORTC classification for primary cutaneous lymphomas: a proposal from the Cutaneous Lymphoma Study Group of the European Organization for Research and Treatment of Cancer. Blood 1997; 90:354–371.

10. Grange F, Bagot M. Prognosis of primary cutaneous lymphomas. Ann Dermatol Venereol 2002; 129:30–40.

11. LeBoit PE, McNutt NS, Reed JA, Jacobson M, Weiss LM. Primary cutaneous immunocytoma. A B-cell lymphoma that can easily be mistaken for cutaneous lymphoid hyperplasia. Am J Surg Pathol 1994; 18:969–978.

12. Duncan LM, LeBoit PE. Are primary cutaneous immunocytoma and marginal zone lymphoma the same disease? Am J Surg Pathol 1997; 21:1368–1372.

31.2. Primary Cutaneous Plasmacytoma (PCP)

Dmitry V. Kazakov, Günter Burg, and Werner Kempf
Department of Dermatology, University Hospital, Zürich, Switzerland

CLASSIFICATION

> WHO/EORTC Classification (2005): Primary cutaneous marginal zone B-cell lymphoma, variant
> WHO Classification (2001): Extraosseous plasmacytoma
> EORTC Classification (1997): Plasmacytoma
> REAL Classification (1997): Plasma cell myeloma/plasmacytoma

DEFINITION

Primary cutaneous plasmacytoma (PCP) is a rare variant of primary cutaneous B-cell lymphoma, derived from clonally expanded, variably matured plasma cells. The first case of true PCP was reported by Stout and Frerichs in 1949 (1). Since then, less than 40 cases have been published under this name (2). In theWHO–EORTC consensus classification, PCP is regarded as a morphologic variant of primary cutaneous marginal zone B-cell lymphoma (MZL).

CLINICAL FEATURES

Elderly or middle-aged persons (mean age approximately 60 years; range from 22 to 88 years) are mainly affected. There is a prominent male preponderance (male:female ratio, 4:1) (2). PCP manifests as solitary or multiple (up to 50), asymptomatic, red–purple nodules or plaques with no predilection site (Fig. 1). Ulceration is rarely observed (3,4).

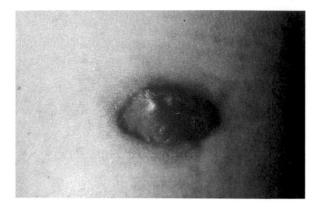

Figure 1 Solitary well-circumscribed nodule on the back.

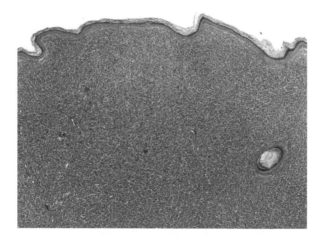

Figure 2 Diffuse dense infiltrate through the entire dermis.

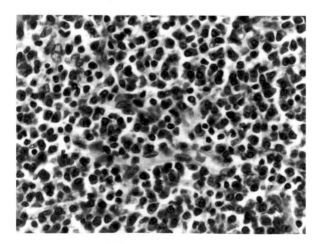

Figure 3 Infiltrate composed of typical and atypical plasma cells.

HISTOLOGY

There is a diffuse or nodular infiltrate (Fig. 2) composed of plasma cells with varying degrees of maturation and pleomorphism. The infiltrate usually spares the epidermis and often shows perivascular and/or periadnexal accentuation. The subcutis may be involved. Sometimes the tumor consists almost exclusively of mature-looking plasma cells with a "clock-face" nuclear chromatin pattern (Fig. 3). In other cases, there are high numbers of pleomorphic and immature cells (plasmablasts). The latter have dispersed chromatin, a high nuclear/cytoplasmic ratio, and prominent nucleoli. A typical finding is the presence of Russell and Dutcher bodies (intracytoplasmic and intranuclear inclusions respectively). Multinucleated plasma cells as well as mitotic figures can be found (3,5,6).

IMMUNOHISTOCHEMISTRY

Neoplastic cells usually demonstrate reactivity with CD79a, CD38, and CD138 antigens as well as with some cytokeratins. Cytoplasmic Ig and monoclonal expression of Ig light chains are usually present. The tumor cells are negative for CD20 and common leukocyte antigen (3–6).

MOLECULAR BIOLOGY

In some cases, clonal rearrangement of IgH genes is detected (7), while the others show no detectable gene rearrangements by PCR notwithstanding the presence of light chain restriction identified immunohistochemically (6).

TREATMENT

Treatment options include surgical removal of the lesions alone or combined with radiation therapy, and chemotherapy alone or in combination with radiation. Systemic or intralesional injections of corticosteroids or tumor necrosis factor-alfa are beneficial in some cases (3–6,8,9).

CLINICAL COURSE AND PROGNOSIS

The clinical course is rather unpredictable and still not clear due to the paucity of cases with long-term follow-up (6). In some patients, the disease runs a benign protracted course with long-term complete remission following treatment. In other instances, the neoplasm progresses rapidly with local or systemic spread. Involvement of lymph nodes, liver, and central nervous system may occur. In addition, PCP may be a precursor of multiple myeloma (MM), even if the complete work-up at the initial presentation is negative. There are no clear-cut prognostic factors which indicate a possible aggressive course of the disease. Cases with multiple skin lesions are thought to show more aggressive behavior, especially if the neoplastic cells produce monoclonal IgA (2,5,10).

Primary cutaneous plasmacytoma

Clinical features
    Middle-aged or elderly patients
    Male predominance
    Multiple or solitary nodules or plaques
Histological features
    Nonepidermotropic diffuse or nodular infiltrate of variably mature and atypical
        plasma cells. Russell and Dutcher bodies
Immunophenotype
    CD79a+, CD20–, CD138+, CKs+, CLA–, Ig (cytoplasmic), monoclonal
        expression of κ or λ
Molecular biology
    IgH rearrangement variably detected
Treatment
    Excision, radiation therapy, or chemotherapy
Clinical course
    Unpredictable

DIFFERENTIAL DIAGNOSIS

The PCP should be distinguished from secondary cutaneous plasmacytoma in MM, secondary skin involvement by extramedullary plasmacytomas (EMP) located elsewhere in mucosae or soft tissue, secondary skin involvement in Waldenström macroglobulinemia (WM), other primary B-cell lymphomas, and a variety of infectious diseases with prominent plasma cell infiltration (e.g., syphilis, borreliosis). In addition, some other inflammatory dermatoses involving the head and neck region are apt to show plasma cell-rich infiltrates—a phenomenon called circumorificial plasmacytosis. They can usually be identified by the polyclonal nature of the infiltrate (immunohistochemistry), identification of the causative agent, clinical features and suggestive history.

Specific involvement of the skin in MM patients occurs in 2% of cases. Differentiation between PCP and specific cutaneous involvement in MM can only be made after additional clinical and laboratory investigations. The cutaneous clinical and histopathological features of PCP and MM are identical. Bone marrow examination, skeletal X-ray, peripheral blood and urine investigations are obligatory during the work-up of a patient with skin lesions consistent with plasmacytoma. Features indicative of MM include bone marrow plasmacytosis of >10%, osteolytic lesions, and detection of a plasma or urine paraprotein.

In the distinction of PCP from skin involvement in WM, clues to the diagnosis of WM include serum monoclonal IgM (>3 gm/dL) and consequent clinical findings (hyperviscosity symptoms, coagulopathies, neuropathies), and bone marrow infiltration by abnormal small to medium-sized lymphocytes showing plasmacytoid features expressing CD20 antigen.

COMMENTS

PCP is a rare disease with relatively limited data on its clinico-pathological presentation, prognosis, and outcome. It is not distinguished as a separate entity from MM in current lymphoma classifications such as the REAL or the WHO classifications. In the EORTC classification for primary cutaneous lymphomas, the condition is included only as a provisional entity within the group of B-cell neoplasms. In the new WHO-EORTC classification PCP is regarded as a variant of MZL, but an analysis of the published material suggests that the two may be different entities.

REFERENCES

1. Stout AP, Frerichs JB. Plasmacytoma of the inframammary region. J Missouri Med Assoc 1949; 46:275–277.
2. Muscardin LM, Pulsoni A, Cerroni L. Primary cutaneous plasmacytoma: report of a case with review of the literature. J Am Acad Dermatol 2000; 43:962–965.
3. Green T, Grant J, Pye R, Marcus R. Multiple primary cutaneous plasmacytomas. Arch Dermatol 1992; 128:962–965.
4. Torne R, Su WP, Winkelmann RK, Smolle J, Kerl H. Clinicopathologic study of cutaneous plasmacytoma. Int J Dermatol 1990; 29:562–566.
5. Wong KF, Chan JK, Li LP, Yau TK, Lee AW. Primary cutaneous plasmacytoma— report of two cases and review of the literature. Am J Dermatopathol 1994; 16:392–397.
6. Kazakov DV, Belousova IE, Muller B, Palmedo G, Samtsov AV, Burg G, Kempf W. Primary cutaneous plasmacytoma: a clinicopathological study of two cases with a long-term follow-up and review of the literature. J Cutan Pathol 2002; 29:244–248.
7. Miyamoto T, Kobayashi T, Hagari Y, Mihara M. The value of genotypic analysis in the assessment of cutaneous plasmacytomas. Br J Dermatol 1997; 137:418–421.
8. Yamamoto T, Katayama I, Nishioka K. Increased plasma interleukin-6 in cutaneous plasmacytoma: the effect of intralesional steroid therapy. Br J Dermatol 1997; 137:631–636.
9. Tsuboi R, Morioka R, Yaguchi H, Shimokawa R, Inaba M, Ogawa H. Primary cutaneous plasmacytoma: treatment with intralesional tumour necrosis factor-alpha. Br J Dermatol 1992; 126:395–397.
10. Kato N, Kimura K, Yasukawa K, Aikawa K. Metastatic cutaneous plasmacytoma: a case report associated with IgA lambda multiple myeloma and a review of the literature of metastatic cutaneous plasmacytomas associated with multiple myeloma and primary cutaneous plasmacytomas. J Dermatol 1999; 26:587–594.
11. Kazakov DV, Michaelis S, Palmedo G, Dummer R, Burg G, Kempf W. IgM-kappa plasmacytomas in a patient with Waldenström macroglobulinemia with monotypic IgM lambda expression [abstr]. J Clin Pathol 2002; 55(suppl 1):A44–45.

31.3. Cutaneous Follicular Lymphoid Hyperplasia with Monotypic Plasma Cells

Dmitry V. Kazakov, Günter Burg, and Werner Kempf
Department of Dermatology, University Hospital, Zürich, Switzerland

DEFINITION

Cutaneous follicular lymphoid hyperplasia with monotypic plasma cells (CFLH-MPC) was reported by Schmid and colleagues in 1995 with a series of 18 patients (1). This disease is considered as a variant of primary cutaneous marginal zone B-cell lymphoma in the WHO/EORTC classification.

CLINICAL FEATURES

Both sexes are equally affected. The median age of patients is 45 years (range 18–83 years). Patients present with solitary or multiple plaques located on the trunk, limbs, and face.

HISTOLOGY

There are nodular infiltrates in the dermis extending into the subcutis with a prominent follicular growth pattern. The interfollicular areas contain high numbers of postcapillary venules similar to those seen in the paracortex as well as mixed infiltrates of macrophages, immunoblasts, and eosinophils. The unique feature is the presence of sheets and strands of plasma cells at the periphery of the lymphoid infiltrates. In some cases the plasma cells can comprise up to 50% of the infiltrate. Russell bodies are not seen. The stroma is markedly sclerotic.

Cutaneous follicular lymphoid hyperplasia with monotypic plasma cells

Clinical features
  Middle-aged adults
  Solitary or multiple plaques
Histological features
  Nodular infiltrates in dermis/subcutis
  Germinal centers
  Sheets and strands of plasma cells
Immunophenotype
  Monoclonal expression of κ or λ by plasma cells, scattered CD30+ blasts
Molecular biology
  IgH rearrangements in majority of cases
Treatment
  Excision
Clinical course
  Favorable

IMMUNOHISTOCHEMISTRY

The plasma cells express monoclonal IgG/λ or IgG/κ. B cells in the germinal centers and mantle zones demonstrate a polyclonal immunoglobulin pattern. T cells have a helper cell phenotype (CD3+, CD4+, CD8–). Variable numbers of CD30+ blasts are scattered within the infiltrate.

MOLECULAR BIOLOGY

Clonal IgH rearrangements are detected in the majority of cases.

TREATMENT

Excision or other destructive methods can be employed.

CLINICAL COURSE AND PROGNOSIS

The clinical course is favorable but persistent disease and local recurrences may be seen on rare occasions.

DIFFERENTIAL DIAGNOSIS

The CFLH-MPC differs from inflammatory pseudotumor (plasma cell granuloma) in having monoclonal plasma cells.

COMMENTS

CFLH-MPC may represent an intermediate step between cutaneous lymphoid hyperplasia and true B-cell lymphoma, sometimes called "clonal cutaneous lymphoid hyperplasia". Nowdays, many consider CFLH-MPC a variant of primary cutaneous marginal zone lymphoma.

REFERENCES

1. Schmid U, Eckert F, Griesser H, Steinke C, Cogliatti SB, Kaudewitz P, Lennert K. Cutaneous follicular lymphoid hyperplasia with monotypic plasma cells. A clinicopathologic study of 18 patients. Am J Surg Pathol 1995; 19:12–20.
2. Medeiros LJ, Picker LJ, Abel EA, Hu CH, Hoppe RT, Warnke RA, Wood GS. Cutaneous lymphoid hyperplasia. Immunologic characteristics and assessment of criteria recently proposed as diagnostic of malignant lymphoma. J Am Acad Dermatol 1989; 21:929–942.

32

Primary Cutaneous Follicle Center Lymphoma

Dmitry V. Kazakov, Werner Kempf, and Günter Burg
Department of Dermatology, University Hospital, Zürich, Switzerland

CLASSIFICATION

> WHO/EORTC Classification (2005): Cutaneous follicle center lymphoma; variants: follicular, follicular and diffuse, diffuse
> WHO Classification (2001): Cutaneous follicle center lymphoma
> REAL Classification (1997): Follicle center lymphoma, follicular
> EORTC Classification (1997): Primary cutaneous follicle center cell lymphoma

DEFINITION

Follicular lymphoma is the most common type of primary cutaneous B-cell lymphomas with a predilection for the scalp, forehead, and trunk (Fig. 1) (1–3). Synonyms for follicular lymphoma include reticulohistiocytoma of the dorsum or Crosti lymphoma (4–9). Follicular lymphoma presenting in cutaneous sites may also be secondary to spread from nodal follicular lymphoma.

CLINICAL FEATURES

Primary cutaneous follicular lymphoma usually presents with localized disease and rarely disseminates. The lesions are usually red-brown papules of nodules, most commonly seen on the scalp, forehead, and trunk (Fig. 1).

HISTOLOGY

In nodal follicular lymphoma as defined by the WHO classification, the majority of cases have a follicular component but may contain diffuse areas, often with sclerosis. Nodal follicular lymphoma is composed of a mixture of centrocytes and centroblasts and graded by the proportion of centroblasts (Grades 1–3), since histologic grading can predict the clinical outcome. Grade 1 has 0–5 centroblasts/high power field; Grade 2, 6–15 centroblasts/high power; Grade 3, >15 centroblasts/high power

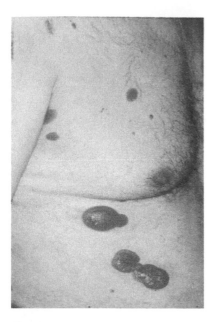

Figure 1 Cutaneous follicular lymphoma: multiple nodules on the trunk.

field. Ten high power fields within different follicles are counted (5). Cutaneous follicular lymphoma shows a **follicular or a follicular and diffuse or a diffuse growth pattern** within the dermis, often extending into the subcutaneous tissue which contains a mixture of centrocytes and centroblasts with a predominantly follicular pattern. Occassionally, a diffuse pattern may be seen. In most cases, there is a Grenz zone (Fig. 2). Neoplastic follicles show a relatively monomorphic cellular composition (Fig. 3). This is in contrast to the polymorphous composition of a reac-

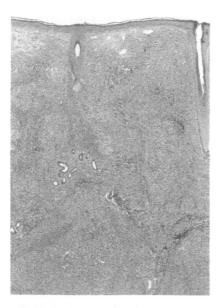

Figure 2 Cutaneous follicular lymphoma: diffuse lymphocytic infiltrate with numerous follicles and Grenz zone.

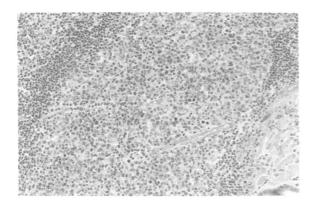

Figure 3 Cutaneous follicular lymphoma: neoplastic follicle with a mixture of small, medium, and large lymphoid cells (Giemsa).

tive follicle in a reactive infiltrate (pseudolymphoma) which is characterized by an admixture of centrocytes, centroblasts, immunoblasts, and tingible body macrophages (10).

Distinguishing between reactive and malignant follicles can be extremely difficult. Reactive follicles have a significantly higher number of mitoses, numerous tingible body macrophages, and often a starry sky pattern. All these features are uncommon in neoplastic follicles. There may be remnants of reactive follicles in follicular lymphoma.

IMMUNOHISTOCHEMISTRY

The neoplastic B cells are usually CD 10+, CD 19+, CD20+, CD22+, CD79a+, CD5−, CD23+/−, and CD43− (5,10). The tumor cells express the nuclear protein bcl-6 (11).

A major difference between primary and secondary follicular lymphoma involving cutaneous sites is the presence of the bcl-2 translocation. The bcl-2 translocation, which is usually present in 75–95% of nodal follicular lymphomas, is less often found in primary cutaneous follicular lymphomas (12). This discrepancy has led to speculation that primary cutaneous follicular lymphoma may be a separate disease (5,6).

TREATMENT

Careful staging is required for proper management. If disease is limited to the skin, treatment consists of local radiotherapy and/or surgical excision if a single lesion or a small number of lesions are present (13,14). A new therapeutic approach, with favorable responses and no severe side effects reported, is the intralesional or systemic use of a monoclonal anti-CD20 antibody [Mabthera (Rituximab®)] (15–19). Treatment of cutaneous lesions of systemic follicular lymphoma should be directed at the underlying disease.

CLINICAL COURSE AND PROGNOSIS

Primary follicular lymphoma presenting in skin has a favorable prognosis (1–4,13,14,20,21) with an estimated 5-year survival of 97% (6).

Cutaneous follicule center lymphoma

Clinical features
  Nodules predominantly in the head and neck region
Histological features
  Nodular or diffuse infiltrates consisting of centrocytes and centroblasts, small lymphocytes. Neoplastic follicles
Immunophenotype
  CD10+, CD19+, CD20+, CD22+, CD79a+, CD5−, CD23+/−, CD43− , bcl-6+,bcl-2 usually negative
Molecular biology
  Clonal IgH rearrangement in majority of cases
Laboratory evaluation
  Search for Borrelia infection
Treatment
  Excision, ionizing radiation, antibiotics, rituximab
Clinical course and prognosis
  Excellent prognosis, tendency to recur

DIFFERENTIAL DIAGNOSIS

The differential diagnosis of primary cutaneous follicular lymphoma includes other B-cell lymphomas such as extranodal marginal zone B-cell lymphoma of MALT type. In this lymphoma, there are usually reactive lymphoid follicles surrounded by a heterogeneous cellular infiltrate composed of centrocyte-like cells, monocytoid B cells, plasma cells, lymphoplasmacytoid cells, and small lymphocytes. The plasma cells usually are monoclonal, immunophenotypic analysis reveals a light-chain restriction for kappa or lambda light chains (10). Some cases of cutaneous mantle-cell lymphoma may morphologically resemble a cutaneous follicular lymphoma. In contrast to follicular lymphoma, the neoplastic cells in mantle-cell lymphoma express CD5 and cyclin D1.

COMMENTS

The excellent prognosis and uncommon progression to extracutaneous disease strongly suggest that primary cutaneous follicular lymphoma is a distinct entity. In addition, differences in expression of bcl-2 and responsiveness to therapy also support this concept. As a consequence, the WHO classification defines a variant termed "cutaneous follicle center lymphoma."

However, there is a controversy in classification of cutaneous *follicle center lymphoma* regarding the current lymphoma classification schemes. Follicular lymphoma as defined in the EORTC classification has a nodular or diffuse infiltrate of cells which contain a mixture of centrocytes and centroblasts. Remnants of reactive follicles may be observed; however, neoplastic follicles are rare (6). This is in contrast to the definition of cutaneous follicle center lymphoma in the WHO classification which is predominantly follicular but may have a partially diffuse pattern (5,9). Most cases *of follicle center cell lymphoma,* as used in the EORTC classification, are mostly diffuse and would thus be considered *diffuse large B-cell lymphomas* in the WHO classification.

REFERENCES

1. Garcia CF, Weiss LM, Warnke RA, Wood GS. Cutaneous follicular lymphoma. Am J Surg Pathol 1986; 10:454–463.
2. Pimpinelli N, Santucci M, Bosi A, Moretti S, Vallecchi C, Messori A, Giannotti B. Primary cutaneous follicular center-cell lymphoma—a lymphoproliferative disease with favourable prognosis. Clin Exp Dermatol 1989; 14:12–19.
3. Rijlaarsdam JU, Meijer CJ, Willemze R. Differentiation between lymphadenosis benigna cutis and primary cutaneous follicular center cell lymphomas. A comparative clinico-pathologic study of 57 patients. Cancer 1990; 65:2301–2306.
4. Berti E, Alessi E, Caputo R, Gianotti R, Delia D, Vezzoni P. Reticulohistiocytoma of the dorsum. J Am Acad Dermatol 1988; 19:259–272.
5. Nathwani BN, Harris NL, Weisenburger D, Isaacson PG, Piris MA, Berger F, Müller-Hermelink HK, Swerdlow SH. In: Jaffe ES, Harris NL, Stein H, Vardiman J, eds. Pathology and Genetics of Tumours of Haematopoietic and Lymphoid Tissues. Lyon: IARC Press, 2001:162–167.
6. Willemze R, Kerl H, Sterry W, Berti E, Cerroni L, Chimenti S, Diaz-Perez JL, Geerts ML, Goos M, Knobler R, Ralfkiaer E, Santucci M, Smith N, Wechsler J, van Vloten WA, Meijer CJ. EORTC classification for primary cutaneous lymphomas: a proposal from the Cutaneous Lymphoma Study Group of the European Organization for Research and Treatment of Cancer. Blood 1997; 90:354–371.
7. Sander CA, Flaig MJ, Kaudewitz P, Jaffe ES. The revised European–American classification of Lymphoid Neoplasms (REAL): a preferred approach for the classification of cutaneous lymphomas. Am J Dermatopathol 1999; 21:274–278.
8. Jaffe ES, Sander CA, Flaig MJ. Cutaneous lymphomas: a proposal for a unified approach to classification using the REAL/WHO classification. Ann Oncol 2000; 11:17–21.
9. Sander CA, Flaig MJ, Jaffe ES. Cutaneous manifestations of lymphoma: a clinical guide based on the WHO classification. Clin Lymphoma 2001; 2:86–100.
10. Sander CA, Flaig MJ. Morphologic spectrum of cutaneous B-cell lymphomas. Dermatol Clin 1999; 17:593–599.
11. Falini B, Fizzotti M, Pileri S, Liso A, Pasqualucci L, Flenghi L. Bcl-6 protein expression in normal and neoplastic lymphoid tissues. Ann Oncol 1997; 8:101–104.
12. Cerroni L, Volkenandt M, Rieger E, Soyer HP, Kerl H. bcl-2 protein expression and correlation with the interchromosomal 14; 18 translocation in cutaneous lymphomas and pseudolymphomas. J Invest Dermatol 1994; 102:231–235.
13. Santucci M, Pimpinelli N, Arganini L. Primary cutaneous B-cell lymphoma: a unique type of low-grade lymphoma. Clinicopathologic and immunologic study of 83 cases. Cancer 1991; 67:2311–2326.
14. Rijlaarsdam JU, Toonstra J, Meijer OW, Noordijk EM, Willemze R. Treatment of primary cutaneous B-cell lymphomas of follicle center cell origin: a clinical follow-up study of 55 patients treated with radiotherapy or polychemotherapy. J Clin Oncol 1996; 14:549–555.

15. Sabroe RA, Child FJ, Woolford AJ, Spittle MF, Russell-Jones R. Rituximab in cutaneous B-cell lymphoma: a report of two cases. Br J Dermatol 2000; 143:157–161.
16. Heinzerling L, Urbanek M, Funk JO, Peker S, Bleck O, Neuber K, Burg G, von den Driesch P, Dummer R. Reduction of tumor burden and stabilization of disease by systemic therapy with anti-CD20 antibody (rituximab) in patients with primary cutaneous B-cell lymphoma. Cancer 2000; 89:1835–1844.
17. Heinzerling L, Dummer R, Kempf W, Schmid MH, Burg G. Intralesional therapy with anti-CD20 monoclonal antibody rituximab in primary cutaneous B-cell lymphoma. Arch Dermatol 2000; 136:374–378.
18. Gellrich S, Muche JM, Pelzer K, Audring H, Sterry W. Der anti-CD20-antikörper bei primär kutanen B-Zell-lymphomen. Erste Erfahrungen in der dermatologischen Anwendung. Hautarzt 2001; 52:205–210.
19. Paul T, Radny P, Krober SM, Paul A, Blaheta HJ, Garbe C. Intralesional rituximab for cutaneous B-cell lymphoma. Br J Dermatol 2001; 144:1239–1243.
20. Cerroni L, Arzberger E, Pütz B, Hofler G, Metze D, Sander CA, Rose C, Wolf P, Rütten A, McNiff JM, Kerl H. Primary cutaneous follicle center cell lymphoma with follicular growth pattern. Blood 2000; 95:3922–3928.
21. Willemze R, Meijer CJ, Sentis HJ, Scheffer E, van Vloten WA, Toonstra J, van der Putte SC. Primary cutaneous large cell lymphomas of follicular center cell origin. A clinical follow-up study of nineteen patients. J Am Acad Dermatol 1987; 16:518–526.

33

Primary Cutaneous Diffuse Large B-cell Lymphoma

Günter Burg and Werner Kempf
Department of Dermatology, University Hospital, Zürich, Switzerland

CLASSIFICATION

> WHO/EORTC Classification (2005): Cutaneous diffuse large B-cell lymphoma leg type and others
> WHO Classification (2001): Diffuse large B-cell lymphoma
> REAL Classification (1997): Diffuse large B-cell lymphoma
> EORTC Classification (1997): Large B-cell lymphoma of the lower leg

DEFINITION

Primary cutaneous diffuse large B-cell lymphomas (DLBCL) are lymphomas composed of large B cells (centroblasts and immunoblasts) and have a rather aggressive course. DLBCL include a variety of different entities, formerly referred to as centroblastic lymphoma, immunoblastic lymphoma, some cases of reticulohistiocytoma of the dorsum (Crosti's disease), anaplastic large B-cell lymphomas, multilobated large B-cell lymphomas, and a variant showing a predominant reactive T-cell infiltrate, which has been referred to as T-cell rich B-cell lymphoma (1,2). Two forms of primary cutaneous large B-cell lymphomas are distinguished in the WHO/EORTC–Consensus Classification: DLBCL, leg-type and DLBCL, other.

33.1. Primary Cutaneous Large B-cell Lymphoma, Leg Type

Clinical Features

Cutaneous DLBCL comprise about 1–3% of all cutaneous lymphomas and approximately 5–10% of cutaneous B-cell lymphomas. People over the age of 70 years are most commonly affected. There are contradictory reports on gender preponderance (3,4). In the vast majority of patients, the tumor(s) are located on the (lower) legs (Fig. 1). They present with solitary or multiple red to violaceous dense nodules of

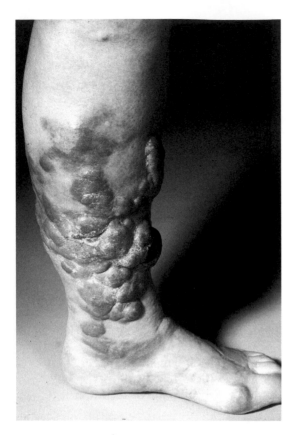

Figure 1 Multiple nodules on the lower leg of an elderly lady.

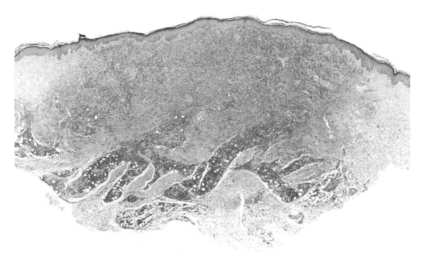

Figure 2 Dense lymphocytic infiltrate in the upper and mid dermis with a more perivascular pattern in the deeper parts.

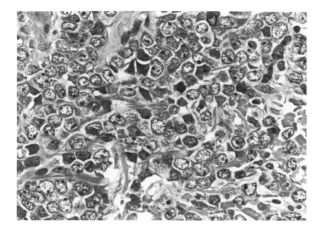

Figure 3 Tumor cells resembling centroblasts.

firm consistency sometimes with ulceration. Occurrence on other sites than the legs is uncommon.

Histology

A diffuse growth pattern is commonly found with a monomorphous infiltrate involving all dermal layers as well as the subcutaneous fat (Fig. 2). The neoplastic cells either resemble centroblasts with large noncleaved nuclei and nucleoli attached to the nuclear membrane (Fig. 3), or immunoblasts with a large vesicular nucleus and a prominent centrally placed nucleolus. In addition, multilobated, anaplastic, or large cleaved cells can be found (5). Mitotic figures can frequently be detected. In some cases, epidermotropism of the infiltrate can be observed and give rise to confusing the tumor with a cutaneous T-cell lymphoma. Small B-cells are not present and only a few reactive T-cells are found.

Immunohistochemistry

The tumor cells express CD19, CD20, CD22, and CD79a. Loss of B-cell markers also occurs (6). Monotypic expression of Ig light chains can be detected on the cell surface (sIg) and/or within the cytoplasm (cIg). In addition, Bcl-2 expression is strongly expressed independent of localization (7). Bcl-6 is expressed in most tumors, but usually weaker than by the tumor cells in follicle centre lymphoma (FCL). CD10 is usually absent or weakly expressed. In contrast to FCL, MUM-1/IRF4 may be expressed (8).

Molecular Biology

In contrast to systemic large B-cell lymphomas, t(14;18) is absent in primary cutaneous DLBCL despite strong expression of bcl-2 (9). Chromosomal translocation (t 8;14), which is found in 75% of Burkitt lymphoma, has also been reported in a cutaneous large B-cell lymphoma (10). The strong expression of bcl-2 which my result from chromosomal amplification of the bcl-2 gene (11) may be one explanation for the more aggressive course of DLBCL compared to other cutaneous B-cell lymphoma, since bcl-2 acts as an antiapoptotic protein. Chromosomal imbalances were recently found in the majority of primary cutaneous LBL of the leg type with translocations of myc, IgH and bcl-6 genes (12).

There are only a few studies on the etiology and the pathogenesis of DLBCL of the skin. Both primary cutaneous FCL and DLBCL of the lower leg descend from germinal center cells (13). Hepatitis C virus RNA has been detected in some cases of DLBCL (14).

Treatment

In localized forms, excision and radiotherapy are the treatment of choice. Remission of Borrelia-associated cases has been observed after antibiotic treatment (15). In patients with multiple tumors involving anatomically separate areas, both radiotherapy and polychemotherapy are preferred modes of treatment (16). Alternatively, intravenous therapy with the anti-CD20 antibody rituximab may be effective treatment for patients with primary cutaneous LBL (17).

Clinical Course and Prognosis

Primary cutaneous DLBCL displays a poor prognosis with 5-year survival rates of 50–60%. Tumors located on the legs appear to be more aggressive than DLBCL located on other sites (18,19). However, the number of tumoral lesions seem to be prognostically even more relevant, since patients with a solitary tumor had a 5-year-survival of 100%, whereas 5-year-survival in patients with multiple tumors on the legs is 36–45% (19). Fas and ICAM-1 expression seem to be strongly related to a favorable prognosis, whereas expression of FasL and Bcl-2 is related to a poor prognosis.

Primary cutaneous diffuse large B-cell lymphoma

Clinical features
   Elderly patients
   Solitary or multiple grouped nodules on the trunk or lower leg
Histological features
   Predominantly diffuse infiltrate of large B-cells resembling centroblasts or
      immunoblasts. Remnants of follicles
Immunophenotype
   CD20+, CD79a+, Ig light chain +, CD5–, CD23–, CD30–
Molecular biology
   Clonal IgH rearrangement
Laboratory evaluation
   Search for Borrelia
Treatment
   Excision, radiation therapy, rituximab, multi agent chemotherapy
Clinical course and prognosis
   Site-related prognosis. Lesions on lower leg exhibit poor prognosis

---

Differential Diagnosis

The primary differential diagnostic consideration is primary cutaneous FCL, especially in cases with diffuse growth pattern and predominance of large cells. In those cases of FCL, the infiltrate consists predominantly of centrocytes with cleaved nuclei, whereas in DLBCL, diffuse infiltrates of centroblasts and immunoblasts with large round nuclei are present. Moreover, bcl-2 is strongly expressed by almost all tumor cells in DLBCL, but not or only weakly by a few cells in FCL. Pleomorphic and anaplastic large cell lymphoma of T- or B-cell lineage do not show centrocytic and centroblastic features. In addition, the cells are CD30+ in most cases.

Comments

Before the introduction of the WHO/EORTC–Consensus Classification, there was a controversy regarding the classification of DLBCL of the skin. In the EORTC classification (1997) only DLBCL of the lower leg was recognized as a distinct entity, whereas the REAL and WHO classifications did not split DLBCL into site-related forms. In addition, some experts consider DLBL on other sites than the lower legs to represent primary cutaneous FCL (20).

OTHER PRIMARY CUTANEOUS LARGE B-CELL LYMPHOMA

This term refers to variants of DLBCL such as T-cell rich B-cell lymphoma characterized by scattered large B-cells embedded in an infiltrate of small T-cells (see Chapter 33.2) and cases with diffuse infiltrates of large B-cells with anaplastic or plasmablastic cytomorphology. There are only very limited data on these forms of CBCL.

REFERENCES

1. Watabe H, Kawakami T, Soma Y, Baba T, Mizoguchi M. Primary cutaneous T-cell-rich B-cell lymphoma in a zosteriform distribution associated with Epstein-Barr virus infection. J Dermatol 2002; 29:748–753.
2. Suarez-Vilela D, Izquierdo-Garcia FM. Histiocyte and T-cell-rich B-cell lymphoma with Langhans giant cells. Histopathology 2003; 42:92–93.
3. Wechsler J, Bagot M. Primary cutaneous large B-cell lymphomas. Semin Cutan Med Surg 2000; 19:130–132.
4. Hembury TA, Lee B, Gascoyne RD, Macpherson N, Yang B, House N, Medeiros LJ, Hsi ED. Primary cutaneous diffuse large B-cell lymphoma: a clinicopathologic study of 15 cases. Am J Clin Pathol 2002; 117:574–580.
5. Nagatani T, Miyazawa M, Matsuzaki T, Hayakawa H, Iemoto G, Kim ST, Ichiyama S, Naito S, Baba N, Sugiyama A, et al. Cutaneous B-cell lymphoma consisting of large cleaved cells with multilobated nuclei. Int J Dermatol 1993; 32:737–739.
6. Joly P, Thomine E, Lauret P. Cutaneous lymphomas other than mycosis fungoides. Semin Dermatol 1994; 13:172–179.
7. Goodlad JR, Krajewski AS, Batstone PJ, et al. Primary cutaneous diffuse large B-cell lymphoma. Prognostic significance and clinicopathologic subtypes. Am J Surg Pathol 2003; 27:1538–1545.
8. Hoefnagel JJ, Dijkman R, Basso K, et al. Distinct types of primary cutaneous large B-cell lymphoma identified by gene expression profiling. Blood 2004; DOI 10.1182.

9. Geelen FA, Vermeer MH, Meijer CJ, Van der Putte SC, Kerkhof E, Kluin PM, Willemze R. bcl-2 protein expression in primary cutaneous large B-cell lymphoma is site-related. J Clin Oncol 1998; 16:2080–2085.

10. Busschots AM, Geerts ML, Mecucci C, Stul M, Cassiman JJ, van den Berghe H. A translocation (8;14) in a cutaneous large B-cell lymphoma. Am J Clin Pathol 1993; 99:615–621.

11. Mao X, Lillington D, Child FJ, Russell-Jones R, Young B, Whittaker S. Comparative genomic hybridization analysis of primary cutaneous B-cell lymphomas: identification of common genomic alterations in disease pathogenesis. Genes, Chromosomes Cancer 2002; 35:144–155.

12. Hallerman C, Kaune KM, Gesk S, et al. Molecular cytogenetic analysis of chromosomal breakpoints in the IGH, MYC, BCL6 and MALT1 gene loci in primary cutaneous B-cell lymphomas. J Invest Dermatol 2004; 123:213–219.

13. Gellrich S, Rutz S, Golembowski S, Jacobs C, von Zimmermann M, Lorenz P, Audring H, Muche M, Sterry W, Jahn S. Primary cutaneous follicle center cell lymphomas and large B cell lymphomas of the leg descend from germinal center cells. A single cell polymerase chain reaction analysis. J Invest Dermatol 2001; 117:1512–1520.

14. Michaelis S, Kazakov DV, Schmid M, Dummer R, Burg G, Kempf W. Hepatitis C and G viruses in B-cell lymphomas of the skin. J Cutan Pathol 2003; 30:369–372.

15. Hofbauer GF, Kessler B, Kempf W, Nestle FO, Burg G, Dummer R. Multilesional primary cutaneous diffuse large B-cell lymphoma responsive to antibiotic treatment. Dermatology 2001; 203:168–170.

16. Rijlaarsdam JU, Toonstra J, Meijer OW, Noordijk EM, Willemze R. Treatment of primary cutaneous B-cell lymphomas of follicle center cell origin: a clinical follow-up study of 55 patients treated with radiotherapy or polychemotherapy. J Clin Oncol 1996; 14:549–555.

17. Heinzerling LM, Urbanek M, Funk JO, Peker S, Bleck O, Neuber K, Burg G, von Den Driesch P, Dummer R. Reduction of tumor burden and stabilization of disease by systemic therapy with anti-CD20 antibody (rituximab) in patients with primary cutaneous B-cell lymphoma. Cancer 2000; 89:1835–1844.

18. Willemze R, Meijer CJ, Scheffer E, Kluin PM, Van VW, Toonstra J, Van der Putte S. Diffuse large cell lymphomas of follicular center cell origin presenting in the skin. A clinicopathologic and immunologic study of 16 patients. Am J Pathol 1987; 126:325–333.

19. Grange F, Bekkenk MW, Wechsler J, et al. Prognostic factors in primary cutaneous large B-cell lymphomas: a European multicenter study. J Clin Oncol 2001; 19:3602–3610.

20. Willemze R, Kerl H, Sterry W, Berti E, Cerroni L, Chimenti S, Diaz-Perez JL, Geerts ML, Goos M, Knobler R, Ralfkiaer E, Santucci M, Smith N, Wechsler J, van Vloten WA, Meijer CJ. EORTC classification for primary cutaneous lymphomas: a proposal from the Cutaneous Lymphoma Study Group of the European Organization for Research and Treatment of Cancer. Blood 1997; 90:354–371.

33.2. Primary Cutaneous Diffuse Large B-cell Lymphomas, Other: T-cell-Rich B-cell Lymphoma

Dmitry V. Kazakov, Günter Burg, and Werner Kempf
Department of Dermatology, University Hospital, Zürich, Switzerland

CLASSIFICATION

WHO/EORTC Classification (2005): Diffuse large B-cell lymphoma, other
WHO Classification (2001): Diffuse large B-cell lymphoma, variant
REAL Classification (1997): Not listed
EORTC Classification (1997): Not listed

DEFINITION

Primary cutaneous T-cell-rich B-cell lymphoma (TCRBCL) in the WHO/EORTC-consensus classification belongs to primary cutaneous diffuse large B-cell lymphoma, other. It is defined by the predominance (75–90%) of non-neoplastic T cells admixed with scattered tumoral B cells. Primary cutaneous TCRBCL is extremely rare, with less than 20 reported cases.

CLINICAL FEATURES

Men are affected more frequently than women (male:female = 14:3). Patients with primary cutaneous TCRBCL are usually middle-aged (mean age 58 years, range 30–87 years) (1–8). The cutaneous lesions are usually solitary nodules or sometimes deep subcutaneous tumors. Multiple lesions are rare (2). The most frequent site of involvement is the head and neck area.

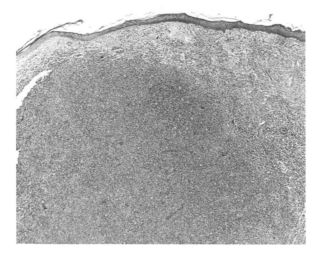

Figure 1   Dense diffuse lymphocytic infiltrate in the entire dermis.

HISTOLOGY

The infiltrate is usually diffuse and consists mainly of small lymphocytes some of which have irregular nuclear contours, epithelioid histiocytes, and plasma cells (Fig. 1). Large neoplastic B cells constitute the minority of the infiltrate and can thus be easily over-looked. The tumor cells are scattered large pleomorphic cells with clear cytoplasm and multilobular nuclei resembling Hodgkin or Reed–Sternberg cells (Fig. 2). Centro-blasts and immunoblasts can be observed. Marked vascular proliferation is found in some cases (3–5).

IMMUNOHISTOCHEMISTRY

The large neoplastic cells express pan-B-cell antigens CD20 and CD79a, but are negative for CD15 and CD30 (Fig. 3). Light chain restriction is usually found.

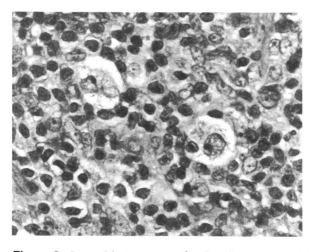

Figure 2   Large blasts representing B cells surrounded by small T lymphocytes.

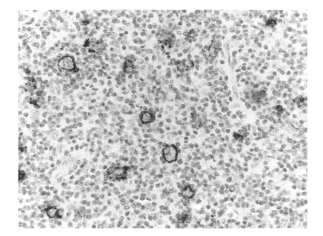

Figure 3 Scattered CD20-positive B cells (red color) in the background of T-cells.

The reactive small cell population represents T-helper cells but small reactive B cells can also be found (6).

MOLECULAR BIOLOGY

IgH gene rearrangements are found in the majority of cases.

TREATMENT

Radiation therapy, chemotherapy, or surgery alone or in various combinations have been administered with good results (4,6,7).

Cutaneous T-cell-rich B-cell lymphoma

Clinical features
  Elderly patients, male predilection
  Solitary nodules in head and neck region
Histological features
  Small lymphocytes and histiocytes (75–90%), few large cells (pleomorphic, immunoblasts,or centroblasts)
Immunophenotype
  Large cells: pan-B-cell antigens+, CD15–, CD30–
  Light chain restriction (not in all cases)
  Small cells: reactive T-helpers
Molecular biology
  IgH rearrangement in majority of cases
Treatment
  Radiation therapy, chemotherapy, or surgery
Clinical course
  Unknown

CLINICAL COURSE AND PROGNOSIS

Long-term follow-up has only been reported for a small number of patients with primary cutaneous TCRBCL. After a median follow-up of two years, most patients were alive. It appears that the prognosis in primary cutaneous TCRBCL is better than in the nodal counterpart.

DIFFERENTIAL DIAGNOSIS

The histological picture in TCRBCL may resemble that seen in the lymphocyte-predominant type of Hodgkin lymphoma or small to medium-sized pleomorphic T-cell lymphoma. The former involves the skin only on very rare occasions and can be differentiated from TCRBCL by expression of CD15 and CD30 on the large cells. The Detection of B-cell clonality allows the distinction of TCRBCL from T-cell lymphomas (8).

COMMENTS

The cause of the prominent T-cell infiltration in primary TCRBCL has not been elucidated. In the nodal disease, it has been explained by increased interleukin-4 production by tumor cells or EBV infection.

REFERENCES

1. Li S, Griffin CA, Mann RB, Borowitz MJ. Primary cutaneous T-cell-rich B-cell lymphoma: clinically distinct from its nodal counterpart? Mod Pathol 2001; 14:10–13.
2. Sander CA, Kaudewitz P, Kutzner H, Simon M, Schirren CG, Sioutos N, Cossman J, Plewig G, Kind P, Jaffe ES. T-cell-rich B-cell lymphoma presenting in skin. A clinico-pathologic analysis of six cases. J Cutan Pathol 1996; 23:101–108.
3. Arai E, Sakurai M, Nakayama H, Morinaga S, Katayama I. Primary cutaneous T-cell-rich B-cell lymphoma. Br J Dermatol 1993; 129:196–200.
4. Dommann SN, Dommann-Scherrer CC, Zimmerman D, Dours-Zimmermann MT, Hassam S, Burg G. Primary cutaneous T-cell-rich B-cell lymphoma. A case report with a 13-year follow-up. Am J Dermatopathol 1995; 17:618–624.
5. Dunphy CH, Nahass GT. Primary cutaneous T-cell-rich B-cell lymphomas with flow cytometric immunophenotypic findings. Report of 3 cases and review of the literature. Arch Pathol Lab Med 1999; 123:1236–1240.
6. Kamarashev J, Dummer R, Schmidt MH, Kempf W, Kurrer MO, Burg G. Primary cutaneous T-cell-rich B-cell lymphoma and Hodgkin's disease in a patient with Gardner's syndrome. Dermatology 2000; 201:362–365.
7. Wollina U. Complete response of a primary cutaneous T-cell-rich B cell lymphoma treated with interferon alpha2a. J Cancer Res Clin Oncol 1998; 124:127–129.
8. Take H, Kubota K, Fukuda T, Shinonome S, Ishikawa O, Shirakura T. An indolent type of Epstein–Barr virus-associated T-cell-rich B-cell lymphoma of the skin: report of a case. Am J Hematol 1996; 52:221–223.

34

Intravascular Large B-cell Lymphoma

Günter Burg, Werner Kempf, and Dmitry V. Kazakov
Department of Dermatology, University Hospital, Zürich, Switzerland

CLASSIFICATION

WHO/EORTC Classification (2005): Intravascular large B-cell lymphoma
WHO Classification (2001): Intravascular large B-cell lymphoma (IV-LBL)
REAL Classification (1997): Diffuse large B-cell lymphoma
EORTC Classification (1997): Intravascular large B-cell lymphoma (provisional
   entity)

DEFINITION

Intravascular large B-cell lymphoma (IV-LBL) belongs to the group of diffuse large B-cell lymphomas, other, and in most of the cases, IVL is a systemic disease from the very beginning. It is a rare high-grade malignant type of extranodal large cell lymphoma, characterized by the presence of tumor cells in the lumina of small vessels, particularly capillaries and venules especially of the skin and the nervous system. The tumor cells express B-cell markers in the vast majority of cases. Rare tumors have a T-cell phenotype (see Comments). Other synonyms include systemic angioendotheliomatosis (1), intravascular lymphomatosis, and Tappeiner–Pfleger syndrome. This rare disease was initially regarded as a neoplastic proliferation of endothelial cells. Neoplastic angioendotheliomatosis has to be differentiated from reactive angioendotheliomatosis, which demonstrates a wide clinicopathologic spectrum in conjunction with a variety of underlying systemic inflammatory or neoplastic diseases (2,3).

CLINICAL FEATURES

Classical IV-LBL shows erythematous or violaceous plaques or nodules on the face, trunk or lower extremities (4,5). Clinically, they closely resemble livedo racemosa. Other lesions mimic erythema nodosum (6). Coexistence with hemangiomas has been reported (7). Neurologic signs and symptoms are also frequent. In contrast, the Asian variant of intravascular large B-cell lymphoma is characterized by

269

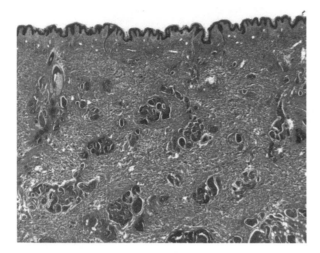

Figure 1 Scattered infiltrates of lymphocytic cells in the mid and deep dermis. (Histologic specimen kindly provided by H. Kutzner)

hemophagocytic syndrome with pancytopenia and hepatosplenomegaly without cutaneous or neurological abnormalities (8).

HISTOLOGY

The microscopic features are very pathognomonic showing a dense proliferation of atypical large lymphoid cells with round or oval nuclei within the lumina of small blood vessels (Figs. 1 and 2).

IMMUNOHISTOCHEMISTRY

In the more prevalent B-cell form, neoplastic cells are positive for CD20 and negative for CD3, CD43, CD23, and cyclin D1 (Bcl-1) protein. Some cases are CD5-positive

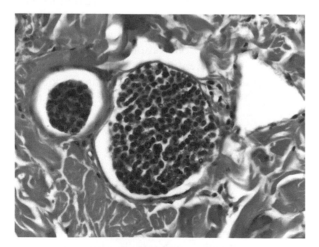

Figure 2 Atypical lymphocytic cells with round or oval nuclei within the lumina of small blood vessels. (Histologic specimen kindly provided by H. Kutzner)

(9). However, the biologic significance of CD5 antigen expression in cases of IV-LBL is uncertain. These neoplasms might arise from a separate lineage of CD5-positive B-cells or from a specific, early stage of B-cell differentiation. Alternatively, some investigators have suggested that CD5 antigen expression by B-cells is a marker of activation (9,10).

MOLECULAR BIOLOGY

IV-LBLL shows rearrangements of IgH family genes. Structural aberrations in chromosomes 1, 6, and 18, especially 1p and trisomy 18 have been found in some cases (11). Mutations of p53, p16, and p21 genes are rarely found in IV-LBL (12). EBV-associated intravascular lymphomatosis has been reported with Kaposi sarcoma in an AIDS patient (13).

CD29 (beta1 integrin subunit), CD43 (leukosialin), CD44 (H-CAM), CD54 (ICAM-1), embryonal N-CAM (e-NCAM), and EMA (episialin) are molecules known to be involved in lymphocyte and endothelial adhesion processes (14). Intravascular neoplastic lymphocytes react for CD44, but are negative for CD29 and for CD54. Considering that CD29 is critical for lymphocyte trafficking in general and for transvascular migration in particular, and that CD54 is also involved in transvascular lymphocyte migration, their absence in intravascular lymphomatosis may contribute to the intravascular and disseminated distribution pattern (14).

THERAPY

Since IV-BCL is a systemic disease with widespread dissemination, thorough staging investigations are mandatory early in the course of the disease. Special emphasis has to be addressed to the involvement of the central nervous system, the lung, kidney, and adrenals (15). Multiagent chemotherapy (CHOP) is the standard treatment (16). Successful treatment with high-dose chemotherapy and autologous peripheral blood stem cell transplantation (17) or autologous bone marrow transplantation (18) has been reported.

CLINICAL COURSE AND PROGNOSIS

In contrast to other cutaneous B-cell lymphomas, the intravascular B-cell lymphoma shows a bad prognosis. The clinical course is variable, but the disease cannot be cured (19). The involvement of the central nervous system is the most important prognostic factor.

DIFFERENTIAL DIAGNOSIS

The most important differential diagnosis is reactive (benign) angioendotheliomatosis, which shares similar histological and ultrastructural features but is clinically distinct from its neoplastic counterpart (2,3). The reactive variant has been associated with subacute bacterial endocarditis, peripheral vascular atherosclerosis, dermal amyloid angiopathy, antiphospholipid syndrome, iatrogenic arteriovenous

---

Intravascular large B-cell lymphoma

Clinical features
  Erythematous or violaceous plaques or nodules on the face, trunk, or lower
    extremities
  Livedo racemosa or erythema nodosum-like features
  Neurologic signs and symptoms
Histological features
  Small dermal vessels filled by large lymphocytes
Immunophenotype
  CD20+, CD23−, and cyclin D1−
  Some cases CD5+
  Rare T-cell cases (CD3+)
Molecular biology
  Clonal IgH rearrangement
Treatment
  Multiagent chemotherapy
Clinical course and prognosis
  Poor prognosis

---

fistulas underlying hepatopathy and hypertensive portal gastropathy, and in chronic
lymphatic leukemia.

Erythema nodosum may be a clinical differential diagnosis in some cases of
IV-BCL (6). Reactive and neoplastic angioendotheliomatosis show some differences
in the immunocytochemical pattern using antibodies to leukocyte common antigen
(LCA), specialized B- and T-lymphocytic determinants, Factor VIII-related antigen
(FVIIIRAG), blood group isoantigens A, B, and H, epithelial antigens, vimentin,
and actin, and Ulex europaeus I lectin (20).

COMMENTS

Rare cases of intravascular lymphomas represent T-cell lymphomas (21–24). These
tumors may be associated with EBV infection (24).

REFERENCES

1. Pfleger L, Tappeiner J. Zur Kenntnis der systemisierten endotheliomatose der cutanen
   blutgefaesse (reticuloendotheliomatose?). Hautarzt 1959; 10:359–363.
2. Lazova R, Slater C, Scott G. Reactive angioendotheliomatosis. Case report and review
   of the literature. Am J Dermatopathol 1996; 18:63–69.
3. McMenamin ME, Fletcher CD. Reactive angioendotheliomatosis: a study of 15 cases
   demonstrating a wide clinicopathologic spectrum. Am J Surg Pathol 2002; 26:685–697.
4. Berger TG, Dawson NA. Angioendotheliomatosis. J Am Acad Dermatol 1988; 18:
   407–412.
5. Perniciaro C, Winkelmann RK, Daoud MS, Su WPD. Malignant angioendotheliomatosis
   is an angiotropic intravascular lymphoma. Immunohistochemical, ultrastructural, and
   molecular genetics studies. Am J Dermatopathol 1995; 17:242–248.

6. Kiyohara T, Kumakiri M, Kobayashi H, Shimizu T, Ohkawara A, Ohnuki M. A case of intravascular large B-cell lymphoma mimicking erythema nodosum: the importance of multiple skin biopsies. J Cutan Pathol 2000; 27:413–418.

7. Rubin MA, Cossman J, Freter CE, Azumi N. Intravascular large cell lymphoma coexisting within hemangiomas of the skin. Am J Surg Pathol 1997; 21:860–864.

8. Murase T, Nakamura S. An Asian variant of intravascular lymphomatosis: an updated review of malignant histiocytosis-like B-cell lymphoma. Leuk Lymphoma 1999; 33: 459–473.

9. Khalidi HS, Brynes RK, Browne P, Koo CH, Battifora H, Medeiros LJ. Intravascular large B-cell lymphoma: the CD5 antigen is expressed by a subset of cases. Mod Pathol 1998; 11:983–988.

10. Kanda M, Suzumiya J, Ohshima K, Tamura K, Kikuchi M. Intravascular large cell lymphoma: clinicopathological, immuno-histochemical and molecular genetic studies. Leuk Lymphoma 1999; 34:569–580.

11. Tsukadaira A, Okubo Y, Ogasawara H, Urushibata K, Honda T, Miura I, Kubo K. Chromosomal aberrations in intravascular lymphomatosis. Am J Clin Oncol 2002; 25:178–181.

12. Abe S, Kumanishi T. Molecular genetic analysis of intravascular malignant lymphomatosis cells. Rinsho Shinkeigaku 1995; 35:1473–1475.

13. Hsiao CH, Su IJ, Hsieh SW, Huang SF, Tsai TF, Chen MY, How SW. Epstein–Barr virus-associated intravascular lymphomatosis within Kaposi's sarcoma in an AIDS patient. Am J Surg Pathol 1999; 23:482–487.

14. Ponzoni M, Arrigoni G, Gould VE, Del Curto B, Maggioni M, Scapinello A, Paolino S, Cassisa A, Patriarca C. Lack of CD 29 (beta1 integrin) and CD 54 (ICAM-1) adhesion molecules in intravascular lymphomatosis. Hum Pathol 2000; 31:220–226.

15. Baumann TP, Hurwitz N, Karamitopolou-Diamantis E, Probst A, Herrmann R, Steck AJ. Diagnosis and treatment of intravascular lymphomatosis. Arch Neurol 2000; 57:374–377.

16. Munakata S, Hirano S, Yoshiyama Y, Koizumi M, Kobayasi T, Hattori T. Beneficial effects of CHOP therapy in a case of intravascular large B-cell lymphoma diagnosed by skin biopsy. Rinsho Shinkeigaku 2000; 40:476–479.

17. Koizumi M, Nishimura M, Yokota A, Munekata S, Kobayashi T, Saito Y. Successful treatment of intravascular malignant lymphomatosis with high-dose chemotherapy and autologous peripheral blood stem cell transplantation. Bone Marrow Transplant 2001; 27:1101–1103.

18. Rose C, Staumont D, Jouet JP. Successful autologous bone marrow transplantation in intravascular lymphomatosis. Br J Haematol 1999; 105:313–314.

19. Bogomolski-Yahalom V, Lossos IS, Okun E, Sherman Y, Lossos A, Polliack A. Intravascular lymphomatosis—an indolent or aggressive entity? Leuk Lymphoma 1998; 29:585–593.

20. Wick MR, Rocamora A. Reactive and malignant "angioendotheliomatosis": a discriminant clinicopathological study. J Cutan Pathol 1988; 15:260–271.

21. Sepp N, Schuler G, Romani N, Geissler D, Gattringer C, Burg G, Bartram CR, Fritsch P. "Intravascular lymphomatosis" (angioendotheliomatosis): evidence for a T-cell origin in two cases. Hum Pathol 1990; 21:1051–1058.

22. Sangueza O, Hyder DM, Sangueza P. Intravascular lymphomatosis: report of an unusual case with T cell phenotype occurring in an adolescent male. J Cutan Pathol 1992; 19: 226–231.

23. Setoyama M, Mizoguchi S, Orikawa T, Tashiro M. A case of intravascular malignant lymphomatosis (angiotropic large-cell lymphoma) presenting memory T cell phenotype and its expression of adhesion molecules. J Dermatol 1992; 19:263–269.

24. Malicki DM, Suh YK, Fuller GN, Shin SS. Angiotropic (intravascular) large cell lymphoma of T-cell phenotype presenting as acute appendicitis in a patient with acquired immunodeficiency syndrome. Arch Pathol Lab Med 1999; 123:335–337.

35

B-cell Lymphomas with Common Secondary Cutaneous Involvement

35.1. Lymphomatoid Granulomatosis

Günter Burg and Werner Kempf
Deptment of Dermatology, University Hospital, Zürich, Switzerland

CLASSIFICATION

WHO/EORTC Classification (2005): Not listed
WHO Classification (2001): Lymphomatoid granulomatosis
REAL Classification (1997): Not listed
EORTC Classification (1997): Not listed

DEFINITION

Lymphomatoid granulomatosis (LYG), originally described by Liebow et al. (1), is a rare multisystemic angiocentric and angiodestructive lymphoproliferative disease involving extranodal sites, especially the lungs, skin, and nervous system. It is EBV+ in most cases and may progress to diffuse large B-cell lymphoma.

CLINICAL FEATURES

Lymphomatoid granulomatosis affects usually adults, but cases have been described in children (2). The most common sites of involvement are the lungs. Almost all patients have pulmonary manifestations during their disease course. The other two commonly involved organs are the brain and kidneys. Malignant lymphoma involving lymph nodes develop in 12% of patients. About 50% of the patients with LYG have skin involvement (3). Exclusive cutaneous involvement is rare and may be associated with a better outcome. The clinical features of cutaneous LYG are extremely diverse (4) and generally transient (5). Multiple erythematous dermal papules and/or subcutaneous nodules, with or without ulceration, facial edema, and folliculitis-like eruptions (5–7) may be present. Frequently, patients who have early cutaneous involvement with LYG, later develop nervous system and joint manifestations (5).

HISTOLOGY

There is a nodular, angiocentric and angiodestructive dense, polymorphous, lympho-histiocytic infiltrate in the dermis and subcutaneous tissue leading to necrosis. Angio-destruction is less evident in the skin compared to other organs. The infiltrate surrounds and invades not only vessels but also nerves and epidermal appendages (8). In some cases, atypical lymphocytes can be present.

IMMUNOHISTOCHEMISTRY

The tumor cells are EBV+, CD20+ B-cells. They are often few in number and obscured by a prominent T-cell rich infiltrate.

MOLECULAR BIOLOGY

Most cases of LYG show clonal rearrangement of immunoglobulin H genes. Although the predominant infiltrating cells are T cells, the T-cell receptor genes are not clonally rearranged. These findings indicate that LYG is an angiocentric T-cell-rich B-cell lymphoproliferative disorder (9,10). EBV sequences can be loca-lized to B cells and are clonal in most cases. Contrarily to the extracutaneous forms of lymphomatoid granulomatosis, it is difficult or impossible to detect Epstein–Barr virus DNA sequences in primary and isolated cutaneous lymphomatoid granulomatosis (11,12).

Recent studies implicate the chemokines IP-10 and Mig in the pathogenesis of the vascular damage. Most patients have defects in cytotoxic T-cell function and reduced levels of CD8+ T cells (13).

TREATMENT

Some cases of LYG regress spontaneously, but most patients require therapy (4). As optimal therapy is unknown, attempts have been made with cyclophosphamide and prednisone, aggressive combination chemotherapy consisting of methotrexate, dox-orubicin, cyclophosphamide, vincristine, prednisone, and bleomycin (MACOP-B) (14) and interferon-alpha 2b (13–15). Surgery and radiation (16) therapy may be helpful in selected patients with localized disease (17).

CLINICAL COURSE AND PROGNOSIS

The prognosis of LYG varies widely. Adverse prognostic factors include neurologic manifestations, and presence of large numbers of atypical lymphoreticular cells within the infiltrates. Unilateral chest lesions and large numbers of small lymphocytes

Lymphomatoid granulomatosis

Clinical features
  Pulmonary involvement
  Skin involvement common, but usually not specific
Histological features
  Angiocentric and angiodestructive infiltrate of polymorphous lymphohistiocytic
    infiltrate
Immunophenotype
  Tumor cells CD20+ and EBV+, reactive cells CD3+
Molecular biology
  Clonal IgH rearrangement, EBV
Treatment
  Multiagent chemotherapy or interferon-alpha
Clinical course and prognosis
  Unfavorable prognosis. In exclusively cutaneous involvement more favorable

and histiocytes within the infiltrate seem to be associated with a better prognosis. Almost two-thirds of patients die and the median survival is only 14 months (18).

DIFFERENTIAL DIAGNOSIS

Lymphomatoid granulomatosis has to be differentiated from extranodal NK/T-cell lymphoma, nasal type that also often is EBV+ and may show an angiocentric, angiodestructive growth pattern. Wegener granulomatosis and midline granuloma are further differential diagnoses to be considered (19).

REFERENCES

1. Liebow AA, Carrington CR, Friedman PJ. Lymphomatoid granulomatosis. Hum Pathol 1972; 3:457–558.
2. Pisani RJ, DeRemee RA. Clinical implications of the histopathologic diagnosis of pulmonary lymphomatoid granulomatosis. Mayo Clin Proc 1990; 65:151–163.
3. Brodell RT, Miller CW, Eisen AZ. Cutaneous lesions of lymphomatoid granulomatosis. Arch Dermatol 1986; 122:303–306.
4. Beaty MW, Toro J, Sorbara L, Stern JB, Pittaluga S, Raffeld M, Wilson WH, Jaffe ES. Cutaneous lymphomatoid granulomatosis: correlation of clinical and biologic features. Am J Surg Pathol 2001; 25:1111–1120.
5. James WD, Odom RB, Katzenstein AL. Cutaneous manifestations of lymphomatoid granulomatosis. Report of 44 cases and a review of the literature. Arch Dermatol 1981; 117:196–202.
6. Wood ML, Harrington CI, Slater DN, Rooney N, Clark A. Cutaneous lymphomatoid granulomatosis: a rare cause of recurrent skin ulceration. Br J Dermatol 1984; 110:619–625.
7. Carlson KC, Gibson LE. Cutaneous signs of lymphomatoid granulomatosis. Arch Dermatol 1991; 127:1693–1698.
8. Jambrosic J, From L, Assaad DA, Lipa M, Sibbald RG, Walter JB. Lymphomatoid granulomatosis. J Am Acad Dermatol 1987; 17:621–631.

9.   Donner LR, Dobin S, Harrington D, Bassion S, Rappaport ES, Peterson RF. Angio-
     centric immunoproliferative lesion (lymphomatoid granulomatosis). A cytogenetic,
     immunophenotypic, and genotypic study. Cancer 1990; 65:249–254.
10. McNiff JM, Cooper D, Howe G, Crotty PL, Tallini G, Crouch J, Eisen RN. Lympho-
     matoid granulomatosis of the skin and lung. An angiocentric T-cell-rich B-cell lympho-
     proliferative disorder. Arch Dermatol 1996; 132:1464–1470.
11. Angel CA, Slater DN, Royds JA, Nelson SN, Bleehen SS. Epstein–Barr virus in
     cutaneous lymphomatoid granulomatosis. Histopathology 1994; 25:545–548.
12. Tas S, Simonart T, Dargent J, Kentos A, Antoine M, Knoop C, Estenne M,
     De Dobbeleer G. Primary and isolated cutaneous lymphomatoid granulomatosis follow-
     ing heart–lung transplantation. Ann Dermatol Venereol 2000; 127:488–491.
13. Jaffe ES, Wilson WH. Lymphomatoid granulomatosis: pathogenesis, pathology and
     clinical implications. Cancer Surv 1997; 30:233–248.
14. Jenkins TR, Zaloznik AJ. Lymphomatoid granulomatosis. A case for aggressive therapy.
     Cancer 1989; 64:1362–1365.
15. Bohle M, Rasche K, Muller KM, Schultze-Werninghaus G, Fisseler-Eckhoff A. Lym-
     phomatoide granulomatose: differentialdiagnose und therapie. Med Klin 1999; 94:
     513–519.
16. Nair BD, Joseph MG, Catton GE, Lach B. Radiation therapy in lymphomatoid granu-
     lomatosis. Cancer 1989; 64:821–824.
17. Patton WF, Lynch JP III. Lymphomatoid granulomatosis. Clinicopathologic study of
     four cases and literature review. Medicine (Baltimore) 1982; 61:1–12.
18. Katzenstein AL, Carrington CB, Liebow AA. Lymphomatoid granulomatosis: a clinico-
     pathologic study of 152 cases. Cancer 1979; 43:360–373.
19. Stamenkovic I, Toccanier MF, Kapanci Y. Polymorphic reticulosis (lethal midline
     granuloma) and lymphomatoid granulomatosis: identical or distinct entities? Virchows
     Arch A Pathol Anat Histol 1981; 390:81–91.

Burkitt Lymphoma

Günter Burg, Werner Kempf, and Dmitry V. Kazakov
Department of Dermatology, University Hospital, Zürich, Switzerland

CLASSIFICATION

WHO/EORTC Classification (2005): Not listed
WHO Classification (2001): Burkitt lymphoma/leukemia
REAL Classification (1997): Burkitt lymphoma
EORTC Classification (1997): Not listed

DEFINITION

Burkitt lymphoma (BL) is an aggressive B-cell lymphoma-associated with Epstein–Barr virus infection (EBV) in most cases and featuring translocation of the c-myc gene (1).

CLINICAL FEATURES

Burkitt lymphoma occurs endemically in children in the "lymphoma belt" of Central Africa and in Papua. The incidence peaks at 4–8 years of age with a male:female ratio of 2:1. Sporadic cases are seen in children and young adults throughout the rest of the world (2,3). It is also seen in association with HIV induced immunodeficiency (4). Because BL is so common in Africa, it accounts for 30–50% of all childhood lymphomas. In the United States and Europe, it makes up only 1–2% of all B-cell lymphomas. The most frequently involved sites are the jaws, ovaries, testes, thyroid, adrenals, and breasts, i.e., tissues that are comparatively poor in lymphoreticular elements. Patients present with large tumors due to the high proliferation rate and rapid growth of BL (Fig. 1). The skin may show secondary involvement (5) or indicates relapse of BL (6,7).

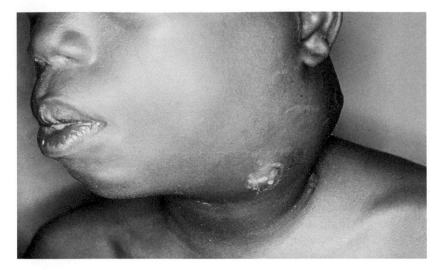

Figure 1 Tumor with fistulation on the neck of a child. (From Ref. 8.)

HISTOLOGY

A cohesive monotonous infiltrate composed of medium-sized cells with round or ovoid nuclei and fine or coarse granular chromatin is seen. The cytoplasm is deeply basophilic and usually contains lipid vacuoles. There are many mitotic figures and a high rate of spontaneous cell death. The apoptotic tumor cells are ingested by macrophages whose scattered distribution creates the typical "starry sky" pattern (Figs. 2 and 3). Variants of this classical histological type have been described. Skin infiltrates display the same histo- and cytomorphological features (8).

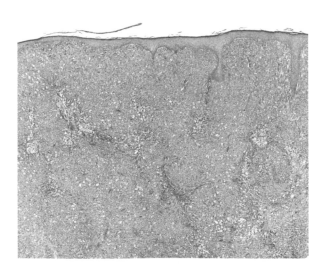

Figure 2 Dense diffuse lympocytic infiltrate in the entire dermis.

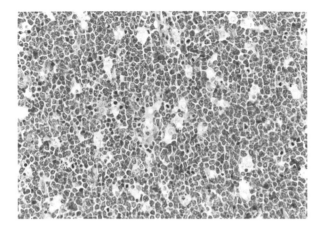

Figure 3 Dense infiltrate of plasmacytoid cells with intermingled tingible body macrophages (starry sky pattern).

IMMUNOHISTOCHEMISTRY

The tumor cells express B-cell associated antigens (CD19, CD20, CD22), are positive for CD10, Bcl-6 (pointing to a germinal center origin), and are negative for CD5, CD23, Bcl-2, and TdT.

MOLECULAR BIOLOGY

There is clonal rearrangement of the immunoglobulin (Ig) heavy and light chain genes. The typical feature is the t(8;14) translocation of the myc-gene, which by this comes under the influence of the Ig-gene promoters on chromosome 14.

Burkitt lymphoma

Clinical features
   Bulky tumors typically involving head and neck with secondary skin involvement
Histological features
   Dense diffuse infiltrate of medium-sized tumor cells with scattered macrophages
      (starry sky pattern)
Immunophenotype
   CD10+, CD19+, CD20+, CD22+, Bcl-6+, CD5–, CD23–, Bcl-2–, and TdT–
Molecular biology
   Clonal IgH rearrangement
      EBV
Treatment
   Multiagent chemotherapy
Clinical course and prognosis
   Favorable prognosis

Epstein–Barr virus is not exclusively essential in the pathogenesis of BL but plays an important role especially in endemic BL inducing a long lasting polyclonal activation of B-lymphocytes, which may favor the development of lymphoma, due to defective T-cell regulation of EBV-infected B-cells. Low socioeconomic status and early EBV infection are associated with a higher prevalence of EBV positive BL (9). HIV infection also predisposes to BL by causing both T- and B-cell alterations (4).

TREATMENT

Intensive polychemotherapy cures up to 90% of children with classic BL (10,11). This treatment may be combined with autologous stem cell (12) or autologous bone marrow transplantation (13,14).

CLINICAL COURSE AND PROGNOSIS

Until the mid-1980, the prognosis was very poor with very few long-term survivors. Failures were mainly due to central nervous system and bone marrow involvement. Today, the outlook for patients with BL, who are properly treated, is favorable.

DIFFERENTIAL DIAGNOSIS

Histologically, "starry sky"-like features are also found in B-cell pseudolymphomas, in T-cell rich B-cell lymphomas of the skin (15), and in lymphocyte-rich Hodgkin lymphoma.

COMMENTS

Some experts use the term "Burkitt-like" lymphoma for either the nonclassical presentation of BL or for tumors lacking association with EBV. Rarely, patients may present with bone marrow involvement and leukemic phase of the disease.

REFERENCES

1. Burkitt D. A sarcoma involving the jaws in African children. Br J Surg 1958; 46:218–223.
2. O'Conor GT, Rappaport H, Smith EB. Childhood lymphoma resembling "Burkitt tumor" in the United States. Cancer 1965; 18:411–417.
3. Mann RB, Jaffe ES, Braylan RC, Nanba K, Frank MM, Ziegler JL, Berard CW. Non-endemic Burkitts's lymphoma. A B-cell tumor related to germinal centers. N Engl J Med 1976; 295:685–691.
4. Raphael M, Gentilhomme O, Tulliez M, Byron PA, Diebold J. Histopathologic features of high-grade non-Hodgkin's lymphomas in acquired immunodeficiency syndrome. The French Study Group of Pathology for Human Immunodeficiency Virus-Associated Tumors. Arch Pathol Lab Med 1991; 115:15–20.
5. Rogge T. Burkitt's lymphoma with skin infiltrates. Hautarzt 1975; 26:379–382.

6. Bonilla Velasco FA, Agud Aparicio J, Martinez Arronte F, Rodriguez Illera E, Durantez Martinez A. Unspecified Burkitt's lymphoma with cutaneous involvement. Rev Clin Esp 1979; 152:399–402.

7. Bachmeyer C, Bazarbachi A, Rio B, Delmer A, Hunault M, Zittoun R, Le Tourneau A, Aractingi S. Specific cutaneous involvement indicating relapse of Burkitt's lymphoma [letter]. Am J Hematol 1997; 54:176.

8. Burg G, Braun-Falco O. Cutaneous lymphomas, pseudolymphomas and related disorders. Berlin, Heidelberg, New York, Tokyo: Springer-Verlag, 1983.

9. Facer CA, Playfair JH. Malaria, Epstein–Barr virus, and the genesis of lymphomas. Adv Cancer Res 1989; 53:33–72.

10. Baruchel A, Schaison G. Recent advances in B cell acute lymphoblastic leukemia (Burkitt leukemia) therapy in childhood. Nouv Rev Fr Hematol 1993; 35:106–108.

11. Patte C, Michon J, Frappaz D, Leverger G, Rubie H, Soussain C, Pico JL. Therapy of Burkitt and other B-cell acute lymphoblastic leukaemia and lymphoma: experience with the LMB protocols of the SFOP (French Paediatric Oncology Society) in children and adults. Baillieres Clin Haematol 1994; 7:339–348.

12. Sweetenham JW, Pearce R, Taghipour G, Blaise D, Gisselbrecht C, Goldstone AH. Adult Burkitt's and Burkitt-like non-Hodgkin's lymphoma-outcome for patients treated with high-dose therapy and autologous stem-cell transplantation in first remission or at relapse: results from the European Group for Blood and Marrow Transplantation. J Clin Oncol 1996; 14:2465–2472.

13. Jost LM, Jacky E, Dommann-Scherrer C, Honegger HP, Maurer R, Sauter C, Stahel RA. Short-term weekly chemotherapy followed by high-dose therapy with autologous bone marrow transplantation for lymphoblastic and Burkitt's lymphomas in adult patients. Ann Oncol 1995; 6:445–451.

14. Weinthal JA, Goldman SC, Lenarsky C. Successful treatment of relapsed Burkitt's lymphoma using unrelated cord blood transplantation as consolidation therapy. Bone Marrow Transplant 2000; 25:1311–1313.

15. Dommann SN, Dommann SC, Zimmerman D, Dours ZM, Hassam S, Burg G. Primary cutaneous T-cell-rich B-cell lymphoma. A case report with a 13-year follow-up. Am J Dermatopathol 1995; 17:618–624.

Mantle Cell Lymphoma

Christian A. Sander and Michael J. Flaig
Department of Dermatology, LMU, Munich, Germany

CLASSIFICATION

WHO/EORTC Classification (2005): Not listed
WHO Classification (2001): Mantle cell lymphoma
REAL Classification (1997): Mantle cell lymphoma
EORTC Classification (1997): Not listed

DEFINITION

Mantle cell lymphoma is a B-cell lymphoma involving the mantle cells in the mantle zone of the lymphoid follicle, not infrequently secondarily involving the skin (1).

CLINICAL FEATURES

Approximately 4–6% of non-Hodgkin lymphomas are mantle cell lymphomas (2,3). Mantle cell lymphoma presenting in skin is a rare event, with only a few cases reported in the literature (4–6). Secondary skin involvement is seen in about 20% of mantle cell lymphoma with stage IV disease (7). Clinically, mantle cell lymphoma usually presents with nodules or plaques.

HISTOLOGY

Nodal mantle cell lymphoma in most cases has a diffuse or vaguely nodular pattern (2,8–10). Additionally, there are mantle cell lymphomas with a nodular growth pattern resembling follicular lymphoma and mantle cell lymphomas with a mantle zone pattern of growth (10). Cytologically, the lymphoid cells are small to medium sized,

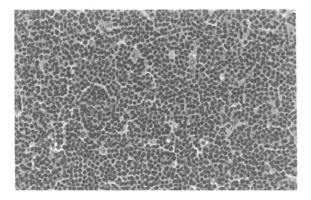

Figure 1 Small sized lymphocytes with scant cytoplasm.

usually slightly larger than normal lymphocytes, with more dispersed chromatin, scant pale cytoplasm, and inconspicuous nucleoli (Fig. 1). The nuclei have an irregular or cleaved configuration in most cases. In a small percentage of cases, the nuclei may be small and resemble those of small lymphocytes (9). Other rare cases are dominated by lymphocytes with features of lymphoblastic lymphoma, with larger nuclei with more finely dispersed chromatin and a high mitotic rate, recongnized as blastoid variant of mantle cell lymphoma in the WHO classification (9,11).

IMMUNOHISTOCHEMISTRY

The most specific marker for mantle cell lymphoma is expression of cyclin D1, as CD5 may also be expressed in rare cases of MALT lymphomas (12,13). Additionally, the lymphoid cells are CD20+, CD79a, CD43+, IgM+, IgD+, CD10–, CD23–, bcl-2+, bcl-6–. The expression of lambda light chains is more frequent than that of kappa light chains (1,14). The cells also show positivity of the cell membrane for alkaline phosphatase.

MOLECULAR BIOLOGY

Nodal mantle cell lymphomas have a characteristic chromosomal translocation, t(11;14). The bcl-1/Prad-1 gene, which is located on chromosome 11q13, is translocated to chromosome 14q32. As a result, cyclin D1 is overexpressed (14,15). By Northern blot analysis, virtually 100% of cases of mantle cell lymphoma show expression of Prad-1 (16). Data regarding the bcl-1 translocation in primary cutaneous mantle cell lymphomas are not available.

TREATMENT

Since primary cutaneous mantle cell lymphoma is extremely rare, our knowledge of therapeutic options is limited. If localized to the skin, therapy of a single lesion may

Mantle cell lymphoma

Clinical features
    Primary cutaneous involvement exceedingly rare. Nodules or plaques
Histological features
    Diffuse or nodular infiltrates of small to medium sized lymphoid cells with scant
        pale cytoplasm
Immunophenotype
    Cyclin D1+, CD5+, CD20+, CD79a+, CD43+, IgM+, IgD+, CD10−, CD23−,
        bcl-2+, bcl-6−
Molecular biology
    Translocation t(11;14)
Treatment
    Unknown
Clinical course and prognosis
    Primary cutaneous form unknown. Secondary form with unfavorable prognosis

consist of local radiotherapy and/or surgery. Treatment of cutaneous lesions of systemic mantle cell lymphoma should directed at the underlying disease.

CLINICAL COURSE AND PROGNOSIS

The prognosis of primary cutaneous mantle cell lymphoma is controversial in the literature. Survival times between 18 months after diagnosis (4) and 17 years (5) have been observed. The prognosis for nodal mantle cell lymphoma is unfavorable; the median survival is 3–5 years and cures are rare.

DIFFERENTIAL DIAGNOSIS

Since mantle cell lymphoma may resemble other B-cell lymphomas, such as follicular lymphoma, B-CLL, extranodal marginal zone B-cell lymphoma of MALT type, or pseudolymphomas with a B-cell immunophenotype, immunophenotypic studies are required for accurate diagnosis (17–19).

REFERENCES

1. Swerdlow SH, Berger F, Isaacson PI, Müller-Hermelink HK, Nathwani BN, Piris MA, Harris NL. In: Jaffe ES, Harris NL, Stein H, Vardiman J, eds. Pathology and Genetics of Tumours of Haematopoietic and Lymphoid Tissues. Lyon: IARC Press, 2001:168–170.
2. Coupland SE, Dallenbach FE, Stein H. Kleinzellige B-Zell Lymphome: differentialdiagnostische Leitlinien. Pathologe 2000; 21:147–161.
3. Bookman MA, Lardelli P, Jaffe ES, Duffey PL, Longo DL. Lymphocytic lymphoma of intermediate differentiation: morphologic, immunophenotypic, and prognostic factors. J Natl Cancer Inst 1990; 82:742–748.
4. Geerts ML, Busschots AM. Mantle-cell lymphomas of the skin. Dermatol Clin 1994; 12:409–417.

5. Bertero M, Novelli M, Fierro MT, Bernengo MG. Mantle zone lymphoma: an immuno-histologic study of skin lesions. J Am Acad Dermatol 1994; 30:23–30.

6. Marti RM, Campo E, Bosch F, Palou J, Estrach T. Cutaneous lymphocyte-associated antigen (CLA) expression in a lymphoblastoid mantle cell lymphoma presenting with skin lesions. Comparison with other clinicopathologic presentations of mantle cell lymphoma. J Cutan Pathol 2001; 28:256–264.

7. Ellison DJ, Turner RR, Van Antwerp R, Martin SE, Nathwani BN. High-grade mantle zone lymphoma. Cancer 1987; 60:2717–2720.

8. Banks PM, Chan J, Cleary ML, Delsol G, De Wolf-Peeters C, Gatter K, Grogan TM, Harris NL, Isaacson PG, Jaffe ES, et al. Mantle cell lymphoma. A proposal for unifica-tion of morphologic, immunologic, and molecular data. Am J Surg Pathol 1992; 16: 637–640.

9. Harris NL, Jaffe ES, Stein H, Banks PM, Chan JK, Cleary ML, Delsol G, De Wolf-Peeters C, Falini B, Gatter KC. A revised European–American classification of lymphoid neoplasms: a proposal from the International Lymphoma Study Group. Blood 1994; 84:1361–1392.

10. Medeiros LJ, Jaffe ES. Low-grade B-cell lymphomas not specified in the Working For-mulation. Jaffe ES, ed. Surgical Pathology of the Lymph Nodes and Related Organs. Philadelphia: WB Saunders, 1995:221–251.

11. Sander CA, Medeiros LJ, Abruzzo LV, Horak ID, Jaffe ES. Lymphoblastic lymphoma presenting in cutaneous sites. A clinicopathologic analysis of six cases. J Am Acad Dermatol 1991; 25:1023–1031.

12. Ferry JA, Yang WI, Zukerberg LR, Wotherspoon AC, Arnold A, Harris NL. CD5+ extranodal marginal zone B-cell (MALT) lymphoma. A low grade neoplasm with a propensity for bone marrow involvement and relapse. Am J Clin Pathol 1996; 105:31–37.

13. Ballesteros E, Osborne BM, Matsushima AY. CD5+ low-grade marginal zone B-cell lymphomas with localized presentation. Am J Surg Pathol 1998; 22:201–207.

14. Barista I, Romaguera EJ, Cabanillas F. Mantle-cell lymphoma. Lancet Oncol 2001; 2:141–148.

15. Raffeld M, Jaffe ES. bcl-1, t(11;14), and mantle cell-derived lymphomas. Blood 1991; 78:259–263.

16. Raffeld M, Sander CA, Yano T, Jaffe ES. Mantle cell lymphoma: an update. Leuk Lym-phoma 1992; 8:161–166.

17. Sander CA, Flaig MJ. Morphologic spectrum of cutaneous B-cell lymphomas. Dermatol Clin 1999; 17:593–599.

18. Sander CA, Flaig MJ, Jaffe ES. Cutaneous lymphomas: a proposal for a unified approach to classification. Clin Lymphoma, 2001: 2:86–100.

19. Flaig MJ, Sander CA. Diagnostik kutaner B-Zell Lymphome. Pathologe 2000; 21: 190–195.

Waldenström Macroglobulinemia

Dmitry V. Kazakov, Günter Burg, and Werner Kempf
Department of Dermatology, University Hospital, Zürich, Switzerland

CLASSIFICATION

WHO/EORTC Classification (2005): Not listed
WHO Classification (2001): Not listed
REAL Classification (1997): Not listed
EORTC Classification (1997): Not listed

DEFINITION

Waldenström macroglobulinemia (WM) is a hematological malignancy characterized by a clonal expansion of lymphocytes with plasmacytoid features that produce
a monoclonal IgM protein and infiltrate bone marrow, lymph nodes, and spleen. The
disease was initially described by Waldenström in 1944 (1).

CLINICAL FEATURES

Most patients with WM are adults in their sixth or seventh decade of life (median age
at the time of diagnosis is 65 years), with a slight male dominance (2,3). The clinical
features are highly variable, but the most common ones include fatigue, weight loss,
lymphadenopathy, anemia, hyperviscosity syndrome, and hepatosplenomegaly (4).
In some patients, the disease may be asymptomatic for a long time or is preceded
by monoclonal gammopathy of undetermined significance (MGUS) (5). Nonspecific
cutaneous changes of WM include urticarial and purpuric eruptions, ulcers, bullous
lesions, and vasculitides; they may be caused by the hyperviscosity syndrome and
paraprotein-associated autoimmune phenomena. Specific lesions result from the
infiltration of the skin by neoplastic cells or a product of these cells and are referred
to as lymphoplasmacytic infiltration of the skin and IgM storage papules, respectively. The IgM storage papules are asymptomatic, small, pearly, skin-colored,

discrete papules situated on the extensor aspects of the limbs, buttocks, or trunk. The papules may have hemorrhagic, crusted, or umbilicated centers. The specific cellular infiltration presents as asymptomatic infiltrative papules, plaques, or nodules (6–13).

HISTOLOGY

The storage papules represent deposits of IgM in the skin; one sees hyaline amorphous material in the dermis more prominent around blood vessels and adnexal structures. The material is PAS-positive and does not stain with Congo red dye and thioflavine-T; thus, it is not amyloid. The specific infiltrates contain a non-epidermotropic proliferation of small to medium-sized lymphocytes showing plasmacytoid features. These hybrid cells are sometimes referred to as "plymphs" (14). Mature plasma cells and small, well-differentiated lymphocytes are also observed.

IMMUNOHISTOCHEMISTRY

The tumor cells possess the immunophenotype consistent with late stage B-cell development with transformation into plasma cells (CD19+, CD20+, CD5−, CD10−, CD23−, CD79a+, CD138+/−) (4,5). The cells produce monoclonal IgM, usually kappa. The IgM deposits can be demonstrated by direct immunofluorescence.

MOLECULAR BIOLOGY

Monoclonal rearrangement of IgH genes has been demonstrated in the skin lesions (9).

Cutaneous involvement in Waldenström macroglobulinemia

Clinical features
   Elderly adults, multiple systemic symptoms including hyperviscosity syndrome
   Specific cutaneous changes with IgM storage papules and neoplastic cell
      infiltration
Histological features
   Storage papules: deposits of IgM as hyaline amorphous material
   Small to medium-sized "plymphs"
Immunophenotype
   CD19+, CD20+, CD5−, CD10−, CD23−, CD79a+, CD138+/−, often IgM-κ
Molecular biology
   Clonal IgH rearrangement
Treatment
   Chemotherapy
Clinical course and prognosis
   Usually chronic relapsing and remitting course
   Median survival 5 years

TREATMENT

Chemotherapy is generally required to treat the systemic manifestations.

CLINICAL COURSE AND PROGNOSIS

WM is currently considered an incurable condition characterized by a chronic relapsing and remitting course in most patients. Median survival is about 5 years. Old age (over 60 years), male sex, anemia (hemoglobin less than 10 g/L), and neutropenia (less than $1.7 \times 10^9/L$) are factors associated with a poorer prognosis (15). Death occurs because of organ failure, tumor spread, or complicating infection. It is not clear whether specific cutaneous infiltrates herald disease progression or not.

DIFFERENTIAL DIAGNOSIS

Clinical investigation is decisive in the differentiation of specific skin infiltrates of WM from primary cutaneous B-cell lymphomas. Neoplastic cells in primary cutaneous plasmacytoma and lesions of secondary skin involvement by multiple myeloma are atypical plasma cells (CD20−, CD79a+), in contrast to the "plymphs" (CD20+, CD79a+) of WM.

COMMENTS

The diagnosis of WM is based on the presence of a peak on serum immunoglobulin electrophoresis consisting of a monoclonal IgM (5,6). The serum M-component often exceeds 10 g/dL. In addition, bone marrow infiltration by the neoplastic cells with corresponding cytological and immunocytological features is required.

REFERENCES

1. Waldenström J. Incipient myelomatosis or essential hyperglobulinemia with fibrinogenopenia—new syndrome? Acta Med Scand 1944; 117:216–247.
2. Dimopoulos MA, Alexanian R. Waldenstrom's macroglobulinemia. Blood 1994; 83:1452–1459.
3. Herrinton LJ, Weiss NS. Incidence of Waldenstrom's macroglobulinemia. Blood 1993; 82:3148–3150.
4. Owen RG, Parapia LA, Richards SJ. Should Waldenstrom's macroglobulinaemia be considered part of the spectrum of marginal zone lymphoma? Blood 1999; 94(suppl 1):85 (Abstract).
5. Owen RG, Johnson SA, Morgan GJ. Waldenstrom macroglobulinaemia: laboratory diagnosis and treatment. Hematol Oncol 2000; 18:41–49.
6. Alexanian R, Weber D, Liu F. Differential diagnosis of monoclonal gammopathies. Arch Pathol Lab Med 1999; 123:108–113.
7. Whittaker SJ, Bhogal BS, Black MM. Acquired immunobullous disease: a cutaneous manifestation of IgM macroglobulinaemia. Br J Dermatol 1996; 135:283–286.
8. Finder KA, McCollough ML, Dixon SL, Majka AJ, Jaremko W. Hypergammaglobulinemic purpura of Waldenstrom. J Am Acad Dermatol 1990; 23:669–676.

9. Libow LF, Mawhinney JP, Bessinger GT. Cutaneous Waldenstrom's macroglobuline-mia: report of a case and overview of the spectrum of cutaneous disease. J Am Acad Dermatol 2001; 45:202–206.

10. Daoud MS, Lust JA, Kyle RA, Pittelkow MR. Monoclonal gammopathies and asso-ciated skin disorders. J Am Acad Dermatol 1999; 40:507–535, quiz 536–508.

11. Mascaro JM, Montserrat E, Estrach T, Feliu E, Ferrando J, Castel T, Mallolas J, Rozman C. Specific cutaneous manifestations of Waldenstrom's macroglobulinaemia. A report of two cases. Br J Dermatol 1982; 106:217–222.

12. Bergroth V, Reitamo S, Konttinen YT, Wegelius O. Skin lesions in Waldenstrom's macroglobulinaemia. Characterization of the cellular infiltrate. Acta Med Scand 1981; 209:129–131.

13. Appenzeller P, Leith CP, Foucar K, Scott AA, Bigler CF, Thompson CT. Cutaneous Wal-denstrom macroglobulinemia in transformation. Am J Dermatopathol 1999; 21:151–155.

14. Grogan TM, Spier CM. The B cell immunoproliferative disorders, including multiple myeloma and amyloidosis. In: Knowles DM, ed. Neoplastic Hematopathology. 1st ed. Baltimore: Williams and Wilkins, 1992:1235–1266.

15. Facon T, Brouillard M, Duhamel A, Morel P, Simon M, Jouet JP, Bauters F, Fenaux P. Prognostic factors in Waldenstrom's macroglobulinemia: a report of 167 cases. J Clin Oncol 1993; 11:1553–1558.

36

Other Forms of Cutaneous B-cell Lymphomas

36.1. Subcutaneous B-cell Lymphoma

Dmitry V. Kazakov, Günter Burg, and Werner Kempf
Department of Dermatology, University Hospital, Zürich, Switzerland

CLASSIFICATION

WHO/EORTC Classification (2005): Not listed
WHO Classification (2001): Not listed
REAL Classification (1997): Not listed
EORTC Classification (1997): Not listed

Exclusive involvement of subcutaneous tissue is the hallmark of subcutaneous panniculitis-like T-cell lymphoma. Primary cutaneous B-cell lymphomas (CBCL) sometimes show involvement of the subcutis but cases where the neoplastic infiltrate is confined to the adipose tissue are extremely rare. We have seen this phenomenon in a case of subcutaneous follicle center cell lymphoma (FCCL) (1). The tumor showed no differences from other primary cutaneous FCCL in regard to its morphology (except the peculiar location of the infiltrate), clinical behavior, and prognosis. A 54-year-old woman presented with a large deep-seated subcutaneous tumor on the scalp. Histologically, a dense infiltrate with a follicular growth pattern confined to the fat tissue with involvement of the underlying galea was seen (Fig. 1). The overlying dermis and epidermis were spared. Surgical removal of the tumor combined with orthovolt radiotherapy resulted in complete remission. Subsequently, a second case of primary subcutaneous FCCL has been identified (H. Kutzner, unpublished data). In addition, a case of primary cutaneous diffuse large B-cell lymphoma associated with the involvement of the subcutis, muscle tissue, and cranial nerves has been described (2).

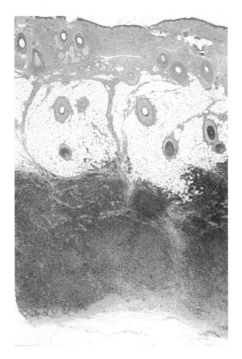

Figure 1 Dense diffuse lymphocytic infiltrate with a follicular growth pattern in the subcutis.

REFERENCES

1. Kazakov DV, Burg G, Dummer R, Palmedo G, Muller B, Kempf W. Primary subcutaneous follicular centre cell lymphoma with involvement of the galea: a case report and short review of the literature. Br J Dermatol 2002; 146:663–666.
2. Amo Y, Tanei R, Yonemoto K, Katsuoka K, Mori M. Diffuse large B-cell lymphoma associated with skin, muscle and cranial nerve involvement. Eur J Dermatol 2000; 10:306–308.

36.2. Cutaneous B-cell Lymphoma with Signet Ring-Cell Morphology

Dmitry V. Kazakov, Günter Burg, and Werner Kempf
Department of Dermatology, University Hospital, Zürich, Switzerland

CLASSIFICATION

WHO/EORTC Classification (2005): Not listed
WHO Classification (2001): Not listed
REAL Classification (1997): Not listed
EORTC Classification (1997): Not listed

DEFINITION

Cutaneous B-cell lymphoma with signet ring-cell morphology is an extremely rare, recently reported morphologic subtype of CBCL typified by high numbers of signet ring lymphoid cells in the neoplastic infiltrate.

CLINICAL FEATURES

The average age of the patients in the original series was 55.5 years (1). Clinically, the patients presented with solitary or multiple skin nodules ranging in size from 2 to 3 cm in diameter. There was no lymphadenopathy or evidence of systemic disease.

HISTOLOGY

There is a diffuse or nodular infiltrate in the dermis (and perhaps subcutis) composed of numerous cells with conventional signet-ring appearance as well as cells with clear cytoplasm and brightly eosinophilic, intracytoplasmic, Russell body-like inclusions displacing the nuclei toward the periphery. The neoplastic cells can be grouped in small clusters.

IMMUNOHISTOCHEMISTRY

The neoplastic cells are positive for leukocyte common antigen and B-cell associated antigens, while also showing monoclonal expression of light chains.

MOLECULAR BIOLOGY

No data are available.

TREATMENT

In the original report, the lesions were excised.

DIFFERENTIAL DIAGNOSIS

Some nodal T-cell lymphomas with signet-ring appearance of neoplastic lymphocytes may involve the skin (2). In addition, one should exclude signet ring-cell melanomas, metastatic carcinomas from the gastrointestinal tract or breast as well as some cutaneous epithelial tumors displaying signet-ring morphology.

COMMENTS

There is not enough data to fully describe cutaneous signet ring-cell B-cell lymphoma. Further observations are needed. An awareness of this morphological variant of CBCL and its recognition is important for the purpose of differential diagnosis, as well as for accumulating enough cases to more accurately characterize the tumor and its prognosis.

REFERENCES

1. Moran CA, Suster S, Abbondanzo SL. Cutaneous B-cell lymphoma with signet ring-cell morphology: a clinicopathologic and immunohistochemical study of three cases. Am J Dermatopathol 2001; 23:181–184.
2. Weiss LM, Wood GS, Dorfman RF. T-cell signet-ring cell lymphoma. A histologic, ultrastructural, and immunohistochemical study of two cases. Am J Surg Pathol 1985; 9: 273–280.

37

Blastic NK-Cell Lymphoma

Werner Kempf, Reinhard Dummer, Dmitry V. Kazakov, and Günter Burg
Department of Dermatology, University Hospital, Zürich, Switzerland

CLASSIFICATION

> WHO/EORTC Classification (2005): CD4+/CD56+hematodermic neoplasm
>   (formerly blastic NK cell lymphoma)
> WHO Classification (2001): Blastic NK-cell lymphoma
> REAL Classification (1997): Not listed
> EORTC Classification (1997): Not listed

DEFINITION

Blastic CD4+ CD56+ NK-cell lymphoma is another recently described entity within the group of CD56+ neoplasms with distinct clinical manifestation and phenotype of the tumor cells (1–3). Recent evidence suggests an origin from a plasmcytoid dendritic cells. The disease is also referred under following synonyms: blastoid NK-cell leukemia/lymphoma, agranular CD4+ CD56+ hematodermic neoplasm.

CLINICAL FEATURES

The disease seems to affect mainly people in their sixth decade (4), but has also been described in children or adolescents (5). Skin involvement occurs in 87% of the patients and manifests with contusiform, brownish infiltrated plaques, or nodules (6,7) (Fig. 1). The oral mucosa is commonly involved (Fig. 2).

HISTOLOGY

Histologically, dense monomorphous infiltrates of tumor cells are located mainly in the upper and mid-dermis, separated from epidermis by a small Grenz zone (Fig. 3). Tumor cells are medium- to large-sized with round or pleomorphic nuclei (Fig. 4). Mitoses are not uncommon. Erythrocyte extravasation is a characteristic feature, explaining the bruise-like appearance (Fig. 5).

297

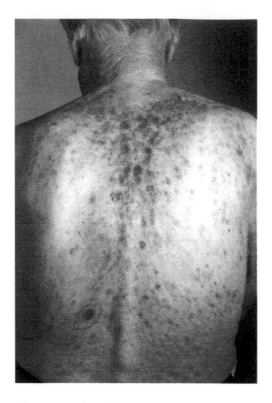

Figure 1 Disseminated red-brown plaques some of which resembling bruising (contusiform).

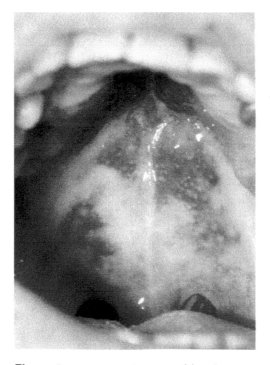

Figure 2 Hemorrhagic mucosal involvement.

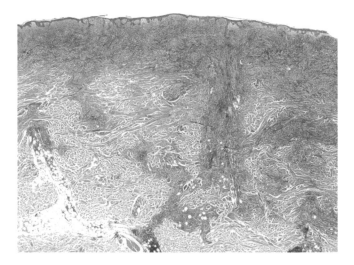

Figure 3 Diffuse dense infiltrate filling in the upper dermis and extending into the deep dermis. Note a thin Grenz zone.

IMMUNOHISTOCHEMISTRY

The cells express CD4, CD56, and CD123, but are negative for other T, B, NK-cell or myeloid markers. The latter distinguishes blastic CD4+ CD56+ NK-cell lymphoma from acute myeloid or monomyelocytic leukemia (AML M4 and M5), which coexpresses CD43 and CD74 in addition to myeloid markers (CD13, CD15, myeloperoxidase, lysozyme). Expression of CD68 or TdT by a minority of tumor cells and cases may be found (8).

MOLECULAR BIOLOGY

Since the tumor cells are not related to T-cells, there is no clonal rearrangement of TCR genes.

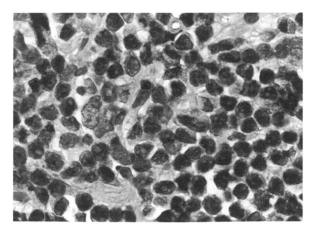

Figure 4 Large tumor cells with almost vesicular nuclei displaying fine chromatin.

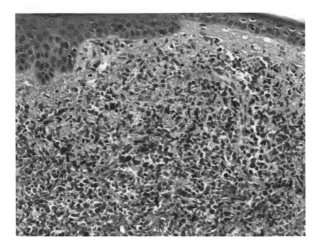

Figure 5 Extravasated erythrocytes admixed with tumor cells, which is the histological correlate for the contusiform clinical aspect.

TREATMENT

Multiagent chemotherapy results in complete remission in 80% of the patients, but the majority of patients experience recurrence in less than 2 years (4).

CLINICAL COURSE AND PROGNOSIS

The course of the disease is rapid with leukemic spread and involvement of bone marrow and CNS. The outcome is fatal without therapeutic intervention.

Blastic NK-cell lymphoma

Clinical features
  Mainly elderly people
  Contusiform, brownish infiltrated plaques or nodules
  Mucosal involvement common
Histological features
  Monomorphous infiltrates of medium- to large-sized blastoid tumor
    cells with round or pleomorphic nuclei
  Erythrocyte extravasation
Immunophenotype
  CD4+, CD56+, and CD123+
Molecular biology
  No clonal rearrangement of TCR genes
Treatment
  Multiagent chemotherapy
Clinical course and prognosis
  Aggressive course

COMMENTS

Although the cell of origin is not yet completely elucidated, the immunophenotypic profile suggests that the tumor cells represent most probably precursor cells related to activated plasmacytoid monocytes (9) and cytogenetically are related to dendritic myeloid and to lymphoid precursor cells.

REFERENCES

1. Chan JK, Sin VC, Wong KF, Ng CS, Tsang WY, Chan CH, Cheung MM, Lau WH. Nonnasal lymphoma expressing the natural killer cell marker CD56: a clinicopathologic study of 49 cases of an uncommon aggressive neoplasm. Blood 1997; 89:4501–4513.
2. DiGiuseppe JA, Louie DC, Williams JE, Miller DT, Griffin CA, Mann RB, Borowitz MJ. Blastic natural killer cell leukemia/lymphoma: a clinicopathologic study. Am J Surg Pathol 1997; 21:1223–1230.
3. Petrella T, Dalac S, Maynadie M, Mugneret F, Thomine E, Courville P, Joly P, Lenormand B, Arnould L, Wechsler J, Bagot M, Rieux C, Bosq J, Avril MF, Bernheim A, Molina T, Devidas A, Delfau-Larue MH, Gaulard P, Lambert D. CD4+ CD56+ cutaneous neoplasms: a distinct hematological entity? Groupe Francais d'Etude des Lymphomes Cutanes (GFELC). Am J Surg Pathol 1999; 23:137–146.
4. Feuillard J, Jacob MC, Valensi F, Maynadie M, Gressin R, Chaperot L, Arnoulet C, Brignole-Baudouin F, Drenou B, Duchayne E, Falkenrodt A, Garand R, Homolle E, Husson B, Kuhlein E, Le Calvez G, Sainty D, Sotto MF, Trimoreau F, Bene MC. Clinical and biologic features of CD4(+) CD56(+) malignancies. Blood 2002; 99:1556–1563.
5. Chang SE, Huh J, Choi JH, Sung KJ, Moon KC, Koh JK. Clinicopathological features of CD56+ nasal-type T/natural killer cell lymphomas with lobular panniculitis. Br J Dermatol 2000; 142:924–930.
6. Dummer R, Potoczna N, Haffner AC, Zimmermann DR, Gilardi S, Burg G. A primary cutaneous non-T, non-B CD4+, CD56+ lymphoma. Arch Dermatol 1996; 132:550–553.
7. Kato N, Yasukawa K, Kimura K, Sugawara H, Aoyagi S, Mishina T, Nakata T. CD2–CD4+ CD56+ hematodermic/hematolymphoid malignancy. J Am Acad Dermatol 2001; 44:231–238.
8. Khoury JD, Medeiros LJ, Manning JT, Sulak LE, Bueso-Ramos C, Jones D. CD56(+) TdT(+) blastic natural killer cell tumor of the skin: a primitive systemic malignancy related to myelomonocytic leukemia. Cancer 2002; 94:2401–2408.
9. Petrella T, Comeau MR, Maynadie M, Couillault G, De Muret A, Maliszewski CR, Dalac S, Durlach A, Galibert L. 'Agranular CD4+ CD56+ hematodermic neoplasm' (blastic NK-cell lymphoma) originates from a population of CD56+ precursor cells related to plasmacytoid monocytes. Am J Surg Pathol 2002; 26:852–862.

38

Precursor Lymphoblastic Leukemia/Lymphoma

38.1. Precursor T-Lymphoblastic Leukemia/Lymphoma

Werner Kempf, Dmitry V. Kazakov, and Günter Burg
Department of Dermatology, University Hospital, Zürich, Switzerland

CLASSIFICATION

WHO/EORTC Classification (2005): Precusor lymphoblastic leukemia/lymphoma (T-cell)

WHO Classification (2005): Precursor T-lymphoblastic leukemia/lymphoma, precursor T-cell acute lymphoblastic leukemia

REAL Classification (1997): Precursor T-lymphoblastic leukemia/ lymphoma

EORTC Classification (1997): Not listed

DEFINITION

A neoplasm of T-lymphoblasts (T-LBL) of unknown etiology, involving bone marrow, peripheral blood, nodal, and, in some cases, extranodal sites. Precursor T-LBL and precursor T-cell acute lymphoblastic leukemia are considered to represent a spectrum of one disease. In lymphoma, a tumor mass can be discerned, whereas in leukemic forms, involvement of bone marrow and peripheral blood is the predominant feature (1). Eighty-five to 90% of lymphoblastic lymphomas are precursor T-LBL (2).

CLINICAL FEATURES

T-lymphoblasts predominantly affects adolescents with a male predominance. Half of the cases manifest as tumor mass in the mediastinum. The skin may be occasionally involved (3). T-lymphoblasts presents with solitary or multiple nodules, just as does B-LBL.

HISTOLOGY

There are nodular or diffuse monomorphous infiltrates of lymphoblasts which are separated by the epidermis by a Grenz zone. The infiltrates display a "cobble stone" or "starry sky" pattern and consist of blasts of various size with condensed or finely dispersed chromatin and prominent nucleoli. Eosinophils are admixed with the lymphoblasts.

IMMUNOHISTOCHEMISTRY

Tumor cells in B-LBL variably express CD2, CD3, CD4, CD5, CD7, CD8, and CD34. The immunophenotypic hallmark of the lymphoblasts is their positivity for terminal deoxynucleotidyl transferase (TdT). Expression of CD79a has been observed in some cases (10%) and may lead to confusion with precursor B-LBL (4). Lymphoblasts are negative for myeloperoxidase, but the myeloid-associated markers CD13 and CD33 may be expressed.

MOLECULAR BIOLOGY

The tumor cells may exhibit clonal rearrangement of TCR genes (5). Various cytogenetic abnormalities in T-LBL have been described (for details, see Ref. 1).

TREATMENT

Treatment of precursor T-ALL in adults is similar to other types of ALL. Survival rates of T-ALL in children is comparable to B-ALL. Multiagent chemotherapy is primary therapy in T-LBL.

CLINICAL COURSE AND PROGNOSIS

T-ALL is a high grade-malignant disease, especially in children (1).

DIFFERENTIAL DIAGNOSIS

Differential diagnosis of T-LBL includes leukemic infiltrates of acute myeloid leukemia and B-cell variants of acute lymphoblastic leukemia. Immunophenotyping in skin infiltrates and tumor cells in peripheral blood with demonstration of T-cell antigens is essential to identify precursor T-cell ALL/LBL.

REFERENCES

1. Jaffe ES, Harris NL, Stein H, Vardiman JW. World Health Organization Classification of Tumors. Pathology and Genetics of Tumours of Hematopoietic and Lymphoid Tissues. Lyon: IARC Press, 2001.
2. Warnke RA, Weiss LM, Chan JKC, Cleary ML, Dorfman RF. Tumors of lymph nodes and spleen. In: Atlas of Tumor Pathology, Atlas of Tumor Pathology. Washington, D.C.: Armed Forces Institute of Pathology, 1995.

3. Chimenti S, Fink-Puches R, Peris K, Pescarmona E, Putz B, Kerl H, Cerroni L. Cutaneous involvement in lymphoblastic lymphoma. J Cutan Pathol 1999; 26:379–385.

4. Pilozzi E, Pulford K, Jones M, Muller-Hermelink HK, Falini B, Ralfkiaer E, Pileri S, Pezzella F, De Wolf-Peeters C, Arber D, Stein H, Mason D, Gatter K. Co-expression of CD79a (JCB117) and CD3 by lymphoblastic lymphoma. J Pathol 1998; 186:140–143.

5. Pilozzi E, Muller-Hermelink HK, Falini B, de Wolf-Peeters C, Fidler C, Gatter K, Wainscoat J. Gene rearrangements in T-cell lymphoblastic lymphoma. J Pathol 1999; 188: 267–270.

6. Sauder CA, Medeiros LJ, Abruzzo LV, Horak ID, Jaffe ES. Lymphoblastic lymphoma presenting in cutaneous sites. A clinico-pathologic analysis of six cases. J Am Acad Dermatol 1991; 25:1023–1031.

38.2. Precursor B-Lymphoblastic Leukemia/Lymphoma

Werner Kempf, Dmitry V. Kazakov, and Günter Burg
Department of Dermatology, University Hospital, Zürich, Switzerland

CLASSIFICATION

WHO/EORTC Classification (2005): Precursor B-lymphoblastic leukemia/lymphoma

WHO Classification (2001): Precursor B-lymphoblastic leukemia/lymphoma, precursor B-cell acute lymphoblastic leukemia

REAL Classification (1997): Precursor B-lymphoblastic leukemia/lymphoma

EORTC Classification: Not listed

DEFINITION

Neoplasm of B-lymphoblasts (B-LBLs) of unknown etiology, involving bone marrow, peripheral blood, nodal and extranodal sites. B-lymphoblast most frequently involves the skin, bone, and lymph nodes (1). Unlike precursor T-cell lymphoblastic lymphoma, which commonly involves lymph nodes and the mediastinum, B-LBL usually involves extranodal sites, most often the skin, and rarely presents as a mediastinal mass (2).

Precursor B-LBL and precursor B-cell acute lymphoblastic leukemia are considered to represent a spectrum of one disease. In lymphoma, a tumor mass can be discerned whereas in leukemic forms involvement of bone marrow and peripheral blood is the predominant feature.

CLINICAL FEATURES

B-lymphoblast predominantly affects children and young adults with a median age of 20 years (1,3,4). A male predominance has been reported (2). Only few cases of cutaneous involvement by B-LBL have been described in detail (5). The most common presentation seems to be multiple reddish nodules, while ulceration is uncommon.

307

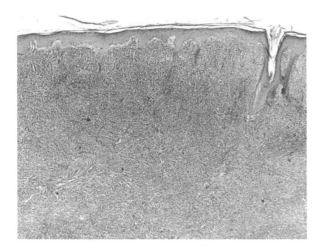

Figure 1 Precursor B-cell lymphoblastic leukemia/lymphoma: Diffuse lymphocytic infiltrate in the entire dermis.

HISTOLOGY

There are nodular or diffuse monomorphous infiltrates of lymphoblasts which may be separated by the epidermis by a Grenz zone (Figs. 1 and 2) (6). The infil trates display a "cobble stone" or "starry sky" pattern and consist of blasts of various size with condensed or finely dispersed chromatin and blue–gray cytoplasm (Fig. 3).

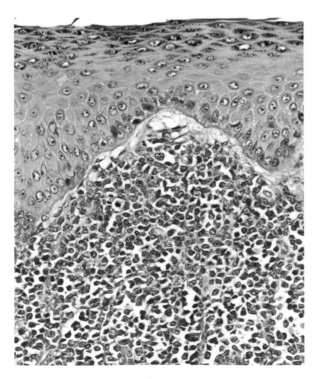

Figure 2 Precursor B-cell lymphoblastic leukemia/lymphoma: Infiltrate of medium-sized pleomorphic cells.

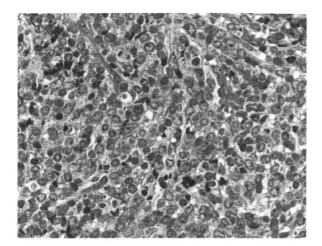

Figure 3 Precursor B-cell lymphoblastic leukemia/lymphoma: Infiltrate of tumor cells in the bone marrow demonstrating nuclei sparse chromatin.

IMMUNOHISTOCHEMISTRY

The tumor cells in B-LBL express CD19, CD79a, but are usually negative for CD20. The immunophenotypic hallmark of the lymphoblasts is their positivity for terminal deoxynucleotidyl transferase (TdT). All neoplasms have been positive for CD99 and bcl-2, and shown a high proliferation rate (5). Although the lymphoblasts are negative for myeloperoxidase, the myeloid-associated markers CD13 and CD33 may be expressed.

MOLECULAR BIOLOGY

Various cytogenetic abnormalities in B-LBL have been described and are of prognostic importance. The translocation t(9;22) is more frequent in adults and associated with a poorer prognosis.

Precursor B-cell lymphoblastic lymphoma/leukemia

Clinical features
  Children and young adults.
  Multiple reddish nodules. Ulceration uncommon
Histological features
  Nodular or diffuse monomorphous infiltrates of lymphoblasts with "starry sky"
Immunophenotype
  CD19+, CD20–, CD79a+, CD99+, TdT+
Molecular biology
  Translocation t(9;22) in some cases
Treatment
  Chemotherapy
Clinical course and prognosis
  Variable prognosis, Good prognosis, especially in children.
  Tendency to relapse.

TREATMENT

Multiagent chemotherapy is the primary therapy in B-LBL. With aggressive chemotherapy, patients with precursor B-LBL rarely develop leukemia and appear to have a better prognosis than do patients with B-ALL (2).

CLINICAL COURSE AND PROGNOSIS

Compared to other acute leukemias, B-ALL exhibits a good prognosis, especially in children. Complete remission rate (CRR) in children is over 90% and over 80% of pediatric patients can be cured. In adults, CRR is lower at 60–85%. The prognosis is related to genetic features. Precursor B-LBL shows a high CRR after multiagent chemotherapy or surgical excision followed by local radiotherapy. Relapses occur in one-third of the patients (2).

DIFFERENTIAL DIAGNOSIS

Cutaneous B-LBL must be included in the differential diagnosis of small blue cell tumors, especially in children. The differential diagnosis of B-LBL includes leukemic infiltrates of acute myeloid leukemia and T-cell variants of acute lymphoblastic leukemia. Immunophenotyping of skin infiltrates and tumor cells in peripheral blood by flow cytometry is essential to distinguish these disorders.

REFERENCES

1. Maitra A, McKenna RW, Weinberg AG, Schneider NR, Kroft SH. Precursor B-cell lymphoblastic lymphoma. A study of nine cases lacking blood and bone marrow involvement and review of the literature. Am J Clin Pathol 2001; 115:868–875.
2. Lin P, Jones D, Dorfman DM, Medeiros LJ. Precursor B-cell lymphoblastic lymphoma: a predominantly extranodal tumor with low propensity for leukemic involvement. Am J Surg Pathol 2000; 24:1480–1490.
3. Millot F, Robert A, Bertrand Y, Mechinaud F, Laureys G, Ferster A, Brock P, Rohrlich P, Mazingue F, Plantaz D, Plouvier E, Pacquement H, Behar C, Rialland X, Chantraine JM, Guilhot F, Otten J. Cutaneous involvement in children with acute lymphoblastic leukemia or lymphoblastic lymphoma. The Children's Leukemia Cooperative Group of the European Organization of Research and Treatment of Cancer (EORTC). Pediatrics 1997; 100:60–64.
4. Kahwash SB, Qualman SJ. Cutaneous lymphoblastic lymphoma in children: report of six cases with precursor B-cell lineage. Pediatr Dev Pathol 2002; 5:45–53.
5. Chimenti S, Fink-Puches R, Peris K, Pescarmona E, Putz B, Kerl H, Cerroni L. Cutaneous involvement in lymphoblastic lymphoma. J Cutan Pathol 1999; 26:379–385.
6. Sauder CA, Medeiros LJ, Abruzzo LV, Horak ID, Jaffe ES. Lymphoblastic lymphoma presenting in cutaneous sites. A clinico-pathologic analysis of six cases. J Am Acad Dermatol 1991; 25:1023–1031.

39

Cutaneous Manifestations of Hodgkin Lymphoma

Marshall E. Kadin
Beth Israel Deaconess Medical Center, Harvard Medical School, Boston, Massachusetts, U.S.A.

Werner Kempf and Günter Burg
Department of Dermatology, University Hospital, Zürich, Switzerland

INTRODUCTION

Secondary involvement of the skin with Hodgkin lymphoma (HL) is an infrequent event, usually occurring as a late manifestation of advanced systemic HL.

In addition, a variety of skin disorders have been associated with systemic HL. Cutaneous lesions of HL can be a presenting feature of HIV infection. Finally, primary cutaneous HL has been observed in immunocompetent patients who may or may not eventually develop systemic HL.

SECONDARY INVOLVEMENT OF THE SKIN BY SYSTEMIC HODGKIN LYMPHOMA

Skin involvement occurs in 0.5–7.5% of patients with nodal HL (1,2). In these patients, skin involvement is thought to be caused by retrograde spread through obstructed lymphatics, by direct extension from underlying lymph nodes, or by hematogenous spread (1). Secondary cutaneous lesions of Hodgkin lymphoma usually present as multiple papules or nodules in areas of direct extension from involved lymph nodes or at distant sites (2). Lesions are most common on the trunk but may occur anywhere on the body.

Secondary cutaneous lesions are nonepidermotropic and contain Reed–Sternberg cells or mononuclear variants surrounded by an inflammatory infiltrate. The distinction from lymphomatoid papulosis can be made by immunophenotype. RS cells in classical Hodgkin lymphoma (H/RS cells) generally do not express leukocyte common antigen (LCA or CD45RA), B- or T-cell antigens and may express CD15 (Lewis-X), whereas Reed–Sternberg like cells in lymphomatoid papulosis are LCA+, CD15–, and express T-cell antigens in most cases (3).

SKIN DISORDERS ASSOCIATED WITH SYSTEMIC HODGKIN LYMPHOMA

A variety of nonspecific erythematous, urticarial, vesicular, and bullous manifestations of Hodgkin lymphoma have been described. These nonspecific lesions are thought to be part of a paraneoplastic syndrome in response to cytokines secreted by H/RS cells (4).

Erythema nodosum has also been described in association with Hodgkin lymphoma (5). The lesions of erythema nodosum may appear several months before systemic relapse and respond to chemotherapy for Hodgkin lymphoma. Icthyosiform changes (acquired ichthyosis) also occur in association with and respond to therapy for Hodgkin lymphoma (6). Other skin disorders which may be associated with Hodgkin lymphoma and regress with therapy include acrokeratosis paraneoplastica (Basex syndrome) (7), erythema annulare centrifugum (8), granulomatous slack skin (9), prurigo nodularis (10), and follicular mucinosis (11).

One of the most common cutaneous changes in Hodgkin lymphoma is pruritus. Intense, often unmanageable pruritus, can be a presenting sign of HL or reflect relapse. Patients may also develop all the stigmata of intense pruritus, including excoriations and prurigo nodularis (10). Gratifyingly, the pruritus is usually one of the first features to disappear with treatment of systemic disease.

Granulomatous slack skin (12) and lymphomatoid papulosis have also been associated with HL, but generally do not respond to chemotherapy for HL. Lymphomatoid papulosis may occur before, simultaneous with, or following Hodgkin lymphoma (13–15). In one of these cases, the LyP and HL appeared to derive from a common T-cell clone (15). It was suggested that subclones of a common T-cell clone acquire further independent genetic abnormalities which can then lead to the development of LyP, Hodgkin disease, and mycosis fungoides in the same patient (15).

HIV-ASSOCIATED HODGKIN LYMPHOMA

In immunocompetent patients, HL involves contiguous lymph node groups, with hematogenous dissemination and extranodal disease usually occurring only as a late manifestation of disease. In contrast, extranodal sites of disease, including the skin, are observed in approximately 60% of HIV-associated HL patients (16–18). The skin lesions in HIV-associated HL contain a paucity of lymphocytes. Patients with HIV-associated HL may also have a variety of infectious diseases or Kaposi sarcoma involving the skin.

PRIMARY CUTANEOUS HODGKIN LYMPHOMA

Although some prior cases reported to be primary cutaneous Hodgkin disease are now thought to be examples of LyP or anaplastic large cell lymphoma, some cases of bona fide Hodgkin lymphoma presenting in the skin are well established (19). About one-half of these patients eventually developed nodal Hodgkin lymphoma (Fig. 1). One patient presented with multiple cutaneous lesions 2 years before the development of nodal Hodgkin disease of mixed cellularity type (20). The Reed–Sternberg cells in both the skin and lymph node contained Epstein–Barr transcripts

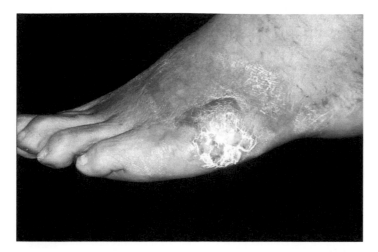

Figure 1 Scaly nodule on the foot of a patient, who many years later developed nodal disease. (From Ref. 21.)

and latent membrane protein. In perhaps the largest series, five patients with primary cutaneous Hodgkin lymphoma were described. They ranged in age from 17 to 54 years; four were men and one a woman (22). The lesions were nodules or tumors with deep dermal and subcutaneous infiltrates containing diagnostic Reed–Sternberg cells (Fig. 2). The Reed–Sternberg cells had a phenotype typical of systemic Hodgkin lymphoma (CD30+, CD15+, CD25+, HLA-DR+, and negative for LCA (CD45R). In one case, the RS cells coexpressed T-cell antigens CD2, CD4, and CD5 in frozen sections. Epstein–Barr viral studies were not done.

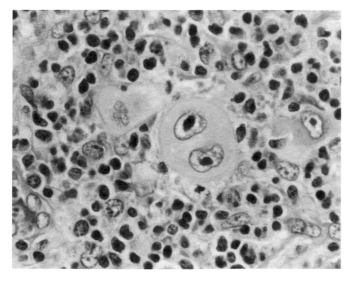

Figure 2 Binucleated Reed–Sternberg cell in an infiltrate of cutaneous Hodgkin lymphoma.

Hodgkin lymphoma—cutaneous manifestations

Clinical features
  Primary cutaneous IIL: exceedingly rare
  Multiple nodules
Histological features
  Deep dermal and subcutaneous mixed cellular infiltrates containing diagnostic
  Reed–Sternberg cells
Immunophenotype
  CD30+, CD15+, CD25+, HLA-DR+, and negative for LCA (CD45R)
Molecular biology
  EBV in some cases
Treatment
  Unknown
Clinical course and prognosis
  Development of nodal disease determines course

REFERENCES

1. White RM, Patterson JW. Cutaneous involvement in Hodgkin's disease. Cancer 1985; 55:1136.
2. Tassies D, Sierra J, Montserrat E, Marti R, Estrach T, Rozman C. Specific cutaneous involvement in Hodgkin's disease. Hematol Oncol 1992; 10:75.
3. Kadin ME, Nasu K, Sako D, Said J, Vonderheid E. Lymphomatoid papulosis. A cutaneous proliferation of activated helper T cells expressing Hodgkin's disease-associated antigens. Am J Pathol 1985; 119:315–325.
4. Milionis HJ, Elisaf MS. Psoriasiform lesions as paraneoplastic manifestions in Hodgkin's disease. Ann Oncol 1998; 9:449.
5. Simon S, Azevedo SH, Byrnes JJ. Erythema nodosum heralding recurrent Hodgkin's disease. Cancer 1985; 56:1470.
6. Ronchese F, Gates DC. Ichthyosioform atrophy of the skin in Hodgkin's disease. N Engl J Med 1956; 255:287.
7. Lucker GPH, Steijlen PM. Acrokeratosis paraneoplastica (Bazex syndrome) occurring with acquired ichthyosis in Hodgkin's disease. Br J Dermatol 1995; 133:322.
8. Leimert JT, Corder MP, Skibba CA, Gingrich RD. Erythema annulare centrifugum and Hodgkin's disease. Arch Intern Med 1979; 139:486.
9. Benisovich V, Papadopoulos E, Amerosis EL, Zucker-Franklin D, Silber R. The association of progressive, atrophying, chronic, granulomatous dermohypodermatitis with Hodgkin's disease. Cancer 1988; 62:2425.
10. Shelnitz LS, Paller AS. Hodgin's disease manifesting as prurigo nodularis. Pediatr Dermatol 1990; 7:136.
11. Ramon DR, Jorda E, Molina I, Galan A, Torres V, Alcacer J, Monzo E. Follicular mucinosis and Hodgkin's disease. Int J Dermatol 1992; 31:791.
12. Noto G, Provata G, Miceli S, Arico M. Granulomatous slack skin: report of a case associated with Hodgkin's disease and review of the literature. Br J Dermatol 1994; 131:275.
13. Lederman J, Sober A, Harrist T, Lederman GS. Lymphomatoid papulosis following Hodgkin's disease. J Am Acad Dermatol 1987; 16:331–335.
14. Kaudewitz P, Stein H, Plewig G, Schwarting R, Gerdes J, Burg G, Kind P, Eckert F, Braun-Falco O. Hodgkin's disease followed by lymphomatoid papulosis: immunopheno-

typic evidence for a close relationship between lymphomatoid papulosis and Hodgkin's disease. J Am Acad Dermatol 1990; 22:999–1006.

15. Davis T, Morton C, Miler-Cassman R, Balk S, Kadin ME. Hodgkin's disease, lymphomatoid papulosis and cutaneous T-cell lymphoma derived from a common T-cell clone. N Engl J Med 1992; 326:1115–1122.

16. Knowles DM, Chamulak GA, Subar M, Burke JS, Dugan M, Wernz J, Slywotzky C, Pelicci G, Dalla-Favera R, Raphael B. Lymphoid neoplasia associated with the acquired immunodeficiency syndrome (AIDS). The New York University Medical Center experience with 105 patients (1981–1986). Ann Intern Med 1988; 108:744–753.

17. Schoeppel JL, Hoppe RT, Dorfman RF, Horning SJ, Collier AC, Chew TG, Weiss LM. Hodgkin's disease in homosexual men with generalized lymphadenopathy. Ann Intern Med 1985; 102:68–70.

18. Shaw MT, Jacobs SR. Cutaneous Hodgkin's disease in a patient with human immunodeficiency virus infection. Cancer 1989; 64:2585.

19. Kumar S, Kingma WQ, Weiss WB, Raffeld M, Jaffe ES. Primary cutaneous Hodgkin's disease with evolution to systemic disease. Association with Epstein–Barr virus. Am J Surg Pathol 1996; 20:754–759

20. Huhn D, Burg G, Mempel W. Spezifische Hartinfietrate Sci Morbus Hodgkin. Dtsch Med Wochenschr 1973; 98:2469–2472

21. Burg G, Braun-Falco O. Cutaneous Lymphomas, Pseudolymphonics and Related Disorders. Berlin: Springer-Verlag. 1983.

22. Sioutus N, Kerl H, Murphy SB, Kadin ME. Primary cutaneous Hodgkin's disease. Unique clinical, morphologic and immunophenotypic findings. Am J Dermatopathol 1994; 16:2–8.

40

Cutaneous Pseudolymphomas

Günter Burg, Werner Kempf, and Dmitry V. Kazakov
Department of Dermatology, University Hospital, Zürich, Switzerland

DEFINITION

Pseudolymphoma (PSL) is a reactive benign lymphoproliferative process, either localized or disseminated, of B- or T-cell predominance, that heals spontaneously and does not recur after elimination of the causative factor (e.g., drugs, bacteria, viruses) or following nonaggressive therapy. There is no evidence for systemic involvement in PSL.

INTRODUCTION

The concept of cutaneous pseudolymphoma (PSL) has been evolving for nearly a century (1). Early descriptions of pseudoleukemic or lymphomatous infiltrates were given by Kaposi (2), who, under the term "sarcoma cutis," included the following groups: (1) "mycosis fungoides"; (2) "lymphodermia cutis" (including "leukemia and pseudoleukemia cutis"); (3) "sarcomatosis cutis" (typical primary solitary sarcoma cutis, such as malignant melanoma); and (4) "sarcoma cutis proprie dictum" (including the two subgroups of sarcoma idiopathicum multiple hemorrhagicum of Kaposi and "sarcoid" tumors).

In 1923, Biberstein coined the term lymphocytoma cutis. Subsequently, Bäfverstedt in 1943 introduced the term lymphadenosis benigna cutis (3). In 1967, Lever introduced the term pseudolymphoma of Spiegler (4) and Fendt (5). Subsequently, Caro and Helwig (6) in 1969 used the term cutaneous lymphoid hyperplasia. Many other terms were proposed. In retrospect, most of these terms were describing cutaneous B-cell pseudolymphomas (B-PSLs). Although actinic reticuloid was first described in 1969 (7), the concept of cutaneous T-cell pseudolymphomas (T-PSL) was not widely accepted until the early 1980s.

Pseudolymphomas are of great clinical relevance because they may be difficult to distinguish from cutaneous lymphomas (CL). For some PSLs, both clinical manifestations and etiology are clearly defined, for example *Borrelia*-associated lymphadenosis benigna cutis. In most cases, however, the etiology of PSL cannot be identified. There are intensive inflammatory (pseudolymphomatous) reactions to stimuli such as insect bite, tattoos, allergen injections (8), physical or microbial irritation, chemicals, or medications (9). Diseases with clonal T-cell populations, but displaying a benign course, are further considered in Chapter 42.2. Lymphomatoid papulosis is currently regarded as cutaneous T-cell lymphoma, but displays features of a T-PSL (10).

Pseudolymphomas are usually divided into *B-cell* and *T-cell forms*, depending on the predominant cell type. In T-PSL, a sleevelike pattern is seen around blood vessels and adnexal structures, while a follicular pattern is common in B-PSL, also known as follicular lymphoid hyperplasia. In addition to routine microscopy, immunohistochemistry and molecular studies aid in distinguishing them from CL. Detection of monoclonal T- or B-cells argues for the presence of a lymphoma, though exceptions exist. However, the final diagnosis should always be based on a clinicopathologic correlation and should never be based on one single criterion.

Treatment of PSL in general is nonaggressive. If the causative agent is identified, it can be specifically treated (for example, antibiotics for *Borrelia* infections) or avoided (removal of contact allergens). In addition, solitary lesions are often excised for diagnostic purposes.

REFERENCES

1. Ploysangam T, Breneman DL, Mutasim DF. Cutaneous pseudolymphomas. J Am Acad Dermatol 1998; 38:877–895.
2. Kaposi M. Idiopathisches multiples Pigmentsarkom der Haut. Arch Dermatol Syphilol 1872; 4:265–273.
3. Baefverstedt B. Ueber Lymphadenosis benigna cutis. Eine klinische pathologisch–anatomische Studie. Acta Derm Venereol (Suppl XI)(Stockh) 1944; 24:1–102.
4. Spiegler E. Über die sogenannte Sarkomatosis cutis. Arch Dermatol Syphilol 1894; 27.
5. Fendt H. Beiträge zur Kenntnis der sogenannten sarcoiden Geschwülste der Haut. Arch Dermatol Syphilol 1900; 53:213–242.
6. Caro WA, Helwig EB. Cutaneous lymphoid hyperplasia. Cancer 1969; 24:487–502.
7. Ive FA, Magnus IA, Warin RP, Jones EW. "Actinic reticuloid"; a chronic dermatosis associated with severe photosensitivity the histological resemblance to lymphoma. Br J Dermatol 1969; 81:469–485.
8. Goerdt S, Spieker T, Wolffer LU. Multiple cutaneous B-cell pseudolymphomas after allergen injections. J Am Acad Dermatol 1996; 34:1072–1074.
9. Harris DW, Ostlere L, Buckley C, Whittaker S, Sweny P, Rustin MH. Phenytoin-induced pseudolymphoma. A report of a case and review of the literature. Br J Dermatol 1992; 127:403–406.
10. Burg G, Braun-Falco O. Cutaneous Lymphomas, Pseudolymphomas and Related Disorders. Berlin: Springer-Verlag, 1983.

40.1. Cutaneous T-cell Pseudolymphoma

Günter Burg, Werner Kempf, and Dmitry V. Kazakov
Department of Dermatology, University Hospital, Zürich, Switzerland

LYMPHOCYTIC INFILTRATION OF JESSNER–KANOF (IDIOPATHIC CUTANEOUS T-CELL PSEUDOLYMPHOMA)

Clinical Features

Jessner and Kanof presented in 1953 at the Bronx Dermatological Society (1) cases designated as "lymphocytic infiltration of the skin." Their description was: "The lesions are flat, discoid, more or less elevated, pinkish to reddish brown, starting as small papules, expanding peripherally, sometimes clearing in the center, sometimes showing a circinate arrangement. The surface is smooth, occasionally uneven. There is no follicular hyperkeratosis. The consistency is firm. There may be only one, a few, or numerous lesions (Fig. 1). They persist for weeks or months or longer, disappear without sequelae, and may return in the same or other areas and cause practically no subjective symptoms. The face is obviously the area of predilection, but other parts of the body may or may not be affected. These cases must be distinguished particularly from cases of chronic discoid lupus erythematosus, under which label they are invariably described; also from sarcoid, tuberserpiginous syphilid, and drug eruption. There are no enlarged lymph nodes. The blood cell count shows only an occasional relative lymphocytosis. The bone marrow smears reveal no abnormalities". This description, given 50 years ago, perfectly reflects the characteristic nosological features of this reaction.

Histology

The pattern is very characteristic and shows a sleeve-like, predominantly lymphocytic infiltrate around the vessels of the upper- and mid-dermis (Figs. 2 and 3). In addition, some macrophages and eosinophils may be found. Usually the histological appearance is rather monomorphous, simulating skin infiltrates in chronic lymphocytic leukemia. In contrast to chronic discoid lupus erythematosus, there is no

319

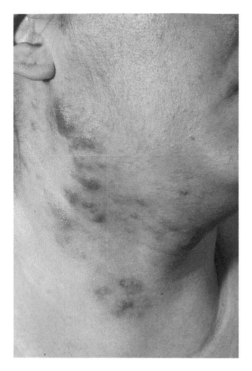

Figure 1 Red papules and nodules on the neck.

vacuolization in the junctional area, no epidermal atrophy or necrotic keratinocytes, and no follicular hyperkeratoses.

Immunohistochemistry

Phenotyping has shown the infiltrate to consist of both B- and T cells (2) even though T cells seem to predominate in most cases (3). Usually, no Ki-1 positive cells can be detected.

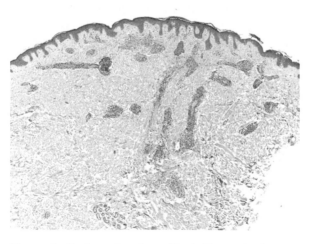

Figure 2 Perivascular sleeve-like infiltrates in the upper- and mid-dermis.

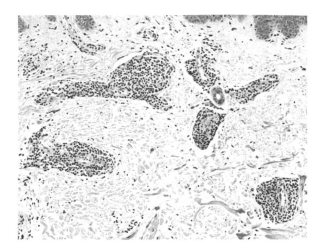

Figure 3 The infiltrates consist predominantly of small lymphocytes.

Comment

Currently there are at least three different concepts about lymphocytic infiltration. We feel that most if not all lesions are due to drugs or other chemicals ingested through food or drinks or even inhaled. Jessner and Kanof differentiated lymphocytic infiltration as "idiopathic" from drug eruptions.

PALPABLE MIGRATORY ARCIFORM ERYTHEMA

Palpable migratory arciform erythema is clinically similar to erythema annulare centrifugum Darier (4). There are circinate or annular slightly elevated erythematous lesions with or without scaling. Histologically, a scant sleeve-like perivascular lymphocytic infiltrate is seen. The disease is characterized by T-helper- and T-suppressor cells in a ratio of 2:1. Immunohistologically, there is no difference from the lymphocytic infiltration of Jessner–Kanof (5).

LYMPHOMATOID CONTACT DERMATITIS

Lymphomatoid contact dermatitis has been reported as a reaction to various allergens including nickel (6,7), cobalt naphthenate (8), isopropyl-diphenylenediamine (9), and others. Genotyping has shown clonal rearrangement in some cases. Such cases may be closely related to "clonal dermatitis" some of which develop into overt CTCL (10). Histologically, epidermotropism of lymphocytes and accumulations of CD1a-positive Langerhans cells may be found (Figs. 4 and 5).

Evolution into cutaneous T-cell lymphoma was observed in four patients with long-standing chronic contact dermatitis (11) present for up to 15 years before clinically and histologically verified mycosis fungoides occurred. Contact allergy was confirmed in these cases by patch testing with sensitization against nickel, potassium dichromate, and formaldehyde. These observations may suggest that at least in some cases, CTCL may be caused by chronic antigenic immunostimulation (12).

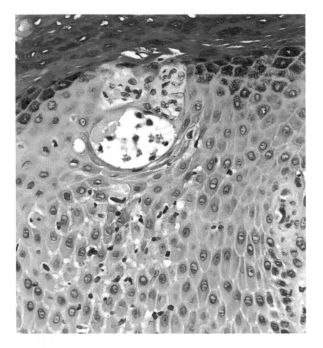

Figure 4 Exocytosis of lymphocytes, spongiosis, and Langerhans cells forming small collections.

ACTINIC RETICULOID

Ive et al. in 1969 (13) first described actinic reticuloid (AR) as a chronic dermatosis associated with severe photosensitivity and bearing a clinical and histological resemblance to malignant lymphoma, especially to Sézary syndrome. Nowadays, AR

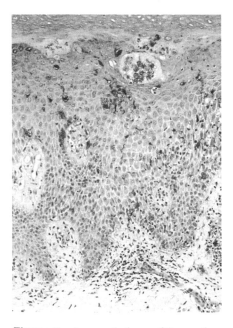

Figure 5 Accumulations of Langerhans cells expressing CD1a.

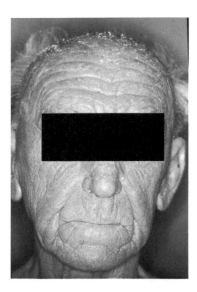

Figure 6 Eczema-like red and scaly infiltration of the sun-exposed skin.

belongs to the group of so-called chronic actinic dermatitis. The clinical presentation is an eczematous and infiltrative dermatitis on light exposed areas with marked thickening and ridging of the skin (Fig. 6). In contrast to Sézary syndrome, nonexposed and palmoplantar areas are not involved.

Histologically, there is a dense infiltrate of lymphocytes mixed with many polyclonal plasma cells, eosinophils, and macrophages. Pathogenetically, AR in most cases primarily is a photoallergic process due to various photosensitizers activated over a wide spectrum of wavelengths. The process persists in typical cases even after removal of the photosensitizer possibly due to the generation of self-antigens. Gene rearrangement analysis, in combination with immunohistochemistry, may be an important adjunct in differentiating between AR and cutaneous T-cell lymphoma (14).

PERSISTENT NODULAR ARTHROPOD-BITE REACTIONS

Following an arthropod bite or sting, persistent itching papules and nodules may develop. In some instances, dermatofibroma develop which have been regarded as an abortive immune reaction involving dermal dendritic cells (15). More commonly, T-PSL develops.

REFERENCES

1. Jessner MK. Lymphocytic infiltration of the skin. Arch Dermatol 1953; 68:447–449.
2. Cerio R, Oliver GF, Jones EW, Winkelmann RK. The heterogeneity of Jessner's lymphocytic infiltration of the skin. Immunohistochemical studies suggesting one form of perivascular lymphocytoma. J Am Acad Dermatol 1990; 23:63–67.
3. Willemze R, Dijkstra A, Meijer CJ. Lymphocytic infiltration of the skin (Jessner): a T-cell lymphoproliferative disease. Br J Dermatol 1984; 110:523–529.
4. Clark WH, Mihm MC Jr, Reed RJ, Ainswarth AM. The lymphocytic infiltrates of the skin. Hum Pathol 1974; 5:25–43.

5. Lohrisch I, Alexandrakis E. Erythema migrans arciforme et palpabile (T-Zell Pseudo-lymphom). Hautarzt 1990; 41:78–82.
6. Danese P, Bertazzoni MG. Lymphomatoid contact dermatitis due to nickel. Contact Dermat 1995; 33:468–469.
7. Houck H, Wirth FA, Kauffman CL. Lymphomatoid contact dermatitis caused by nickel. Am J Contact Dermat 1997; 8:175–176.
8. Schena D, Rosina P, Chieregato C, Colombari R. Lymphomatoid-like contact dermatitis from cobalt naphthenate. Contact Dermat 1995; 33:197–198.
9. Marliere V, Beylot-Barry M, Doutre MS, Furioli M, Vergier B, Dubus P, Merlio JP, Beylot C. Lymphomatoid contact dermatitis caused by isopropyl-diphenylenediamine: two cases. J Allergy Clin Immunol 1998; 102:152–153.
10. Wood GS. Lymphocyte activation in cutaneous T-cell lymphoma. J Invest Dermatol 1995; 105:105S–109S.
11. Fransway AF, Winkelmann RK. Chronic dermatitis evolving to mycosis fungoides: report of four cases and review of the literature. Cutis 1988; 330–335.
12. Schuppli R. Is mycosis fungoides an "immunoma"? Dermatologica 1976; 153:1–6.
13. Ive FA, Magnus IA, Warin RP, Jones EW. "Actinic reticuloid": a chronic dermatosis associated with severe photosensitivity the histological resemblance to lymphoma. Br J Dermatol 1969; 81:469–485.
14. Bakels V, van-Oostveen JW, Preesman AH, Meijer CJ, Willemze R. Differentiation between actinic reticuloid and cutaneous T cell lymphoma by T cell receptor gamma gene rearrangement analysis and immunophenotyping. J Clin Pathol 1998; 51:154–158.
15. Nestle FO, Nickoloff BJ, Burg G. Dermatofibroma. An abortive immunoreactive process mediated by dermal dendritic cells? Dermatology 1995; 190:265–268.

40.2. Cutaneous B-cell Pseudolymphoma

Günter Burg, Werner Kempf, and Dmitry V. Kazakov
Department of Dermatology, University Hospital, Zürich, Switzerland

The prototype of B-cell pseudolymphoma (B-PSL) is *Borrelia*-associated lymphadenosis benigna cutis (LABC). Other B-PSL includes tattoo-induced lymphocytoma cutis and postzoster scar lymphocytoma cutis. In some cases, the cause cannot be identified and are thus referred as "idiopathic" lymphocytoma cutis. There is a considerable overlap between T- and B-PSL as in persistent nodular arthropod bite reactions and nodular scabies. Acral pseudolymphomatous angiokeratoma of children (APACHE) is a plasma cell rich B-PSL which is described in detail in Chapter 40.3.

LYMPHADENOSIS BENIGNA CUTIS

The tongue-twister term of LABC was coined by Bäfverstedt in 1944 (1) and is synonymous with lymphocytoma cutis. In Europe, it is most commonly caused by infection with *Borrelia burgdorferi* (B. Garinii and B. Cefzelii) after a tick bite (*Ixodes ricinus*). Different microbiological, physical, or chemical agents may cause cases lacking association with Borrelia infection. One fascinating trigger appears to be the use of medicinal leeches (*Hirudo medicinalis*) (2).

CLINICAL FEATURES

Two-thirds of all lesions are situated on the head, tending to occur on the ear lobes (Fig. 1). Other predilections are the nose as well as the nipples, the inguinal area and scrotum. Usually, the lesion is a solitary papule or nodule, but several disseminated lesions may occur as well (3).

325

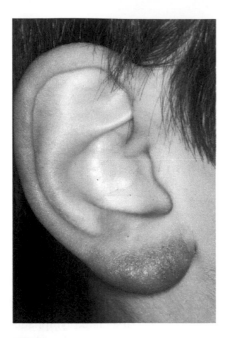

Figure 1 Lymphadenosis benigna cutis: infiltration on the ear lobe.

HISTOLOGY

Microscopic examination shows a nodular dermal infiltrate with reactive follicles (Fig. 2). In addition, there is a rather diffuse infiltrate containing T cells, histiocytes, eosinophils, and polyclonal plasma cells. The presence of macrophages containing ingested nuclear material (Flemming's tingible body macrophages) within the follicles producing a "starry sky" pattern is a common feature in B-PSL (Fig. 3). The infiltrate is predominantly located in the upper and middermis, but may extend

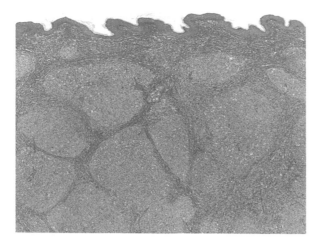

Figure 2 Lymphadenosis benigna cutis: dense lymphocytic infiltrate with follicular pattern.

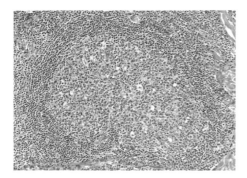

Figure 3 Lymphadenosis benigna cutis: reactive follicle with germinal center and tingible body macrophages containing ingested nuclear material.

into the deep dermis. Small groups of lymphoid cells between collagen bundles may be observed at the periphery of the lesions. This is a helpful histological criterion in the differentiation from cutaneous B-cell lymphoma (CBCL), in which the nodular infiltrate shows convex rather than concave sharply demarcated borders. Measuring microvessel density and vessel distribution may provide another helpful criterion to discriminate between CBCL and B-PSL (4).

IMMUNOHISTOCHEMISTRY

Important techniques for discriminating B-PSL from CBCL are immunophenotyping and genotyping. Phenotypically (5) a polyclonal B-lymphocytic infiltrate without heavy or light chain restriction of the infiltrate is found in most cases. The cells express the phenotype of mature B-cells (CD20, CD79a). However, monotypic expression of kappa or lambda chains can be identified in some cases. In B-PSL, regular and sharply demarcated networks of CD21+ follicular dendritic cells are present, whereas in CBCL, these networks are irregularly shaped (Fig. 4) (6). There

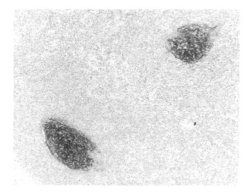

Figure 4 Lymphadenosis benigna cutis: regular and sharply demarcated network of CD21-positive follicular dendritic cells in a germinal center.

Table 1 Differentiation Between Pseudolymphoma (PSL) and Cutaneous B-cell Lymphoma (CBCL)

	CBCL	PSL
Clinical features		
Number of lesions	Solitary or multiple	Usually solitary
Extracutaneous involvement	Possible	Absent
Recurrences	Likely	Usually no recurrences
Survival time	Affected	Not affected
Histological features		
Pattern of infiltrate	Diffuse or nodular, "bottom-heavy"	Nodular (>90%), "top-heavy"
Additional cells	Usually absent	Eosinophils, plasma cells
Transformation	May occur	Never occurs
Immunophenotype		
Immunoglobulin light chains	Monotypic (kappa or lambda)	Polytypic expression
B-cell marker expressing cells	>50% cells	≤50% cells
T-cell marker expressing cells	Few	>50% cells
CD21-positive dendritic cells	Mostly absent Irregular pattern	Mostly present Regular pattern
Genotype		
Ig heavy chain rearrangement	Present in most cases	Absent in most cases

may be rare instances of cutaneous follicular lymphoid hyperplasia, in which sheets of monotypic plasma cells are found (7).

MOLECULAR BIOLOGY

Molecular studies reveal a polyclonal B-cell infiltrate in most cases.

DIFFERENTIAL DIAGNOSIS

The most relevant differential diagnosis of B-cell pseudolymphoma is cutaneous B-cell lymphoma. Several features in combination may be useful for discrimination as listed in Table 1.

COMMENTS

Giant follicular forms of LABC with "inverted follicular pattern" (dark chromatin rich cells in the center and clear border zone) (8,9) are today regarded as marginal zone B-cell lymphomas.

REFERENCES

1. Bäfverstedt B. Ueber lymphadenosis benigna cutis. Eine klinische pathologisch-anatomische studie. Acta Derm Venereol (Stockh) 1944; 24(suppl XI):1–102.

2. Smolle J, Cerroni L, Kerl H. Multiple pseudolymphomas caused by *Hirudo medicinalis* therapy. J Am Acad Dermatol 2000; 43:867–869.
3. Höfer W. Lymphadenosa benigna cutis. Arch Klin Exp Dermatol 1956; 203:23–40.
4. Schaerer L, Schmid MH, Mueller B, Dummer RG, Burg G, Kempf W. Angiogenesis in cutaneous lymphoproliferative disorders: microvessel density discriminates between cutaneous B-cell lymphomas and B-cell pseudolymphomas. Am J Dermatopathol 2000; 22:140–143.
5. Cerroni L, Kerl H. Diagnostic immunohistology: cutaneous lymphomas and pseudolymphomas. Semin Cutan Med Surg 1999; 18:64–70.
6. Burg G, Hess M, Küng E, Dommann SNW, Dummer R. Semimalignant ("Pseudolymphomatous") cutaneous B-cell lymphomas. Derm Clin 1994; 12:399–407.
7. Schmid U, Eckert F, Griesser H, Steinke C, Cogliatti SB, Kaudewitz P, Lennert K. Cutaneous follicular lymphoid hyperplasia with monotypic plasma cells. A clinicopathologic study of 18 patients. Am J Surg Pathol 1995; 19:12–20.
8. Duncan SC, Evans HL, Winkelmann RK. Large cell lymphocytoma. Arch Dermatol 1980; 116:1142–1146.
9. Burg G, Braun-Falco O. Cutaneous Lymphomas, Pseudolymphomas and Related Disorders. Berlin: Springer-Verlag, 1983.

40.3. Acral Pseudolymphomatous Angiokeratoma of Children

Dmitry V. Kazakov, Günter Burg, and Werner Kempf
Department of Dermatology, University Hospital, Zürich, Switzerland

DEFINITION

Acral pseudolymphomatous angiokeratoma of children (APACHE) is a rare pseudolymphomatous disorder occurring mainly in children. It was described by Ramsay and colleagues in 1983 (1). In 1980, Crow (2) published a case report describing a very similar condition. About 20 cases of this disorder have been reported.

CLINICAL FEATURES

Occurrences of APACHE are seen mostly in children, although adults can also be affected (3–6). The typical clinical presentation is multiple (up to 40), asymptomatic, small (1–7 mm), irregularly shaped papules located unilaterally on the fingers, toes, and hands (Fig. 1). The lesions have a scaly, keratotic surface with a collarette. Their color is usually red-violet, accounting for their angiomatous appearance (1,3). Coalescence of the lesions has been noted. Longitudinal splitting of the nails, onycholysis, and nail deformities may occur (3,7). Two cases with solitary lesions have also been reported (5,8).

HISTOLOGICAL FEATURES

The dermis contains a moderately to very dense, non-epidermotropic lymphoid infiltrate that, in some cases, extends into the subcutis (Fig. 2). In addition, thick-walled, gaping blood vessels with prominent plump endothelial cells are found (3) (Fig. 3). In some instances, the vascular component is less prominent, featuring a proliferation of postcapillary venules with swollen endothelial cells within and around the infiltrate (5). The cellular infiltrate is composed of small, well-differentiated lymphocytes admixed with a few plasma cells, histiocytes, and giant cells. In some instances, a few eosinophils may be present (5,6) (Fig. 4). There are no abnormal mitotic figures or

331

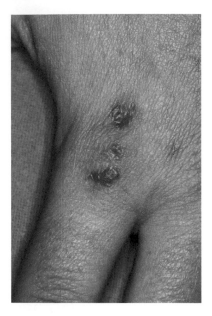

Figure 1 Papules on the back of a child's hand. (Courtesy of S. Lautenschlager, Switzerland.)

cellular pleomorphism. The epidermis overlying the infiltrate is intact, slightly atrophic, or shows acanthotic changes at the margins. Subtle vacuolar alteration of the basal layer may be present (6).

IMMUNOHISTOCHEMISTRY

The cellular infiltrate represents a mixture of mature T and B cells in variable proportions. The ratio of CD4 to CD8 lymphocytes is also variable (3,5–7). B cells are apt to form small clusters vaguely reminiscent of lymphoid follicles, but these aggregations do not contain CD21-positive follicular dendritic cells (5). The B cells demonstrate polyclonal expression of Ig light chains (4,6,9).

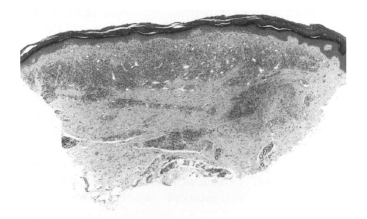

Figure 2 Bandlike infiltrate in the mid-dermis and perivascular pattern in the deep dermis.

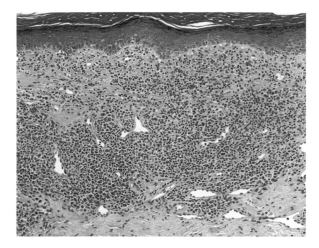

Figure 3 Prominent vessels within the infiltrate.

MOLECULAR BIOLOGY

Both B and T cells appear to be polyclonal (6).

DIFFERENTIAL DIAGNOSIS

The histological differential diagnosis of APACHE includes lymphomatoid drug eruptions, arthropod bite reactions, lichen nitidus, and lymphadenosis benigna cutis. The infiltrate in lymphomatoid drug eruptions (lymphoid vascular reaction pattern) contains lymphocytes with irregular nuclei and is usually angiocentric, obscuring the vessel architecture but without fibrinoid necrosis. Arthropod bite reactions show a wedge-shaped infiltrate with high numbers of eosinophils. The infiltrate in lichen nitidus is usually confined to a single widened dermal papilla. The presence of

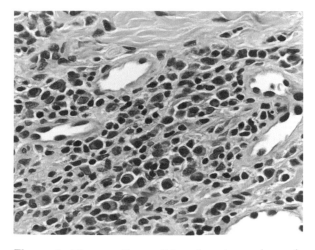

Figure 4 Plasma cells, small lymphocytes, and prominent vessels.

germinal centers in lymphadenosis benigna cutis makes its distinction from APACHE straightforward.

TREATMENT

Destruction of the lesions by curettage, intralesional triamcinolone, or high potency topical corticosteroids under occlusion has been tried and has resulted in complete remission (3,4,6).

CLINICAL COURSE AND PROGNOSIS

APACHE is a benign process. No recurrences have been reported following treatment. When left untreated, the lesions can regress, show a waning and waxing course, or remain unchanged for months or years (3–5).

Acral pseudolymphomatous angiokertoma of children (APACHE)

Clinical features
  Mostly children
  Small red-violet, unilateral acral papules
Histological features
  Non-epidermotropic infiltrate of small lymphocytes admixed with a few
    plasma cells
  Thick-walled gaping blood vessels with prominent plump endothelium
Immunophenotype
  Variable numbers of mature T and B cells
Molecular biology
  Polyclonal T and B cells
Treatment
  Excision, laser surgery
Clinical course and prognosis
  Benign

COMMENTS

Because the pseudolymphomatous component is often more prominent than the vascular component and the disorder also occurs in adulthood, it has been proposed to alter the term APACHE to "acral angiokeratomatous pseudolymphoma" (4) or "small papular pseudolymphoma" (5) or "papular angiolymphoid hyperplasia" (6).

REFERENCES

1. Ramsay D, Dahl MGC, Malcolm A, Soyer HP, Wilson Jones E. Acral pseudolymphomatous angiokeratoma of children (APACHE). Br J Dermatol 1983; 119 (suppl 33):13 (abstract).
2. Crow KD. Case for diagnosis. Br J Dermatol 1980; 103 (suppl 18):78–80.

3. Ramsay D, Dahl MGC, Malcolm A, Soyer HP, Wilson Jones E. Acral pseudolymphomatous angiokeratoma of children (APACHE). Arch Dermatol 1990; 126:1524–1525.

4. Okada M, Funayama M, Tanita M, Kudoh K, Aiba S, Tagami H. Acral angiokeratoma-like pseudolymphoma: one adolescent and two adults. J Am Acad Dermatol 2001; 45:209–211.

5. Kaddu S, Cerroni L, Pilatti A, Soyer HP, Kerl H. Acral pseudolymphomatous angiokeratoma. A variant of the cutaneous pseudolymphomas. Am J Dermatopathol 1994; 16:130–133.

6. Hagari Y, Hagari S, Kambe N, Kawaguchi T, Nakamoto S, Mihara M. Acral pseudolymphomatous angiokeratoma of children: immunohistochemical and clonal analyses of the infiltrating cells. J Cutan Pathol 2002; 29:313–318.

7. Hara M, Matsunaga J, Tagami H. Acral pseudolymphomatous angiokeratoma of children (APACHE): a case report and immunohistological study. Br J Dermatol 1991; 124:387–388.

8. Fernandez-Figueras MT, Puig L. Of APACHEs and PALEFACEs. Am J Dermatopathol 1995; 17:209–211.

9. Ito K, Fujiwara H, Ito M. Acral pseudolymphomatous angiokeratoma of children (APACHE). Hifubyo-Shinryoh 2000; 22:979 (in Japanese).

40.4. Pseudolymphomatous Folliculitis

Dmitry V. Kazakov, Günter Burg, and Werner Kempf
Department of Dermatology, University Hospital, Zürich, Switzerland

CLINICAL FEATURES

This disease occurs in both sexes with a slight male predominance. The median age of patients is 41 years (range 2–66 years). They tend to present with a solitary, dome-shaped or flat, nonulcerated, red to violaceous nodule usually less than 1.5 cm in diameter. While the site of predilection is the face, the scalp and trunk may also be affected (1,2).

HISTOLOGICAL FEATURES

There is a diffuse or nodular dense infiltrate in the dermis and/or in the subcutis that surrounds and invades pilosebaceous units. The latter are irregularly enlarged and show deformation of the follicular walls. Destruction of the hair follicles and sebaceous glands can occur. The infiltrate is composed of either atypical lymphocytes with cerebriform nuclei showing high mitotic activity or monocytoid/centrocyte-like B-cells intermingled with a few plasma cells. A typical finding is the presence of small clusters of histiocytes in the perifollicular areas. Granulomas with foreign body reactions are seen rarely (2).

IMMUNOHISTOCHEMISTRY

The infiltrate is usually a mixture of B cells and T cells in varying proportions. In some cases a striking predominance of one lineage is seen. In cases with a dominant B-cell population, no monoclonal expression of Ig light chains is seen. The perifollicular histiocytes are positive for S-100 and CD1a, and negative for CD68, and lysozyme (T-cell-associated dendritic cells) (2).

MOLECULAR BIOLOGY

Neither TCRγ-chains nor IgH genes are clonally rearranged. All cases have been negative for EBER-1.

DIFFERENTIAL DIAGNOSIS

Folliculotropic mycosis fungoides differs from pseudolymphomatous folliculitis in many ways; clinically, the lesions are more superficial (patches and plaques), cerebriform cells dominate the infiltrate, follicular mucinosis can be seen, and clonal TCR gene rearrangements are found.

TREATMENT

Excision of the lesions results in complete cure.

Pseudolymphomatous folliculitis

Clinical features
   Solitary nodule usually on the face of adults
Histological features
   Folliculotropic diffuse or nodular infiltrate composed of cerebriform cells or
      centrocyte-like or monocytoid cells with mitotic activity
   Enlargment and deformation of pilosebaceous units
Immunophenotype
   No monoclonal expression of κ or λ
Molecular biology
   IgH and TCR in germline configuration
   EBER-1 negative
Treatment
   Excision
Clinical course
   Benign

CLINICAL COURSE

The clinical course is favorable and recurrences are very unlikely. Many cases show prompt resolution even after an incisional biopsy.

COMMENTS

The cause of pseudolymphomatous folliculitis in not known. Searches for EBV and herpes simplex virus have been negative.

REFERENCES

1. Kibbi AG, Scrimenti RJ, Koenig RR, Mihm MC Jr. A solitary nodule of the left cheek. Pseudolymphomatous folliculitis. Arch Dermatol 1988; 124:1272–1273, 1276.
2. Arai E, Okubo H, Tsuchida T, Kitamura K, Katayama I. Pseudolymphomatous folliculitis: a clinicopathologic study of 15 cases of cutaneous pseudolymphoma with follicular invasion. Am J Surg Pathol 1999; 23:1313–1319.

40.5. Cutaneous Inflammatory Pseudotumor

Dmitry V. Kazakov, Günter Burg, and Werner Kempf
Department of Dermatology, University Hospital, Zürich, Switzerland

Inflammatory pseudotumor (IPT) (plasma cell granuloma, inflammatory myofibro-blastic pseudotumor) refers to a spectrum of idiopathic benign conditions with unknown etiology that can develop in various organs and deep tissues, particularly in the lung. Whatever the anatomic location, the lesions share common histological features, namely good circumscription, proliferation of myofibroblasts/fibroblasts, a mixed cell infiltrate containing high numbers of plasma cells, and often reactive germinal centers (1). There are only a few reports on cutaneous IPT.

CLINICAL FEATURES

Cutaneous IPT occurs as a solitary, slowly growing, tender nodule measuring 1–3 cm in diameter. There is no site of predilection or gender predominance (2,3).

HISTOLOGICAL FEATURES

The deep dermis and/or subcutis are usually involved. The histopathological features may vary depending on the duration of the lesion (4). In early stages, at scanning magnification, IPT resembles a lymph node (Fig. 1). The lesion is well circumscribed but nonencapsulated. Germinal centers are prominent and usually dispersed throughout the lesion. Numerous plasma cells are seen in the interfollicular areas (plasma cell granuloma) (Fig. 2). There are only a few, if any, spindle cells either scattered or arranged in small clusters. Over time, the spindle/stellate cells start to dominate the infiltrate and become arranged in a fascicular or storiform pattern (IPT) (Fig. 1). Even later stages are characterized by predominant proliferation of fibroblasts and marked fibrosis/sclerosis with thick collagen bundles arranged in concentric whorls (targetoid collagenosis). Histological variations include presence

341

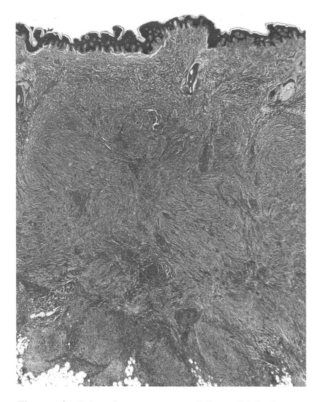

Figure 1 Sclerotic area arranged in a fascicular or storiform pattern surrounded by a lymphocytic infiltrate and formation of germinal centers. (Specimen courtesy of H. Kutzner, Germany.)

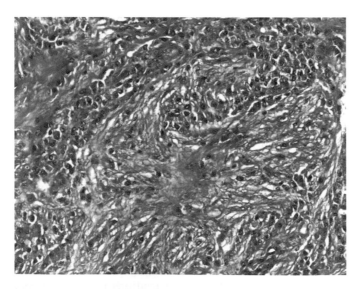

Figure 2 The infiltrate is mainly composed of plasma cells. (Specimen courtesy of H. Kutzner, Germany.)

of high endothelial venules, admixture of eosinophils, calcification, psammoma bodies, and presence of large polygonal cells with single, double or multiple nuclei and prominent eosinophilic nucleoli resembling Reed–Sternberg cells (2–7).

IMMUNOHISTOCHEMISTRY

The plasma cells are polyclonal. The spindle/stellate cells are myofibroblasts expressing SMA and vimentin (inflammatory myofibroblastic pseudotumor). In later stages, SMA reactivity is no longer observed (2,3). The large polygonal cells resembling Reed–Sternberg cells also appear to be myofibroblasts (vimentin+, CD15–, CD30–) (3).

MOLECULAR BIOLOGY

No information is available purely cutaneous lesions.

DIFFERENTIAL DIAGNOSIS

The differential diagnostic spectrum for cutaneous IPT is quite broad, primarily because of the highly variable histological patterns. IPT differs from subcutaneous lymph nodes because it lacks subcapsular and medullary sinuses. The polyclonal nature of the infiltrate allows one to exclude a lymphoma. Angiolymphoid hyperplasia with eosinophilia and Kimura disease both have a more prominent vascular component and eosinophils. Infectious dermatoses (mycobacteria, deep fungal infections) are not well circumscribed, have large numbers of neutrophils, and often display pseudocarcinomatous hyperplasia. In addition, special stains may help to identify

---

Cutaneous inflammatory pseudotumor

Clinical features
  Solitary, slowly growing, tender nodule
Histological features
  Well-circumscribed nodular infiltrates in deep dermis/subcutis
    with reactive germinal centers, plasma cells, eosinophils.
  Proliferation of spindle/stellate myofibroblasts, sclerotic stroma
    in later stages
Immunophenotype
  Polyclonal expression of κ or λ on plasma cells
  Spindle/stellate cells: SMA+
Treatment
  Excision
Clinical course
  Benign

---

a causative pathogen. The later stages of cutaneous IPT should be distinguished from erythema elevatum diutinum and granuloma faciale, both of which usually contain vasculitic changes. Dermatofibroma with lymphoid follicles and perivascular plasmacytosis differs from cutaneous IPT because the germinal centers are unevenly distributed and concentrated at the periphery of the infiltrate.

TREATMENT

Surgical excision is recommended.

CLINICAL COURSE

No recurrences have been described after complete surgical removal.

COMMENTS

The cause of cutaneous IPT is not known. Some investigators believe that the condition represents a persistent hypersensitivity reaction to an unknown antigen (1,3). Klebsiella, Gram-positive cocci, and mycobacteria (mycobacterial spindle-cell proliferations) have been detected in some cases of extracutaneous IPT.

REFERENCES

1. Coffin CM, Humphrey PA, Dehner LP. Extrapulmonary inflammatory myofibroblastic tumor: a clinical and pathological survey. Semin Diagn Pathol 1998; 15:85–101.
2. Hurt MA, Santa Cruz DJ. Cutaneous inflammatory pseudotumor. Lesions resembling "inflammatory pseudotumors" or "plasma cell granulomas" of extracutaneous sites. Am J Surg Pathol 1990; 14:764–773.
3. MacSweeney F, Desai SA. Inflammatory pseudotumour of the subcutis: a report on the fine needle aspiration findings in a case misdiagnosed cytologically as malignant. Cytopathology 2000; 11:57–60.
4. Carlson JA, Ackerman AB, Fletcher CDM, Zelber B. A cutaneous spindle cell lesion. Am J Dermatopathol 2001; 23:62–66.
5. Ramachandra S, Hollowood K, Bisceglia M, Fletcher CD. Inflammatory pseudotumour of soft tissues: a clinicopathological and immunohistochemical analysis of 18 cases. Histopathology 1995; 27:313–323.
6. Yang M. Cutaneous inflammatory pseudotumor: a case report with immunohistochemical and ultrastructural studies. Pathology 1993; 25:405–409.
7. Schurch W, Seemayer TA, Gabbiani G. The myofibroblast: a quarter century after its discovery. Am J Surg Pathol 1998; 22:141–147.

40.6. Castleman Disease

Dmitry V. Kazakov, Günter Burg, and Werner Kempf
Department of Dermatology, University Hospital, Zürich, Switzerland

DEFINITION

Castleman disease (CAD) is an unusual lymphoid hyperplasia of unknown etiology first described by Castleman in 1956. The disease may be systemic or localized and can involve lymph nodes (more often mediastinal ones) or extranodal sites. Three histological subtypes have been identified: the hyaline-vascular (HV) variant (~90% of cases), the plasma cell (PC) variant, and the intermediate variant (1). The HV type occurs in younger persons with few systemic symptoms. The PC type is seen in an older population often with systemic symptoms. The PC type may be associated with POEMS syndrome [polyneuropathy, organomegaly, endocrinopathy, monoclonal gammopathy, skin changes (hyperpigmentation and hypertrichosis)] (2,3). Specific cutaneous involvement is extremely rare, with only a few cases reported (4–6). In rare instances, CAD can be confined to the skin without evidence of lymph node involvement.

CLINICAL FEATURES

Patients with CAD are usually young or middle-aged. The specific skin changes featured solitary or multiple (up to 20), asymptomatic nodules located on the trunk, measuring 2–6 cm in size. A variety of non-specific skin lesions (maculopapular eruptions, pemphigus vulgaris, Kaposi sarcoma, necrotizing vasculitis, paraneoplastic pemphigus, and xanthomas) has been described in patients with CAD (7,8).

HISTOLOGY

All the histological types may occur in the skin. There is a nodular, well-circumscribed infiltrate involving the dermis and subcutaneous tissue with a prominent follicular

345

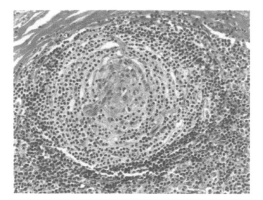

Figure 1   Castleman disease: onion skin-like arrangement of lymphocytes around a central vessel.

growth pattern. Most of the follicles demonstrate atrophic germinal centers and concentric rings of small lymphocytes penetrated by interfollicular capillaries. Multinucleated giant cells resembling the Warthin–Finkeldey cells seen in measles can be observed in some germinal centers. There is also a mixed infiltrate of epithelioid histiocytes and lymphoplasmacytoid cells and large numbers of small vessels with thickened hyalinized walls. The PC type is distinguished by abundant sheets of mature plasma cells in the interfollicular areas and displays little hyalinization of vessels. The HV variant is typified by marked perivascular hyalinization of collagen which can be radially arranged around vessels with thick hyalinized walls (Fig. 1). The HV type seems to predominate in cases with subcutaneous involvement (9).

IMMUNOHISTOCHEMISTRY

The contracted lymphoid follicles are visualized with CD21 and CD35 antibodies (often as a CD21/CD35 antibody cocktail) directed against the C3d and C3b receptors, respectively. Other markers specific for follicular dendritic cells, namely KiM4p, KiM4, KiFDClp, and R4/23 may be used (10–12). The small lymphocytes around the germinal centers are polyclonal B cells. The interfollicular histiocytes stain for CD68 and MAC 387. In addition, clusters of S-100+, CDla, T cells, and occasional CD30+ cells are seen in the interfollicular zones.

MOLECULAR BIOLOGY

No TCR or IgH gene rearrangements have been demonstrated in the skin lesions.

TREATMENT

In solitary CAD, resection is the treatment of choice. Radiation and/or chemotherapy have been used in multicentric disease with inconsistent results.

CLINICAL COURSE AND PROGNOSIS

The impact of skin involvement on the prognosis is not known due to the paucity of observations. In general, patients with localized disease and extranodal lesions have a benign course. Patients with CAD may develop overt lymphomas or follicular dendritic cell sarcomas (11,12).

DIFFERENTIAL DIAGNOSIS

Angiolymphoid hyperplasia with eosinophilia differs from cutaneous CAD because it lacks contracted lymphoid follicles with onion-like mantle zones and perivascular hyalinization, while the infiltrate usually contains large numbers of eosinophils. Cutaneous sinus histiocytosis with massive lymphadenopathy (SHML) demonstrates a more prominent proliferation of epithelioid histiocytes (S-100+, CDla−), some of which have abundant granular, eosinophilic cytoplasm. Hyalinized vessels and abundant plasma cells may be seen in SHML but onion-like structures are lacking. Another clue to SHML is emperipolesis of histiocytes. Study of TCR rearrangements is helpful in distinguishing CAD from skin involvement by angioimmunoblastic T-cell lymphoma. The neoplastic follicles in cutaneous follicular center cell lymphoma and marginal zone lymphoma are usually larger than those seen in CAD, with an expanded irregular meshwork of follicular dendritic cells. Collagen and vascular hyalinization is absent. Light-chain restriction and clonal IgH rearrangements are found in many instances, facilitating the differential diagnosis.

Cutaneous Castleman disease

Clinical features
  Elderly people
  Multiple or solitary nodules
Histological features
  Onion-like follicles with reduced mantle zone and gerninal centers depleted of
    follicular dendritic cells
  Hyalinized collagen and vessels
  Plasma cells
Immunophenotype
  Follicles: CD21+, CD35+, KiM4p+, KiM4+, KiFDClp+, R4/23+
  Mantle zone: polyclonal B cells
Molecular biology
  No TCR or IgH rearrangements
Laboratory evaluation
  Relevant only in POEMS syndrome
Treatment
  Excision, radiation and/or chemotherapy
Clinical course
  Benign

COMMENTS

The cause of the disease is not known. It has been suggested that the PC type may represent an immunologic reaction to EBV and HHV-8 virus, whereas the HV type might be a hamartomatous proliferation. In addition, overproduction of IL-6 by lymphoid cells may account for increased vascular proliferation (13).

REFERENCES

1. Palestro G, Turrini F, Pagano M, Chiusa L. Castleman's disease. Adv Clin Path 1993; 3:11–22.
2. Soubrier MJ, Dubost JJ, Sauvezie BJ. POEMS syndrome: a study of 25 cases and a review of the literature. French Study Group on POEMS Syndrome. Am J Med 1994; 97:543–553.
3. Weichenthal M, Stemm AV, Ramsauer J, Mensing H, Feller AC, Meigel W. POEMS syndrome: cicatricial alopecia as an unusual cutaneous manifestation associated with an underlying plasmacytoma. J Am Acad Dermatol 1999; 40:808–812.
4. Kubota Y, Noto S, Takakuwa T, Tadokoro M, Mizoguchi M. Skin involvement in giant lymph node hyperplasia (Castleman's disease). J Am Acad Dermatol 1993; 29:778–780.
5. Skelton HG, Smith KJ. Extranodal multicentric Castleman's disease with cutaneous involvement. Mod Pathol 1998; 11:983–989.
6. Sleater J, Mullins D. Subcutaneous Castleman's disease of the wrist. Am J Dermatopathol 1995; 17:174–178.
7. Kingsmore SF, Silva OE, Hall BD, Sheldon EA, Cripe LD, St Clair EW. Presentation of multicentric Castleman's disease with sicca syndrome, cardiomyopathy, palmar and plantar rash. J Rheumatol 1993; 20:1588–1591.
8. Wolff H, Kunte C, Messer G, Rappersberger K, Held E, Lohrs U, Plewig G, Meurer M. Paraneoplastic pemphigus with fatal pulmonary involvement in a woman with a mesenteric Castleman tumour. Br J Dermatol 1999; 140:313–316.
9. Kazakov DV, Fanburg-Smith JC, Suster S, Neuhauster TS, Palmedo G, Zamecnik M, Kempf W, Michal M. Castleman disease of the subcutis and underlying skeletal muscle: report of 6 cases. Am J Surg Pathol 2004; 28:569–777.
10. Menke DM, Tiemann M, Camoriano JK, Chang SF, Madan A, Chow M, Habermann TM, Parwaresch R. Diagnosis of Castleman's disease by identification of an immunophenotypically aberrant population of mantle zone B lymphocytes in paraffin-embedded lymph node biopsies. Am J Clin Pathol 1996; 105:268–276.
11. Chan JK, Fletcher CD, Nayler SJ, Cooper K. Follicular dendritic cell sarcoma. Clinicopathologic analysis of 17 cases suggesting a malignant potential higher than currently recognized. Cancer 1997; 79:294–313.
12. Chan AC, Chan KW, Chan JK, Au WY, Ho WK, Ng WM. Development of follicular dendritic cell sarcoma in hyaline-vascular Castleman's disease of the nasopharynx: tracing its evolution by sequential biopsies. Histopathology 2001; 38:510–518.
13. Kinney MC, Hummell DS, Villiger PM, Hourigan A, Rollins-Smith L, Glick AD, Lawton AR. Increased interleukin-6 (IL-6) production in a young child with clinical and pathologic features of multicentric Castleman's disease. J Clin Immunol 1994; 14:382–390.

Pseudolymphomatous Infiltrates in the Context of Other Skin Disorders

Günter Burg and Werner Kempf
Department of Dermatology, University Hospital, Zürich, Switzerland

There are reactive lymphocytic infiltrates that can be referred to as pseudolymphomatous reactions in an even broader sense. These infiltrates have been observed in infestations such as scabies, viral infections (e.g., molluscum contagiosum), after use of *Hirudo medicinalis* (Fig. 1), or in neoplasms, especially those of epithelial origin, which can be accompanied by a significant lymphocytic infiltrate, sometimes with follicular formation, reflecting cell mediated immune response against the tumor cells (Fig. 2). The infiltrate may be composed of T cells or of B cells, especially

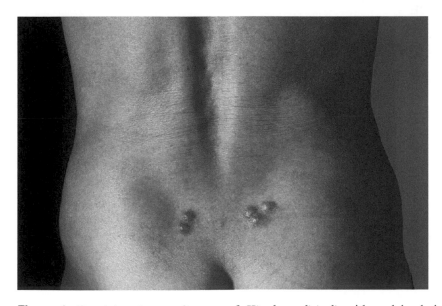

Figure 1 Pseudolymphoma after use of *Hirudo medicinalis* with nodular lesions on the lumbosacral area.

349

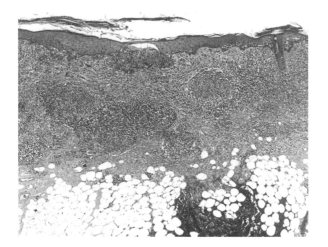

Figure 2   Pseudolymphomatous infiltrate in actinic keratosis with formation of follicles.

with squamous cell carcinoma, basal cell carcinoma, and malignant melanoma, as well as in halo (Sutton) nevi. Polyclonal plasma cells may be numerous especially in head and neck localizations (Fig. 3).

The inflammatory infiltrate can even contain atypical lymphocytes such as in some cases of molluscum contagiosum which may harbor atypical hyperchromatic mononuclear cells with abundant mitotic figures, predominantly composed of T lymphocytes (1), some of them even exhibiting Ki-1/CD30 positivity. Similar reactions may be seen in other viral infections such as verrucae or parapox virus infections.

REFERENCE

1.   de Diego J, Berridi D, Saracibar N, Requena L. Cutaneous pseudolymphoma in association with molluscum contagiosum. Am J Dermatopathol 1998; 20:518–521.

41

Parapsoriasis

Günter Burg, Werner Kempf, Reinhard Dummer, and Dmitry V. Kazakov
Department of Dermatology, University Hospital, Zürich, Switzerland

HISTORICAL PERSPECTIVES

The term "parapsoriasis" is confusing and requires explanation. It encompasses a number of different pathologic states clinically manifested by chronic recalcitrant erythematous scaling lesions.

About 100 years ago, Unna et al. (1) described two cases of the so-called parakeratosis variegata. Brocq (2), some years later, saw one of Unna and colleagues' cases, as well as some similar cases, and described it as "érythrodermies pityriasiques en plaques disséminées."

Brocq (1856–1928) in his article in 1902 reviewed the American, French, and German cases and reported 10 cases of his own (3). He coined the term "parapsoriasis" because of the similarities of the disease to psoriasis, seborrhoic eczema, and lichen ("paralichen").

The common features of the subgroups described by Brocq are: (i) long duration of the disease; (ii) good general health; (iii) absence of itching; (iv) erythema and pityriasiform scaling; (v) control of disease without cure by topical treatment; and (vi) round cell infiltrate in the papillary dermis.

The three conditions depicted in Brocq's scheme (Fig. 1) are:

1. "Parapsoriasis en gouttes" (guttate parapsoriasis). Today, this disease usually is referred to as pityriasis lichenoides chronica or as parapsoriasis guttata of Jadassohn and Juliusberg. It resembles papular syphilis or guttate psoriasis. Nosologically, it is completely unrelated to mycosis fungoides even though otherwise stated by some authors (4). Pityriasis lichenoides et varioliformis acuta (Mucha–Habermann's disease) is an acute variant of this form, which has to be differentiated from lymphomatoid papulosis. These diseases—except lymphomatoid papulosis—are not related to mycosis fungoides or other CTCLs.

2. "Parapsoriasis lichenoide," featuring a network of "pseudopapular" lesions with atrophy exhibiting a poikilodermatous appearance and the cases of parakeratosis variegata, described by Unna (1) and poikilodermia vasculare atrophicans (Jacobi) are most likely variants of the inflammatory form of parapsoriasis en plaques.

351

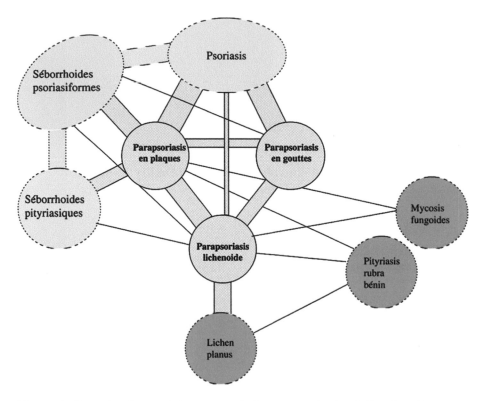

Figure 1 Brocq's scheme of the parapsoriasis group and related disorders (3).

3. "Parapsoriasis en plaques" (Brocq's disease), characterized by round or
   oval well-circumscribed macules ("plaques" in the French terminology),
   is usually 2–6 cm in diameter.

MODERN PERSPECTIVES

Today two groups of parapsoriasis can be differentiated. The benign form ["parapsoriasis en plaques" (Brocq's disease)] and large plaque forms with or without
poikiloderma. The small plaque form never evolves into mycosis fungoides or
CTCL, whereas the large plaque forms after several decades may evolve into mycosis
fungoides or CTCL in up to 50% of the cases. Table 1 summarizes criteria for differentiation of benign and premalignant forms of parapsoriasis en plaques. The relationship between benign and the premalignant forms of parapsoriasis en plaques
in terms of biologic behavior is depicted schematically in Fig. 2.

COMMENTARY

Clinicians have to deal with patients, not just with their diseases. In some instances,
it may be difficult to differentiate benign from premalignant parapsoriasis, as clear-
cut criteria for early diagnosis are lacking. In such situations, the patient may be
faced with a normal life expectancy or the risk of disease progression with tumor

Table 1 Most Useful Criteria for Distinguishing Between Benign and Premalignant Forms of Parapsoriasis en Plaques

	Benign form (small patch type)	Premalignant form (large patch type) with or without poikiloderma
Age distribution	Adults	All ages
Sex incidence (male:female)	5:1	2:1
Clinical features	Small (2–6 cm in diameter), mostly oval, or finger-like patches, slightly erythematous (pseudoatrophy) and wrinkled surface uniformly pinkish or yellowish with pityriasiform scaling	Few large patches pityriasiform scaling with or without telangiectases and netlike pigmentation
Preferential localizations	Trunk and upper extremities	Breast and buttocks
Histological features	Patchy parakeratosis, slight perivascular patchy infiltrate, no edema, no epidermotropism	Slight epidermal atrophy with loss of rete ridges, significant band-like dermal lymphocytic infiltrate sparing the subepidermal zone, no epidermotropism, no edema; telangiectases either prominent (poikilodermatous variant) or absent
Prognosis	Life expectancy normal; no progress to mycosis fungoides	Life expectancy normal in most cases; progress to mycosis fungoides may occur

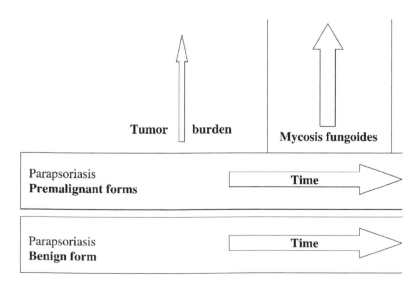

Figure 2 Biologic behavior of the benign and the premalignant forms of parapsoriasis en plaques. The latter have the potential of evolving into mycosis fungoides.

spread and death, even though the clinician cannot adequately assess the risk. Only the dynamic evolution of the disease allows a retrospective diagnosis.

Malignant melanoma, squamous cell carcinoma, mycosis fungoides, or other cutaneous T-cell lymphomas are malignant neoplastic diseases. Lentigo maligna (Hutchinson's freckle, Dubreuilh's disease) and parapsoriasis en plaques are premalignant conditions, just as some adenomas may progress to colon cancer or angioimmunoblastic lymphadenopathy may evolve into lymphoma (5,6). Progress into frank neoplasia usually requires a period of time in these conditions. Changes in the clinical presentation and—more importantly—in the histological, phenotypical or genotypical features indicate this progression. The new molecular technologies such as gene profiling, genomics, and proteomics may allow an even more precise tracking of the disease status. This progression is coupled with a change in prognosis from normal or almost normal life expectancy to reduced survival time.

Those diseases that clearly have clinical and histological changes and cannot be regarded as normal, but also do not fulfill criteria of malignancy, deserve to be labeled with a term, which reflects this intermediate situation and as distinct nosologic entities. This term since the days of Brocq has been "parapsoriasis," and there is no reason for changing it (7). Otherwise, there will be a bias in epidemiologic data on frequencies, mortality rates, and other parameters.

REFERENCES

1. Unna PG, Santi S, Pollitzer S. Ueber die Parakeratosen im allgemeinen und eine neue Form derselben Parakeratosis variegata. Monatsschr Prakt Dermatol 1890; 10:404–412, 444–459.
2. Brocq L. Les érythrodermies pityriasiques en plaques disséminées. Rev Gen Clin J Pract 1897; 11:577–590.
3. Brocq L. Les parapsoriasis. Ann Dermatol Syphilol 1902; 3:433–468.
4. King ID, Ackerman AB. Guttate parapsoriasis/digitate dermatosis (small plaque parapsoriasis) is mycosis fungoides (see comments). Am J Dermatopathol 1992; 14:518–530.
5. Frizzera G, Kaneko Y, Sakurai M. Angioimmunoblastic lymphadenopathy and related disorders: a retrospective look in search of definitions. Leukemia 1989; 3:1–5.
6. Smith JL, Hodges E, Quin CT, McCarthy KP, Wright DH. Frequent T and B cell oligoclones in histologically and immunophenotypically characterized angioimmunoblastic lymphadenopathy. Am J Pathol 2000; 156:661–669.
7. Burg G, Dummer R. Small plaque (digitate) parapsoriasis is an 'abortive cutaneous T-cell lymphoma' and is not mycosis fungoides [editorial; comment]. Arch Dermatol 1995; 131(3):336–338.

41.1. Small Plaque Parapsoriasis

Günter Burg, Werner Kempf, Reinhard Dummer, and Dmitry V. Kazakov
Department of Dermatology, University Hospital, Zürich, Switzerland

CLASSIFICATION

WHO/EORTC Classification (2005): Not listed
WHO Classification (2001): Not listed
REAL Classification (1997): Not listed
EORTC Classification (1997): Not listed

DEFINITION

Benign disorder of unknown etiology and little tendency to progress. Synonyms: parapsoriasis, small patch (digitiform) type (Brocq's disease); parapsoriasis en plaques, benign type; digitate dermatosis, xanthoerythrodermia perstans; chronic superficial dermatitis.

CLINICAL FEATURES

Small (2–6 cm in diameter), mostly oval or finger-like patches, slightly erythematous. The color is brown red, fine and powdery (pityriasiform) scaling (Fig. 1). The surface is wrinkled. These lesions are extraordinarily stable in shape and size over years and decades. They are preferentially located on the trunk and upper extremities, following skin lines.

HISTOLOGY

Patchy parakeratosis. Epidermis normal or slightly spongiotic. Patchy loose perivascular and disseminated lymphocytic infiltrate in the dermis (Fig. 2). No edema in the dermis. Epidermotropism of lymphoid cells is lacking.

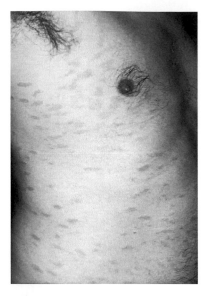

Figure 1 Small plaque parapsoriasis: multiple small finely scaling oval macules and patches.

IMMUNOHISTOCHEMISTRY

Inflammatory pattern, exhibiting mostly CD4+ and some CD8+ cells (1).

MOLECULAR BIOLOGY

Clonal rearrangement for the T-cell receptor genes is not detectable. There may be however clonal rearrangement of undetermined significance in the peripheral blood of patients (2).

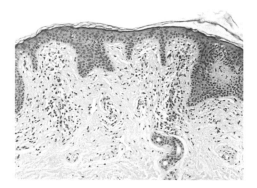

Figure 2 Small plaque parapsoriasis: sparse predominantly perivascular lymphocytic infiltrate in the upper dermis.

TREATMENT

Heliotherapy, topical glucocorticosteroids, or PUVA treatment are effective in clearing skin lesions (3). However, recurrences regularly occur after weeks or months (4).

CLINICAL COURSE AND PROGNOSIS

Life expectancy is normal. Progression into mycosis fungoides or other CTCLs does not occur.

DIFFERENTIAL DIAGNOSIS

Eczema and early stage mycosis fungoides are less stable with respect to size and distribution of skin lesions (5).

REFERENCES

1. Haeffner AC, Smoller BR, Zepter K, Wood GS. Differentiation and clonality of lesional lymphocytes in small plaque parapsoriasis. Arch Dermatol 1995; 131:321–324.
2. Muche JM, Lukowsky A, Asadullah K, Gellrich S, Sterry W. Demonstration of frequent occurrence of clonal T cells in the peripheral blood of patients with primary cutaneous T-cell lymphoma. Blood 1999; 90:1636–1642.
3. Gambichler T, Manke-Heimann A. Balneophototherapy in small plaque parapsoriasis— four case reports. J Eur Acad Dermatol Venereol 1998; 10:179–181.
4. Westphal HJ, Walther A. Phototherapie der Parapsoriasis. Dermatol Monatsschr 1989; 175:555–560.
5. Burg G, Dummer R. Small plaque (digitate) parapsoriasis is an 'abortive cutaneous T-cell lymphoma' and is not mycosis fungoides [editorial; comment]. Arch Dermatol 1995; 131(3):336–338.

41.2. Large Plaque Parapsoriasis *With* and *Without* Poikiloderma

Günter Burg, Werner Kempf, Reinhard Dummer, and Dmitry V. Kazakov
Department of Dermatology, University Hospital, Zürich, Switzerland

LARGE PATCH TYPE *WITHOUT* POIKILODERMA

Classification

> WHO/EORTC Classification (2005): Not listed
> WHO Classification (2001): Not listed
> REAL Classification (1997): Not listed
> EORTC Classification (1997): Not listed

Definition

Premalignant inflammatory disorder with tendency to evolve into mycosis fungoides or other CTCLs. Synonyms: parapsoriasis en plaques, premalignant type, parapsoriasis en grandes plaques simples.

Clinical Features

Few large patches showing pityriasiform scaling. Lesions tend to grow slowly in size. They are preferentially located on the breast and buttocks.

Histology

Patchy parakeratosis, the epidermis is normal or slightly atrophic. There is a significant band-like lymphocytic infiltrate sparing the subepidermal zone. Epidermotropism and edema of the upper dermis usually is missing.

Immunohistochemistry

Inflammatory eczematous pattern with CD4+ and some CD8+ cells (1).

Molecular Biology

Clonal gene rearrangement of T-cell receptors has been found in 50% of the cases (2).

Treatment

Heliotherapy, PUVA or topical glucocorticosteroids usually are effective in clearing skin lesions (3). However, recurrences occur after weeks or months.

Clinical Course and Prognosis

Most cases are stable over years and decades with temporary remissions due to non-aggressive topical therapy. However, up to 50% of the cases may show progression into mycosis fungoides (4–6).

Differential Diagnosis

Early stages of mycosis fungoides or other CTCLs in which skin lesions are less stable and tend to grow in size and thickness within a few weeks.

LARGE PATCH TYPE *WITH* POIKILODERMA

Classification

> WHO/EORTC Classification (2005): Not listed
> WHO Classification (2001): Not listed
> REAL Classification (1997): Not listed
> EORTC Classification (1997): Not listed

Definition

Premalignant form of parapsoriasis with a tendency to evolve into mycosis fungoides or other CTCLs in up to 50% of the cases. Synonyms: Prereticulotic poikiloderma, parapsoriasis en grandes plaques poikilodermiques; poikiloderma vasculare atrophicans; parapsoriasis lichenoides; parakeratosis variegata.

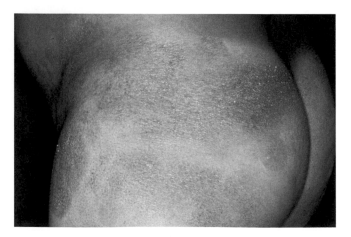

Figure 1 Large plaque parapsoriasis: large erythematous and scaling plaques with slight poikiloderma on the buttocks.

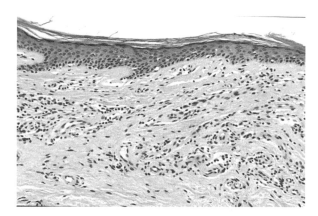

Figure 2 Large plaque parapsoriasis with poikiloderma (also referred to as poikilodermia vasculare atrophicans): atrophic epidermis, telangiectatic vessels, and sparse lymphocytic infiltrate.

Clinical Features

Large patches with net-like telangiectasia and pigmentation rendering the feature of poikilodermia. The localization is preferentially on the breast and buttocks (Fig. 1).

Histology

Parakeratosis. Slight epidermal atrophy with loss of rete ridges. Significant band-like lymphocytic infiltrate, which spares the subepidermal zone and does not invade the epidermis. Dilatation of blood vessels especially in the papillary dermis (Fig. 2).

Immunohistochemistry

The inflammatory infiltrate contains mostly CD4+ lymphocytes and some CD8+ cells (7–9).

Molecular Biology

Lack of clonal T-cell-receptor gene rearrangement.

Treatment

Heliotherapy, PUVA and topical glucocorticosteroids lead to temporary remission of symptoms. The poikilodermatous aspect however remains unchanged. Recurrences occur regularly within weeks or months.

Clinical Course and Prognosis

Evolving into mycosis fungoides or other CTCLs may occur in up to 50% of the cases after years and decades (10).

Differential Diagnosis

Early stages of cutaneous T-cell lymphomas, which progress more rapidly and show clonality of the infiltrate.

REFERENCES

1. Buechner SA. Parapsoriasis en plaques. Characterization of the cellular infiltrate using monoclonal antibodies. Z Hautkr 1988; 63:423–424.
2. Simon M, Flaig MJ, Kind P, Sander CA, Kaudewitz P. Large plaque parapsoriasis: clinical and genotypic correlations. J Cutan Pathol 2000; 27:57–60.
3. Rosenbaum MM, Roenigk HJ, Caro WA, Esker A. Photochemotherapy in cutaneous T cell lymphoma and parapsoriasis en plaques. Long-term follow-up in forty-three patients. J Am Acad Dermatol 1985; 13:613–622.
4. Graciansky PD, Leclercq R, Boulle M. Parapsoriasis en plaques for over 10 years. Evolution towards mycosis fungoides. Appearance of alopecia areas on the plaques and in the extended peripheral zones. Bull Soc Fr Dermatol Syphiligr 1969; 76:301–302.
5. Lazar AP, Caro WA, Roenigk HJ, Pinski KS. Parapsoriasis and mycosis fungoides: the Northwestern University experience, 1970 to 1985. J Am Acad Dermatol 1989; 21:919–923.
6. Kikuchi A, Naka W, Harada T, Sakuraoka K, Harada R, Nishikawa T. Parapsoriasis en plaques: its potential for progression to malignant lymphoma. J Am Acad Dermatol 1993; 29:419–422.
7. McMillan EM, Wasik R, Martin D, Everett MA. T cell nature of exocytic and dermal lymphoid cells in atrophic parapsoriasis demonstrated by monoclonal Leu 1 and affinity isolated antibodies. J Cutan Pathol 1981; 8:355–360.
8. McMillan EM, Peters S, Jackson I, Wasik R, Stoneking L, Everett MA, Hamzavi SL. Immunoperoxidase examination of cutaneous infiltrates of mycosis fungoides and large-plaque atrophic parapsoriasis with OKT10. J Am Acad Dermatol 1984; 10: 457–461.
9. Lindae ML, Abel EA, Hoppe RT, Wood GS. Poikilodermatous mycosis fungoides and atrophic large-plaque parapsoriasis exhibit similar abnormalities of T-cell antigen expression. Arch Dermatol 1988; 124:366–372.
10. Samman PD. The natural history of parapsoriasis en plaques (chronic superficial dermatitis) and prereticulotic poikiloderma. Br J Dermatol 1972; 87:405–411.

42

Cutaneous T-cell Lymphoproliferative Disorders of Unknown Significance

42.1. Papuloerythroderma of Ofuji

Günter Burg and Werner Kempf
Department of Dermatology, University Hospital, Zürich, Switzerland

DEFINITION

Papuloerythroderma of Ofuji (1) is a rare intensely pruritic erythrodermic dermatosis with a polymorphous etiology which frequently includes an association with CTCL, visceral malignancy or immunodeficiency. Since papuloerythroderma has differential diagnostic implications in the context of malignant lymphoma, it is briefly discussed here. It is not listed in any of the major lymphoma classifications.

CLINICAL FEATURES

This rare and nosologically heterogeneous disease was originally described in Japanese patients (1) but similar cases have been reported from western countries (2–4). The median age is 70 years. It occurs more frequent in males than in females (5). The original report describes extensive erythroderma, plaques and solid papules (Figs. 1,2). The coalescing brownish papules are flat-topped and observed mainly on the flexor surfaces of the extremities. The axillae, inguinal regions, antecubital and popliteal fossae, and big furrows on the abdomen are spared (the "deckchair" sign) (1,4,5). The most common abnormal laboratory findings were eosinophilia and an elevated serum IgE level (3,5). Associations with Hodgkin lymphoma (6), visceral malignancies (7), and immunodeficiency syndromes (8,9) have been reported.

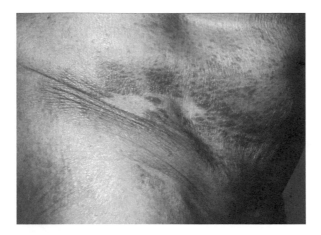

Figure 1 Follicular and plaque-like infiltration of the skin on the trunk with islands of clinically uninvolved skin.

HISTOLOGY

Cutaneous biopsies show eczematous features with dermal lymphocytic and plasmacytic infiltrates, as well as exocytosis of eosinophils and neutrophils in some cases (2,5).

IMMUNOHISTOCHEMISTRY

Staining for S-100 and UCHL-1 (CD45 RO) shows numerous dendritic cells and mature T cells in the dermis (3,10).

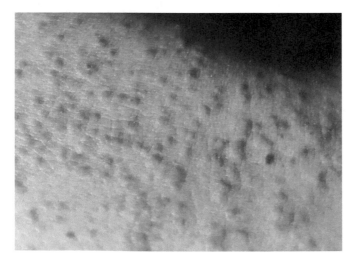

Figure 2 Flat topped lichenoid papules.

TREATMENT

Both PUVA and bath PUVA (11), UVB in combination with topical steroids, etretinate (12), Re-PUVA (13) oral steroids and cyclosporine (14) all appear to be effective therapeutic modalities (5) with both improvement in skin findings and reduction in pruritus.

CLINICAL COURSE AND PROGNOSIS

The prognosis is good, if there is no underlying malignancy.

DIFFERENTIAL DIAGNOSIS

The clinical differential diagnoses include Sézary syndrome and other erythrodermas including paraneoplastic ones. Immunodeficiency disorders have to be excluded.

COMMENTS

Papuloerythroderma associated with follicular mucinosis in mycosis fungoides (MF) and transition to CTCL (5,15), also have been described, raising the possibility that papuloerythroderma may be a precursor or manifestation of CTCL (13).

REFERENCES

1. Ofuji S, Furukawa F, Miyachi Y, Ohno S. Papuloerythroderma. Dermatologica 1984; 169:125–130.
2. Bettoli V, Mantovani L, Altieri E, Strumia R. Ofuji papuloerythroderma: report of a European case. Dermatology 1993; 186:187–189.
3. Tay YK, Tan KC, Wong WK, Ong BH. Papuloerythroderma of Ofuji: a report of three cases and review of the literature. Br J Dermatol 1994; 130:773–776.
4. Aste N, Fumo G, Conti Biggio P. Ofuji papuloerythroderma. J Eur Acad Dermatol Venereol 2000; 14:55–57.
5. Bech-Thomsen N, Thomsen K. Ofuji's papuloerythroderma: a study of 17 cases. Clin Exp Dermatol 1998; 23:79–83.
6. de Vries HJ, Koopmans AK, Starink TM, Mekkes JR. Ofuji papuloerythroderma associated with Hodgkin's lymphoma. Br J Dermatol 2002; 147:186–187.
7. Nazzari G, Sabattini C. Ofuji's papuloerythroderma. An association with early gastric cancer. Eur J Dermatol 1999; 9:317–318.
8. Garcia-Patos V, Repiso T, Rodriguez-Cano L, Castells A. Ofuji papuloerythroderma in a patient with the acquired immunodeficiency syndrome. Dermatology 1996; 192: 164–166.
9. Just M, Carrascosa JM, Ribera M, Bielsa I, Ferrandiz C. Dideoxyinosine-associated Ofuji papuloerythroderma in an HIV-infected patient. Dermatology 1997; 195:410–411.
10. Wakeel RA, Keefe M, Chapman RS. Papuloerythroderma. Another case of a new disease. Arch Dermatol 1991; 127:96–98.
11. Michel S, Hohenleutner U, Landthaler M. Ofuji papuloerythroderma: PUVA bath treatment. Hautarzt 1999; 50:360–362.

12. Fujii K, Kanno Y, Ohgo N. Etretinate therapy for papuloerythroderma. Eur J Dermatol 1999; 9:610–613.
13. Suh KS, Kim HC, Chae YS, Kim ST. Ofuji papuloerythroderma associated with follicular mucinosis in mycosis fungoides. J Dermatol 1998; 25:185–189.
14. Sommer S, Henderson CA. Papuloerythroderma of Ofuji responding to treatment with cyclosporin. Clin Exp Dermatol 2000; 25:293–295.
15. Dwyer CM, Chapman RS, Smith GD. Papuloerythroderma and cutaneous T cell lymphoma. Dermatology 1994; 188:326–328.

Clonal T-cell Disorders

Werner Kempf, Dmitry V. Kazakov, and Günter Burg
Department of Dermatology, University Hospital, Zürich, Switzerland

The T-cell receptor (TCR) is the antigen-specific receptor for T cells. During its differentiation, each T cell undergoes rearrangement of its TCR genes. This constitutes a unique signature or fingerprint for each T cell and all its clonal progeny (1).

In the past, detection of clonal rearrangement of TCR genes by Southern blot or PCR was widely used for differentiation between a malignant lymphoma and a benign reactive infiltrate (pseudolymphoma). Recently, several studies have demonstrated that clonal rearrangement of T cells can be found in more than 90% of CTCL skin biopsies (1–3). Moreover, TCR gene rearrangement studies by Southern blot and PCR techniques are consistently positive regardless of tissue fixation (formalin-fixed, paraffin-embedded vs. fresh-frozen tissue) and biopsy site when the histologic degree of diagnostic confidence is very high (4). Recently, several studies have described the detection of dominant clonal T-cell populations in cutaneous lymphoid hyperplasia, i.e., pseudolymphomas, various inflammatory disorders such as psoriasis, lichen planus, and pityriasis lichenoides, and potential precursor lesions of CTCL such as clonal dermatitis. In part, the detection of clonal T cells in these disorders is due to a higher sensitivity of new PCR-based techniques such as PCR combined with temperature or denaturing gradient gel electrophoresis (TGGE and DGGE, respectively). Due to the high sensitivity of PCR–DGGE and automated high resolution fragmenet analysis (AHRFA), these lymphocytes may comprise as little as 1% of all infiltrating cells. The significance of such a small clone is unclear at the present time. As a consequence, detection of a dominant clonal T-cell population can no longer be used as a single and independent diagnostic criterion to diagnose malignant T-cell lymphoma, much less to grade its level of malignancy. Clonality of lesional lymphocytes cannot be considered synonymous with malignant potential or overt malignancy. Nevertheless, these findings can shed a new light on the pathogenetic aspects of selected lymphoid disorders, such as angiolymphoid hyperplasia with eosinophilia (see below). The presence of clonal T cells may indicate (i) an early phase or precursor of a cutaneous T-cell lymphoma or (ii) involvement of a superantigen in the pathogenesis which could lead to a dominant mono- or oligoclonal T-cell reaction.

These findings underline the necessity to always correlate the results of molecular studies for clonality with clinical, histologic, and immunophenotypic data to achieve the correct diagnosis and nosologic assignment of a disease.

CLONAL DERMATITIS

Clonality studies employing PCR techniques led to the identification of cases with chronic, nonspecific dermatitis harboring T-cell clones. These cases have been referred to as "clonal dermatitis" (1). Some of these patients progressed to overt CTCL. About 25% of clonal dermatitis cases progress to overt CTCL within five years (1). These observations indicate that at least some cases of "clonal dermatitis" represent CTCL precursor lesions. Clonal dermatitis would thus be one of the earliest manifestations of CTCL, harboring a dominant T-cell clone but lacking histologic features diagnostic for CTCL.

LICHEN PLANUS AND PSORIASIS

Clonal T-cell populations have been found in inflammatory skin diseases such as lichen planus and psoriasis. Preferential usage of V beta 3 and/or V beta 13.1 genes by the lesional CD8+ T cells has been found in psoriatic lesions (5). Various clones of T cells have been isolated from mucosal lichen planus (6). Preferential use of V alpha 2 and V beta 3 of TCR was found on lymphocytes in mucosal lichen planus, whereas T-cells in *Candida*-induced lesions did not show a restricted TCR pattern (7). These data reflect the dominance of certain clones in the infiltrating T cells of lichen planus and psoriasis.

PITYRIASIS LICHENOIDES

Pityriasis lichenoides (PL) is a papulosquamous inflammatory skin disorder. Two clinical variants can be distinguished, pityriasis lichenoides et varioliformis acuta (PLEVA) and pityriasis lichenoides chronica (PLC) (Fig. 1). Although PL is regarded as reactive dermatosis, some cases may precede or evolve into large plaque parapsoriasis and mycosis fungoides (MF). Histologically, epidermotropism of lymphocytes, necrotic keratinocytes, and parakeratosis are characteristic features of PL. Some larger and occasionally atypical lymphoid cells are admixed. Immunohistochemically, the lymphocytes are CD4+, CD8+ or CD4– CD8– double negative. Clonal T cells can be found in the majority of PLEVA and PLC by PCR-based techniques (8–12). Although most cases of PL show a benign, self-limiting course, aggressive cases of PLEVA with a foudroyant and fatal course with disseminated erosive skin lesions have been observed (13,25). Such rare patients add support to the hypothesis that PL belong to a spectrum of cutaneous T-cell lymphoproliferative disorders with potential for malignant transformation (14).

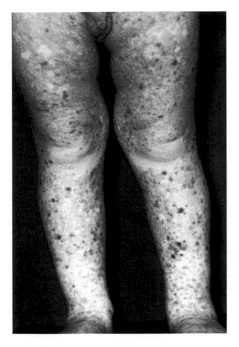

Figure 1 PLEVA: Disseminated hemorrhagic and crusted papules and macules in a child. Occasional detection of clonal T-cell receptor gamma gene rearrangement by PCR has been described.

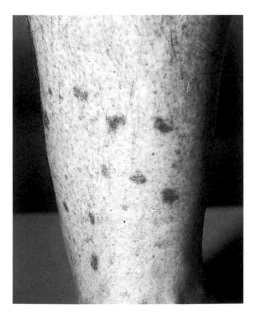

Figure 2 PPD with monoclonality: Multiple red–brown macules on the lower leg.

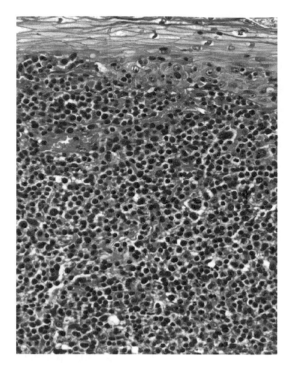

Figure 3 PPD with monoclonality: dense lichenoid lymphocytic infiltrate with occassional atypical cells and extravasated erythrocytes. Detection of clonal T-cell receptor gamma gene rearrangement by PCR.

PERSISTENT PIGMENTED PURPURIC DERMATITIS (PPPD)

Clinically, the disease manifests with multiple purpuric skin lesions (Fig. 2). In one study, half of the biopsies of PPPD showed features typically seen in MF, such as lymphocytes aligned along the junctional zone (15) (Fig. 3). The lymphocytes in MF, but not in PPPD, displayed markedly atypical nuclei. A clonal T-cell population with rearranged TCR genes detected by PCR was present in three of three and one of two specimens from patients with both PPPD and MF, but also in 8 of 12 (66%) specimens typical of lichenoid patterns of PPPD (15). Crowson et al. (16) proposed the term "atypical pigmentary purpura" (APP) for cases of pigmented purpura in which individual lesions, although clinically presenting as PP, show morphological features of MF including atypical lymphocytes and epidermotropism of lymphoid cells. Also, APP should not be equated with purpuric MF; it is not necessarily a precursor lesion of MF, and may be of drug-induced. Moreover, detection of clonality does not imply the necessity for different or more aggressive treatment of clonal PPPD than in nonclonal cases, as we have seen a patient with clonal PPPD showing complete remission after PUVA (17). Clinical features are critical to the final diagnosis because there is an overlap histologically in MF and PPPD.

ANGIOLYMPHOID HYPERPLASIA WITH EOSINOPHILIA AND KIMURA DISEASE

Angiolymphoid hyperplasia with eosinophilia (ALHE) was first described in 1969 (18). It is characterized by solitary or multiple red–brown dermal and subcutaneous nodules usually located on the head and neck (19). Also, ALHE is commonly regarded to be an angioproliferative process due to the presence of prominent, bizarrely-shaped blood vessels, which have been described as epithelioid (20). The relationship of ALHE to Kimura disease, a condition occurring in male Orientals and sharing some of the same clinical and histological features, remains uncertain. Both the cell of origin and the pathogenesis of ALHE remain controversial (21). Histologically, ALHE lesions show irregularly shaped blood vessels and an inflammatory infiltrate dominated by lymphocytes and eosinophils. Immunohistochemical studies demonstrate that the majority of lymphocytes are of T-cell lineage. Occasionally, admixed B cells may form lymphoid follicles (22).

We detected clonally rearranged T-cell receptor genes in ALHE by two independent methods, namely by PCR and DGGE as well as AHFRA. Five of seven patients displayed a clonal T-cell population and proliferative activity of T-cells in lesional tissue (23). The majority of these cases showed a protracted and therapy-resistant course with recurrences. Detection of T-cell clonality has also been reported in cases with Kimura disease (24). These data suggest that some cases of ALHE and Kimura disease harboring a clonal T-cell population may represent a T-cell lymphoproliferative disorder of benign or low-grade malignant nature.

REFERENCES

1. Wood GS. Analysis of clonality in cutaneous T cell lymphoma and associated diseases. Ann N Y Acad Sci 2001; 941:26–30.
2. Flaig MJ, Schuhmann K, Sander CA. Impact of molecular analysis in the diagnosis of cutaneous lymphoid infiltrates. Semin Cutan Med Surg 2000; 19:87–90.
3. Holm N, Flaig MJ, Yazdi AS, Sander CA. The value of molecular analysis by PCR in the diagnosis of cutaneous lymphocytic infiltrates. J Cutan Pathol 2002; 29:447–452.
4. Li N, Bhawan J. New insights into the applicability of T-cell receptor gamma gene rearrangement analysis in cutaneous T-cell lymphoma. J Cutan Pathol 2001; 28:412–418.
5. Chang JC, Smith LR, Froning KJ, Schwabe BJ, Laxer JA, Caralli LL, Kurland HH, Karasek MA, Wilkinson DI, Carlo DJ et al. CD8+ T cells in psoriatic lesions preferentially use T-cell receptor V beta 3 and/or V beta 13.1 genes. Proc Natl Acad Sci USA 1994; 91:9282–9286.
6. Sugerman PB, Savage NW, Seymour GJ. Phenotype and suppressor activity of T-lymphocyte clones extracted from lesions of oral lichen planus. Br J Dermatol 1994; 131:319–324.
7. Simark-Mattsson C, Bergenholtz G, Jontell M, Tarkowski A, Dahlgren UI. T cell receptor V-gene usage in oral lichen planus; increased frequency of T cell receptors expressing V alpha 2 and V beta 3. Clin Exp Immunol 1994; 98:503–507.
8. Weiss LM, Wood GS, Ellisen LW, Reynolds TC, Sklar J. Clonal T-cell populations in pityriasis lichenoides et varioliformis acuta (Mucha–Habermann disease). Am J Pathol 1987; 126:417–421.
9. Dereure O, Levi E, Kadin ME. T-Cell clonality in pityriasis lichenoides et varioliformis acuta: a heteroduplex analysis of 20 cases. Arch Dermatol 2000; 136:1483–1486.

10. Shieh S, Mikkola DL, Wood GS. Differentiation and clonality of lesional lymphocytes in pityriasis lichenoides chronica. Arch Dermatol 2001; 137:305–308.

11. Magro C, Crowson AN, Kovatich A, Burns F. Pityriasis lichenoides: a clonal T-cell lymphoproliferative disorder. Hum Pathol 2002; 33:788–795.

12. Weinberg JM, Kristal L, Chooback L, Honig PJ, Kramer EM, Lessin SR. The clonal nature of pityriasis lichenoides. Arch Dermatol 2002; 138:1063–1067.

13. Yanaba K, Kamide R, Niimura M. A case of febrile ulceronecrotic Mucha–Habermann disease requiring debridement of necrotic skin and epidermal autograft. Br J Dermatol 2002; 147:1249–1253.

14. Kadin ME. T-cell clonality in pityriasis lichenoides: evidence for a premalignant or reactive immune disorder? Arch Dermatol 2002; 138:1089–1090.

15. Toro JR, Sander CA, LeBoit. Persistent pigmented purpuric dermatitis and mycosis fungoides: simulant, precursor, or both? A study by light microscopy and molecular methods. Am J Dermatopathol 1997; 19:108–118.

16. Crowson AN, Magro CM, Zahorchak R. Atypical pigmentary purpura: a clinical, histopathologic, and genotypic study. Hum Pathol 1999; 30:1004–1012.

17. Lor P, Krueger U, Kempf W, Burg G, Nestle FO. Monoclonal rearrangement of the T cell receptor gamma-chain in lichenoid pigmented purpuric dermatitis of gougerot-blum responding to topical corticosteroid therapy. Dermatology 2002; 205:191–193.

18. Wells GC, Whimster IW. Subcutaneous angiolymphoid hyperplasia with eosinophilia. Br J Dermatol 1969; 81:1–14.

19. Olsen TG, Helwig EB. Angiolymphoid hyperplasia with eosinophilia. A clinicopathologic study of 116 patients. J Am Acad Dermatol 1985; 12:781–796.

20. Requena L, Sangueza OP. Cutaneous vascular proliferation. Part II. Hyperplasias and benign neoplasms. J Am Acad Dermatol 1997; 37:887–919.

21. Kung IT, Gibson JB, Bannatyne PM. Kimura's disease: a clinico-pathological study of 21 cases and its distinction from angiolymphoid hyperplasia with eosinophilia. Pathology 1984; 16:39–44.

22. Helander SD, Peters MS, Kuo TT, Su WP. Kimura's disease and angiolymphoid hyperplasia with eosinophilia: new observations from immunohistochemical studies of lymphocyte markers, endothelial antigens, and granulocyte proteins. J Cutan Pathol 1995; 22:319–326.

23. Kempf W, Haeffner AC, Zepter K, Sander CA, Flaig MJ, Mueller B, Panizzon RG, Hardmeier T, Adams V, Burg G. Angiolymphoid hyperplasia with eosinophilia: evidence for a T-cell lymphoproliferative origin. Hum Pathol 2002; 33:1023–1029.

24. Chim CS, Fung A, Shek TW, Liang R, Ho WK, Kwong YL. Analysis of clonality in Kimura's disease. Am J Surg Pathol 2002; 26:1083–1086.

25. Cozzio A, Hafuer J, Kempf W, Haeffer A, Palueddo G, Nidiaelis S, Gilliet R, Zimmermann D, Burg G. Febrile ulcerouecrotic Nudia–Habemann disease with clonality: a cutaneous T-cell lymphoma entity ? J Am Surg Pathol 2004; 51:1014–1017.

43

Skin Involvement in Leukemias

Stanislaw Buechner
Department of Dermatology, University of Basel, Basel, Switzerland

INTRODUCTION

Specific and nonspecific skin lesions are associated with many hematopoietic malignancies. Specific skin lesions result from direct infiltration of the dermis or subcutaneous fat by malignant leukemic cells. Nonspecific lesions are much more common and may be due to marrow failure that is the result of replacement of hematopoietic tissue by neoplastic cells. Petechiae, purpura, and ecchymoses may occur as a result of severe thrombocytopenia. The immunocompromised state of patients with leukemia is often associated with an enhanced susceptibility to bacterial, fungal, and viral infections. Specific skin lesions may be the initial clue to the presence of an underlying hematologic malignancy. Although the majority of specific lesions occur in the setting of established hematologic malignancy, the skin infiltrates may present concomitantly with systemic leukemia, or in some cases, precede the development of systemic disease (1–3). Patients with suspicious clinical lesions should have a skin biopsy performed. The diagnosis of specific skin infiltrates is based on the recognition of the preponderant cell type and pattern of infiltration in the skin and on correlation with clinical and hematologic findings. In the large majority of cases, an objective diagnosis of specific cutaneous infiltrate in patients with leukemia can be made based on distinctive clinicopathologic features. Immunohistochemical studies are helpful for distinguishing lymphoid and nonlymphoid cells, identifying subsets of these cells based on their immunophenotype. Improvements in cell identification by molecular biologic techniques are also essential for the increased precision in the diagnosis and classification of leukemias. Dermatologists must approach cutaneous leukemic infiltrates by being aware of the morphological diversity expressed by these neoplastic proliferations and of the difficulty in differentiating leukemic skin infiltrates from those of lymphomas, nonhematopoietic neoplasms, and numerous nonspecific skin lesions.

The French–American–British (FAB) classification of leukemias is based on the morphologic appearance of bone marrow and blood leukemic blasts, supplemented by cytochemical and immunohistochemical stains (4–6). The FAB type serves as an important basis for classification and in some cases prognosis and therapy of the

Table 1 Classification of Leukemias

French–American–British (FAB) classification of acute leukemias
M0 Acute myeloid leukemia with minimal evidence of myeloid differentiation
M1 Acute myeloid leukemia without maturation
M2 Acute myeloid leukemia with maturation
M3 Acute promyelocytic leukemia
M4 Acute myelomonocytic leukemia
M5 Acute monocytic leukemia
M6 Acute erythroleukemia
M7 Acute megakaryoblastic leukemia
Acute lymphoblastic leukemias

Chronic leukemias
Chronic myeloid leukemia
Chronic lymphocytic leukemia, B-cell type
Chronic lymphocytic leukemia, T-cell type
T-cell prolymphocytic leukemia
Adult T-cell leukemia/lymphoma
Hairy cell leukemia
Chronic myelomonocytic leukemia

---

individual leukemias. The classification of leukemias in which specific skin infiltrates have been reported is shown in Table 1.

REFERENCES

1. Longacre TA, Smoller BR. Leukemia cutis. Analysis of 50 biopsy-proven cases with an emphasis on occurrence in myelodysplastic syndromes. Am J Clin Pathol 1993; 100: 276–284.
2. Su WPD, Buechner SA, Li CY. Clinicopathologic correlations in leukemia cutis. J Am Acad Dermatol 1984; 11:121–128.
3. Ratnam KV, Khor CJL, Su WPD. Leukemia cutis. Dermatol Clin 1994; 12:419–431.
4. Benett JM, Catovsky D, Daniel MT, Flandrin G, Galton DAG, Gralnick HR. Proposals for the classification of the acute leukemias. Br J Haematol 1976; 33:451–458.
5. Bennett JM, Catovsky D, Daniel MT. Proposed revised criteria for the classification of acute myeloid leukemia: a report of the French–American–British cooperative group. Ann Intern Med 1985; 103:620–625.
6. Bennett JM, Catovsky D, Daniel MT, Flandrin G, Galton DAG, Gralnick HR. Proposals for the classification of chronic (mature) B and T lymphoid leukaemias. J Clin Pathol 1989; 42:567–584.

43.1. Chronic Lymphocytic Leukemia, B-cell Type (B-CLL)

Stanislaw Buechner
Department of Dermatology, University of Basel, Basel, Switzerland

Daniel W.P. Su
Department of Dermatology, Mayo Clinic, Rochester, Minnesota, U.S.A.

B-CLL is the most common leukemia of the elderly people in the western world, with only 10–15% of patients diagnosed while less than 50 years of age. There is an average incidence of 2.7 persons with CLL per 100,000 in the United States (1). The disease affects men twice as frequently as women. B-CLL is an accumulative disease of long-lived, mature, monoclonal CD5+ B cells that express high levels of the antiapoptotic protein bcl-2 (1,2). The marrow is invariably involved with leukemia cells. Cellular and humoral defects are common in patients with B-CLL. Patients with B-CLL have a greater susceptibility to infection because of numerous factors, including hypogammaglobulinemia, low complement levels, and abnormal T-cell function.

CLINICAL FEATURES

Specific skin lesions occur in approximately 8% of patients with B-CLL. The reported incidence of cutaneous lesions ranges from 4% to 45% (3), if one takes account of nonspecific findings including purpura, ecchymoses, and maculopapular eruptions. Specific lesions usually present as red or violaceous macules, papules, or nodules (4–7). Single or multiple lesions may be present. Lesions are typically seen on the face, particularly the ears, but may also frequently be seen on the scalp, trunk, and the extremities. Generalized lesions were seen in 17 of 42 patients with specific cutaneous infiltrates of B-CLL (8). The lesions may appear at the sites of herpes simplex and herpes zoster scars; they may be temporary regressing without treatment (9–11) (Fig. 1). Infection with *Borrelia burgdorferi* can trigger the development of specific cutaneous infiltrates which may occur at the sites typical for borrelial lymphocytoma such as the nipple, scrotum, and earlobe (12). In addition, a predilection for specific infiltrates to arise at the site of squamous cell carcinoma, basal cell

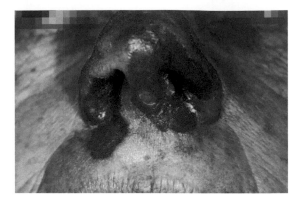

Figure 1 Specific ulcerative lesions at the site of herpes simplex infection.

carcinoma, and actinic keratosis has been observed (13). Atypical manifestations of cutaneous B-CLL have included chronic paronychia (14), subungual erythematous nodules involving several fingers (15), dystrophy of toenails resembling onychomycosis (16), finger clubbing with periosteal bone destruction of the distal digits (17), and papulovesicular eruption of the face (18). The prognosis varies, depending upon clinical stage; the presence of specific skin lesions in patients with B-CLL does not seem to be an independent poor prognostic sign (8).

HISTOLOGY

Three main patterns of skin infiltrates can be observed in B-CLL: superficial and deep perivascular and periadnexal infiltrate, nodular–diffuse infiltrates and band-like infiltrate (8). The infiltrate is typically separated from the epidermis by a narrow Grenz zone of normal collagen although isolated epidermotropic cells may be observed (Fig. 2). Usually, the infiltrate extends through the full thickness of the dermis and into the subcutaneous fat (8,19). The density of the infiltrate varies, and may be limited in a small proportion of cases. Rarely, a subepidermal bullous separation, accompanied by edema of the superficial dermis, may be present. A granulomatous component to the leukemic infiltrates, with epithelioid cells and giant cells can be observed in those specific lesions occurring in herpes simplex and herpes zoster scars

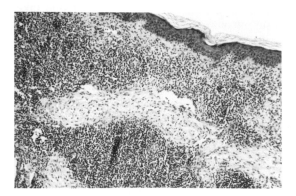

Figure 2 Nodular–diffuse specific infiltrates in the superficial and deep dermis.

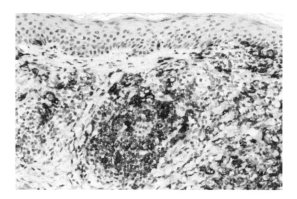

Figure 3   Positivity of neoplastic cells for CD20. The tumor cells also express CD5.

(9,10). The infiltrate is typically monomorphous and consists of small- to medium-sized lymphocytes with a round nucleus, dense nuclear chromatin, small nucleoli, and scant cytoplasm (8,19). Variable numbers of eosinophils, neutrophils, and plasma cells are also present.

IMMUNOHISTOCHEMISTRY

B-CLL cells are characterized by an aberrant immunophenotype CD20+, CD43+, CD5+ (8) (Fig. 3). In addition, B-CLL cells label with CD19, CD23 and CD79a. The neoplastic cells express monoclonal sIgM or sIgM and sIgD. The detection of a monoclonal restriction to either κ or λ is an important feature of B-CLL cells. Demonstration of light-chain restriction may be difficult in formalin-fixed tissue and frozen sections are usually required for optimal analysis.

MOLECULAR BIOLOGY

Clonal rearrangement of Ig heavy (IgH) is demonstrable.

REFERENCES

1. Kipps T. Chronic lymphocytic leukemia. Curr Opin Hematol 2000; 7:223–234.
2. Wierda WG, Kipps T. Chronic lymphocytic leukemia. Curr Opin Hematol 1999; 6:253–261.
3. Ratnam KV, Khor CJL, Su WPD. Leukemia cutis. Dermatol Clin 1994; 12:419–431.
4. Su WPD, Buechner SA, Li CY. Clinicopathologic correlations in leukemia cutis. J Am Acad Dermatol 1984; 11:121–128.
5. Su WPD. Clinical, histopathologic, and immunohistochemical correlations in leukemia cutis. Semin Dermatol 1994; 13:223–230.
6. Buechner SA, Su WPD. Leukemia cutis. In: Arndt KA, Robinson JK, LeBoit PE, Wintroub BU, eds. Cutaneous Medicine and Surgery. Philadelphia: W.B. Saunders Company, 1996:1670.
7. Varkonyi J, Zalatnai A, Timar J, Matolcsi A, Falus A, Bencsath M, Laszlo V, Pocsik E, Kotlan B, Csaszar A. Secondary cutaneous infiltration in B cell chronic lymphocytic leukemia. Acta Haematol 2000; 103:116–121.

8. Cerroni L, Zenahlik P, Hofler G, Kaddu S, Smolle J, Kerl H. Specific cutaneous infiltrates of B-cell chronic lymphocytic leukemia: a clinicopathologic and prognostic study of 42 patients. Am J Surg Pathol 1996; 20:1000–1010.

9. Pujol RM, Matias-Guiu X, Planaguma M, de Moragas JM. Chronic lymphocytic leukemia and cutaneous granulomas at sites of herpes zoster scars. Int J Dermatol 1990; 29:652–654.

10. Cerroni L, Zenahlik P, Kerl H. Specific cutaneous infiltrates of B-cell chronic lymphocytic leukemia arising at the site of herpes zoster and herpes simplex scars. Cancer 1995; 76:26–31.

11. Wakelin S, Young E, Kelly S, Turner M. Transient leukemia cutis in chronic lymphocytic leukemia. Clin Exp Dermatol 1997; 22:37–40.

12. Cerroni L, Höfler G, Bäck B, Wolf P, Maier G, Kerl H. Specific cutaneous infiltrates of B-cell chronic lymphocytic leukemia (B-CLL) at sites typical for *Borrelia burgdorferi* infection. J Cutan Pathol 2002; 29:142–147.

13. Smoller B, Warnke R. Cutaneous infiltrate of chronic lymphocytic leukemia and relationship to primary cutaneous epithelial neoplasms. J Cutan Pathol 1998; 25:160–164.

14. High DA, Luscombe HA, Kauh YC. Leukemia cutis masquerading as chronic paronychia. Int J Dermatol 1985; 24:595–597.

15. Simon CA, Su WPD, Li CY. Subungual leukemia cutis. Int J Dermatol 1990; 29: 636–639.

16. Moller Pedersen L, Nordin H, Nielsen H, Lisse I. Non-Hodgkin malignant lymphoma in the nails in the course of a chronic lymphocytic leukaemia. Acta Derm Venereol (Stockh) 1992; 72:277–278.

17. Calvert RJ, Smith E. Metastatic acropachy in lymphatic leukemia. Blood 1955; 10: 545–549.

18. Desvignes V, Bosq J, Guillaume J, Charpentier P, Carde P, Jasmin C, Avril MF. Eruption papulo-vésiculeuse du visage au cours des leucémies lymphoides chronique. Ann Dermatol Venereol 1990; 117:880–882.

19. Buechner SA, Li CY, Su WPD. Leukemia cutis. A histopathologic study of 42 cases. Am J Dermatopathol 1985; 7:109–119.

43.2. Chronic Lymphocytic Leukemia, T-cell Type (T-CLL)

Stanislaw Buechner
Department of Dermatology, University of Basel, Basel, Switzerland

Daniel W.P. Su
Department of Dermatology, Mayo Clinic, Rochester, Minnesota, U.S.A.

T-CLL is a rare small T-cell disorder. The median age of onset is 57 years. Patients usually present with high lymphocyte count, mild to moderate splenomegaly, and lymphadenopathy. Chromosomal abnormalities of 14q11, 14q32, 7p15 have been found in most cases (1). T-CLL probably represents a small cell variant of prolymphocytic leukemia (T-PLL). T-PLL is characterized by lymphocyte counts greater than 100×10^9/L, marked hepatosplenomegaly, anemia, thrombocytopenia, and lymphadenopathy. Typical T-PLL shows medium-sized lymphocytes with a high nuclear-cytoplasmic ratio and round to oval nuclei, and prominent nucleoli. In a series of 92 patients with T-PLL, 26 (28%) had cutaneous involvement (2). T-PLL is probably the most common form of mature T-cell leukemia, usually with CD4+, CD8–, or, less frequently, CD4+/CD8+ immunophenotype (3). T-PLL is aggressive and has a median survival of less than 1 year.

CLINICAL FEATURES

The most commonly reported skin lesions are a diffuse maculopapular eruption, nodules, and erythroderma (Fig. 1) (2,4,5). Clinically, erythroderma in T-CLL may simulate Sézary syndrome. A localized erythematous lesion involving only the face and ears may be observed. In one instance, T-CLL mimicked dermatomyositis presenting with a violaceous periorbital eruption and poikilodermatous plaques on the arms and chest (6).

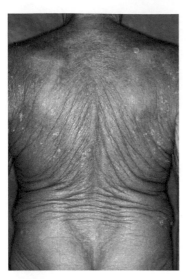

Figure 1 A generalized infiltrated erythroderma.

HISTOLOGY

There is a dense dermal infiltrate of lymphoid cells which is predominantly localized around the blood vessels and appendages. The epidermis is normal, and there is no epidermotropism of lymphoid cells (Fig. 2). The infiltrate is separated from the epider-

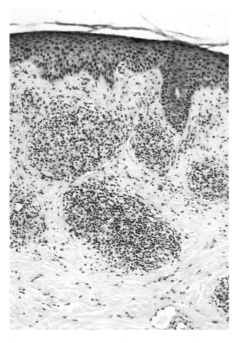

Figure 2 Dermal infiltrate of medium-sized lymphoid cells concentrated around the blood vessels.

mis by a zone of normal collagen. Occasionally, involvement of the subcutaneous fat may be seen. The infiltrate is composed of medium-sized lymphocytes with prominent nucleoli (2,5). There is no evidence of destruction of blood vessels and appendages.

IMMUNOHISTOCHEMISTRY

The immunophenotype is CD2+, CD3+, CD4+. Less frequently, the cells express CD4+, CD8+. Cases that are CD4– and CD8+ are rare, and cases with CD4– and CD8– are exceptional (3,5–7).

REFERENCES

1. Bartlett N, Longo D. T-small lymphocyte disorders. Semin Hematol 1999; 36:164–170.
2. Mallett RB, Matutes E, Catovsky D, Maclennan K, Mortimer PS, Holden CA. Cutaneous infiltration in T-cell prolymphocytic leukaemia. Br J Dermatol 1995; 132:263–266.
3. Catovsky D. CLL variants and T-cell-related issues. Hematol Cell Ther 2000; 42:15–19.
4. Thomas A, Dompmartin A, Troussard X, Moreau A, Mandard C, Leroy D. Localisation cutanée de la leucémie prolymphocytaire T. Ann Dermatol Venereol 1995; 122:526–529.
5. Serra A, Estrach M, Marti R, Villamor N, Rafel M, Montserrat E. Cutaneous involvement as the first manifestation in a case of T-cell prolymphocytic leukaemia. Acta Derm Venereol 1998; 78:198–200.
6. Nousari H, Kimyai-Asadi A, Huang C, Tausk F. T-cell chronic lymphocytic leukemia mimicking dermatomyositis. Int J Dermatol 2000; 39:144–146.
7. Kishimoto H, Mamada A, Katayama I, Nishioka K. Leukaemia cutis in chronic CD8+ T lymphocytic leukaemia. Dermatology 1996; 192:134–135.

43.3. Chronic Myeloid Leukemia (CML)

Stanislaw Buechner
Department of Dermatology, University of Basel, Basel, Switzerland

Daniel W.P. Su
Department of Dermatology, Mayo Clinic, Rochester, Minnesota, U.S.A.

Chronic myeloid leukemia (CML) is a disorder of hematopoietic stem cells accounting for 15% of adult leukemias. The median age at presentation is between 50 and 60 years. Chronic myeloid leukemia has a consistent annual incidence of about 1 per 100,000 people with no known geographic variation. The majority of patients present in the chronic phase with relatively stable disease. Unpredictably, the disease eventually transforms into accelerated and blastic phases, becoming more resistant to treatment. The final and fatal blastic phase has features of an acute leukemia. Chronic myeloid leukemia was one of the first diseases in which a specific chromosomal abnormality was identified, a Philadelphia (Ph') chromosome resulting from the t(9;22)(q34;q11) chromosomal translocation (1–4).

CLINICAL FEATURES

Specific skin lesions in CML are uncommon, with a reported incidence of 2–8%. The lesions are erythematous papules, plaques, or nodules that may become purpuric and ulcerated. The lesions occur anywhere on the skin and may affect the trunk, head, and neck (Fig. 1). Occasionally, the lesions are generalized in distribution. On occasion, only a single lesion is present (5). One patient with an unusual manifestation of CML developed edematous, purpuric areas of induration on the lower leg resembling stasis dermatitis (6). In a case of acute febrile neutrophilic dermatosis (Sweet syndrome) in association with CML, the leukemic cells were demonstrated within the lesions of Sweet syndrome. Juvenile CML, a rare malignancy in childhood, is characterized by a rapidly progressive course and a poor response to therapy. Specific skin lesions have been only rarely reported in juvenile CML. The lesions may present as annular, erythematous, urticarial plaques with central clearing (7).

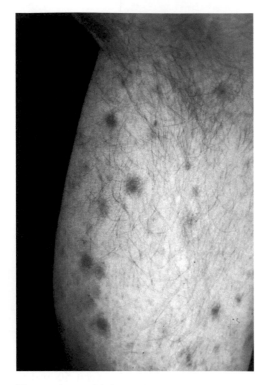

Figure 1 Multiple erythematous papules on the lower leg.

HISTOLOGY

A dense nodular to diffuse infiltrate is present. The infiltrate is most often concentrated in the dermis, but may also involve the subcutaneous fat. The infiltrate is pleomorphic and dominated by mature and immature cells of the granulocytic series, including atypical myelocytes, metamyelocytes, eosinophilic metamyelocytes, and neutrophils (5,8).

IMMUNOHISTOCHEMISTRY

The CML cells stain for CD43, CD45, CD68, myeloperoxidase, and lysozyme (5). Staining for naphthol AS-D chloracetate esterase (NASDCE) may be positive in some cases. In addition, the presence of CD56 expression (neural-cell adhesion molecule) in specific skin infiltrates of CML has been reported (5,9). The presence of the natural killer cell marker, CD56, correlates with aggressive biologic behavior (10).

REFERENCES

1. Kalidas M, Kantarjian H, Talpaz M. Chronic myelogenous leucemia. JAMA 2001; 286: 895–898.
2. Cortes J, Talpaz M, Kantarjian H. Chronic myelogenous leukemia: a review. Am J Med 1996; 100:555–570.

3. Holyoake T. Recent advances in the molecular and cellular biology of chronic myeloid leukaemia: lessons to be learned from the laboratory. Br J Haematol 2001; 113:11–23.

4. Tefferi A, Litzow M, Noel P, Dewald G. Chronic granulocytic leukemia: recent information on pathogenesis, diagnosis, and disease monitoring. Mayo Clin Proc 1997; 72: 445–452.

5. Kaddu S, Zenahlik P, Beham-Schmid C, Kerl H, Cerroni L. Specific cutaneous infiltrates in patients with myelogenous leukemia: a clinicopathologic study of 26 patients with assessment of diagnostic criteria. J Am Acad Dermatol 1999; 40:966–978.

6. Butler DF, Bagor TGJ, Rodman OG. Leukemia cutis mimicking stasis dermatitis. Cutis 1985; 35:47–48.

7. Sres U, Mallory S, Hess J, Keating J, Blomberg G, Dehner L. Cutaneous presentation of juvenile chronic myelogenous leukemia: a diagnostic and therapeutic dilemma. Pediatr Dermatol 1995; 12:364–368.

8. Buechner SA, Li CY, Su WPD. Leukemia cutis. A histopathologic study of 42 cases. Am J Dermatopathol 1985; 7:109–119.

9. Kaddu S, Beham-Schmid C, Zenahlik P, Kerl H, Cerroni L. CD56+ blastic transformation of chronic myeloid leukemia involving the skin. J Cutan Pathol 1999; 26:497–503.

10. Kuwabara H, Nagai M, Yamaoka G, Ohnishi H, Kawakami K. Specific skin manifestations in CD56 positive acute myeloid leukemia. J Cutan Pathol 1999; 26:1–5.

43.4. Hairy-Cell Leukemia (HCL)

Stanislaw Buechner
Department of Dermatology, University of Basel, Basel, Switzerland

Daniel W.P. Su
Department of Dermatology, Mayo Clinic, Rochester, Minnesota, U.S.A.

Hairy-cell leukemia (HCL) is a rare chronic lymphoproliferative disorder character-ized by the presence of circulating monoclonal B lymphocytes that have prominent cytoplasmic projections. Hairy-cell leukemia accounts for 2–3% of all adult leuke-mias. There is a 4:1 male to female predominance with the median age at presenta-tion being 52 years. Hairy cells are slightly larger than regular lymphocytes and show distinct round-to-oval nuclei that are centrally placed within a pale staining cyto-plasm with multiple hair-like projections.

CLINICAL FEATURES

Patients usually present with fatigue, weakness, weight loss and a history of repeated infections, and splenomegaly on physical examination. Lymphadenopathy is an inconsistent finding and may be observed in about 26% of patients (1). Specific skin lesions are considered to be uncommon in contrast to nonspecific skin lesions such as recurrent infections and ecchymoses (2,3). One or more cutaneous infections (includ-ing cellulitis, abscess, herpetic lesions, tinea, candidiasis, and verrucae) were observed in 47 of 113 (42%) patients (2). Infections are the most common cutaneous changes in HCL, accounting for approximately 60% of cases (4). Hairy-cell leukemia is also frequently associated with vasculitis (2,5). Specific skin lesions were seen in 48 (8%) of the 600 cases reported in the literature, but only eight cases were proven by skin biopsy (6). Patients usually present with multiple papules, pustules, or indurated plaques (Figs. 1 and 2). Deep infiltrated nodules may also be present. Lesions are most often located on the trunk and extremities. One patient had macrocheilitis mimicking Melkersson–Rosenthal syndrome that resulted from specific infiltration

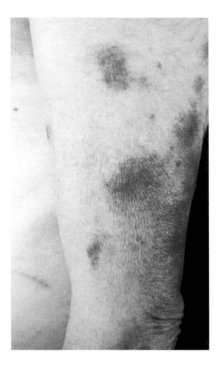

Figure 1 Hairy-cell leukemia: Erythematous indurated plaques on the arm.

of the lips by HCL cells (7). In another puzzling case, a widespread specific skin eruption of HCL was transient, disappearing spontaneously (8).

HISTOLOGY

A dense, diffuse, or patchy infiltrate of uniform, mononuclear cells is found
predominantly in the upper dermis but occasionally involves the entire dermis.

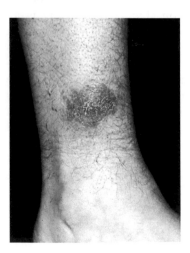

Figure 2 Hairy-cell leukemia: Infiltrated brownish plaque on the leg.

The infiltrate usually surrounds dermal blood vessels and skin appendages. The epidermis is not involved and is separated from the infiltrates by a thin layer of normal upper papillary dermis. The infiltrate consists of small-to-medium sized cells with round or indented hyperchromatic nuclei. The HCL cells exhibit a moderate amount of pink, lacy cytoplasm that tends to leave clear spaces between the nuclei, resulting in a "spongy" appearance (6,9).

IMMUNOHISTOCHEMISTRY

Hairy cells exhibit diffuse cytoplasmic positivity of tartrate-resistant acid phosphatase. The cells usually express CD19, CD20, CD22 and are negative for CD5 and CD21.

REFERENCES

1. Damasio EE, Spriano M, Repetto M, Vimercati AR, Rossi E, Occhini D, Marmont AM. Hairy cell leukemia: a retrospective study of 235 cases by the Italian Cooperative Group (ICGHCL) according to Jansen's clinical staging system. Acta Haematol 1984; 72: 326–334.
2. Finan MC, Su WPD, Li CY. Cutaneous findings in hairy cell leukemia. J Am Acad Dermatol 1984; 11:788–797.
3. Ausubel H, Levine ML, Shapiro L. Leukemia cutis manuum. N Y State J Med 1970; 70:2835–2837.
4. Carsuzaa F, Pierre C, Jaubert D, Viala JJ. Cutaneous findings in hairy cell leukemia. Review of 84 cases. Nouv Rev Fr Hematol 1993; 35:541–543.
5. Kurzrock R, Cohen PR. Mucocutaneous paraneoplastic manifestations of hematologic malignancies. Am J Med 1995; 99:207–216.
6. Arai E, Ikeda S, Itoh S, Katayama I. Specific skin lesions as the presenting symptom of hairy cell leukemia. Am J Clin Pathol 1988; 90:459–464.
7. Connelly TJ, Kauh YC, Luscombe HA, Becker G. Leukemic macrocheilitis associated with hairy-cell leukemia and the Melkersson–Rosenthal syndrome. J Am Acad Dermatol 1986; 14:353–358.
8. Bilsland D, Shahriari S, Douglas WS, Chaudhuri AKR, Todd WTA. Transient leukaemia cutis in hairy-cell leukaemia. Clin Exp Dermatol 1991; 16:207–209.
9. Lawrence DM, Sun NCJ, Mena R, Moss R. Cutaneous lesions in hairy-cell leukemia. Case report and review of the literature. Arch Dermatol 1983; 119:322–325.

43.5. Acute Lymphoblastic Leukemia (ALL)

Stanislaw Buechner
Department of Dermatology, University of Basel, Basel, Switzerland

Daniel W.P. Su
Department of Dermatology, Mayo Clinic, Rochester, Minnesota, U.S.A.

Acute lymphoblastic leukemia (ALL) is the most common malignancy in children, accounting for approximately 30% of childhood cancers. Beyond childhood, the age distribution of the disease is relatively uniform, with a median age of 30–40 years. In adults, ALL represents 20% of all leukemias. In all ages, the incidence is higher in males than in females (1,2).

CLINICAL FEATURES

Patients with ALL have lymphadenopathy in up to 80% and hepatomegaly and/or splenomegaly in up to 75% of the cases (1). Skin involvement is rare and almost always associated with pre-B-cell phenotype. Most commonly, when specific lesions of ALL occur in the skin, they present as multiple red to violaceous papules, plaques, or nodules, which may occasionally ulcerate. The most frequent location of specific skin lesions in children is on the head (3). Cutaneous involvement can be an early manifestation of ALL; skin lesions may be present during weeks to several months before the diagnosis of hematologic disease (3,4).

HISTOLOGY

There are diffuse infiltrates within the dermis extending into the subcutaneous fat. The infiltrate consists of medium to large atypical lymphocytes with pleomorphic nuclei, many of which are in mitosis.

IMMUNOHISTOCHEMISTRY

Acute lymphoblastic leukemia cells are usually CD19+, CD10+, CD20+, CD24+, and HLA-DR+ and may lack CD21.

REFERENCES

1. Cortes JE, Kantarjian HM. Acute lymphoblastic leukemia. Cancer 1995; 76:2393–2417.
2. Lukens JN. Acute lymphocytic leukemia. In: Lee GR, Bithell TC, Foerster J, Athens JW, Lukens JN, eds. Wintrobe's Clinical Hematology. Philadelphia, London: Lea & Febiger, 1993:1892.
3. Millot F, Robert A, Bertrand Y, Mechinaud F, Laureys G, Ferster A, Brock P, Rohrlich P, Mazingue F, Plantaz D, Plouvier E, Pacquement H, Behar C, Rialland X, Chantarine J, Guilhot F, Otten J. Cutaneous involvement in children with acute lympho-blastic leukemia or lymphoblastic lymphoma. Pediatrics 1997; 100:60–64.
4. Zengin N, Kars A, Özisik Y, Canpinar H, Türker A, Ruacan S. Aleukemic leukemia cutis in a patient with acute lymphoblastic leukemia. J Am Acad Dermatol 1998; 38:620–621.

43.6. Acute (Myelo-) Monocytic Leukemia (AMoL, AMMoL)

Stanislaw Buechner
Department of Dermatology, University of Basel, Basel, Switzerland

Daniel W.P. Su
Department of Dermatology, Mayo Clinic, Rochester, Minnesota, U.S.A.

Acute myelomonocytic leukemia (AMMoL, M4) and acute monocytic leukemia (AMoL, M5) account for approximately 25% and 10% of all cases of acute nonlymphocytic leukemia, respectively (1). In AMMoL, both granulocytic and monocytic precursors are present in varying proportions, and each cell line accounts for at least 20% of nucleated bone marrow cells. Early cutaneous involvement occurs more frequently in AMoL and AMMoL than in most other leukemias. Those cases have formerly been diagnosed as "reticuloses" (2). The incidence of specific mucocutaneous lesions in patients with AMoL and AMMoL is approximately 10–30% and 13–27%, respectively (3–6). In a large series of 381 patients with AML in which 14 patients had specific skin involvement, 10 of them were diagnosed as having M4 and M5 subtypes (7).

CLINICAL FEATURES

Specific skin lesions of AMoL and AMMoL present as violaceous to red-brown papules, nodules, and plaques (Figs. 1 and 2) (4,5,8). They are most commonly located on the trunk and extremities, but they can occur anywhere in either a grouped or a generalized pattern. Occasionally, a solitary red, sometimes, necrotic or ulcerated, nodule is found. The eruption may also involve the face and scalp. Mucocutaneous leukemic infiltrates were found in 24 of 81 patients with AMMoL (6). Leukemic gingival hyperplasia is a striking feature of AMoL and AMMoL. The infiltrated gingiva appear swollen, glazed, firm in consistency, and bright red to deep purple in color (6,8). The gums may completely cover the teeth. Deep oral ulcerations may occur in areas subjected to trauma such as the hard palate and tongue (Fig. 3). Specific skin lesions tend to localize at sites of trauma, burns, herpes zoster scars, and catheter placement (3,4,9). Unusual manifestations of AMoL and AMMoL include hemorrhagic bulla (10), conjunctival lesions (11), and a vesicular skin rash mimicking chickenpox (12). The leukemic cells of AMMoL can be found within psoriatic skin plaques (13). Aleukemic leukemia cutis is a rare condition in

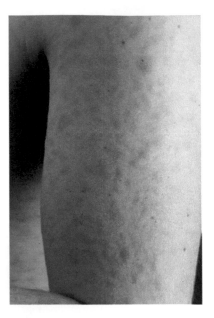

Figure 1   Acute monocytic leukemia (AMoL, M5) presenting as disseminated pale-red papules.

which leukemic cells invade the skin in the absence of peripheral blood and bone marrow involvement. Such lesions may be present several months before diagnosis, but the prognosis is poor after the full leukemic disease develops. Aleukemic skin lesions present as solitary or multiple red or violaceous papules or cutaneous and subcutaneous nodules (14–19). Specific skin lesions are considered to be a poor prognostic sign, and most patients die within a few months (8,20–22).

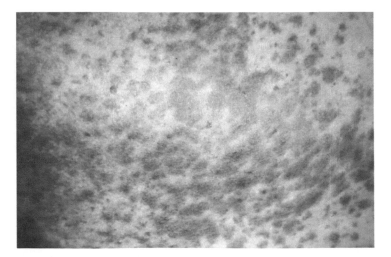

Figure 2   Acute myelomonocytic leukemia (AMMoL, M4). Multiple indurated pink-red papules on the trunk.

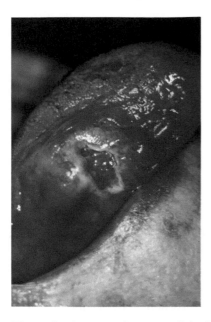

Figure 3 Acute myelomonocytic leukemia (AMMoL, M4). Leukemic infiltrate presenting as a painful and deep ulceration on the tongue.

HISTOLOGY

There is a moderate or dense diffuse or nodular infiltrate in the dermis that extends into the subcutaneous fat (Fig. 4). The epidermis is uninvolved. Perivascular and periadnexal aggregates of neoplastic cells are present in a majority of cases. Usually, there is a concentric layering of neoplastic cells around blood vessels and adnexal structures. A characteristic feature in most cases is the presence of rows of atypical cells migrating between collagen bundles (Fig. 5) (20,23). Mitotic figures vary in number but may be frequent. Infiltration and disruption of the adnexal structures may occur. The infiltrate is composed of medium-sized round to oval neoplastic cells

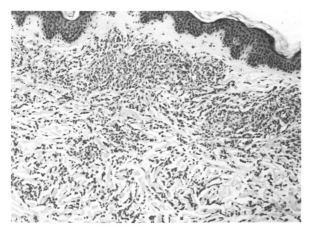

Figure 4 Acute monocytic leukemia (AMoL, M5). Dense dermal infiltrate of medium-sized atypical mononuclear cells. Note sparing of the upper papillary dermis.

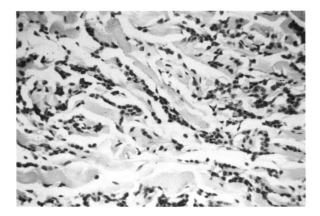

Figure 5 Acute myelomonocytic leukemia (AMMoL, M4). Note rows of atypical cells between collagen bundles forming linear arrays.

with irregularly shaped, hyperchromatic nuclei, surrounded by a rim of faintly eosinophilic cytoplasm. Occasionally, an accompanying granulomatous reaction composed of lymphocytes, histiocytes, and giant cells may be present within the malignant infiltrate (24,25).

IMMUNOHISTOCHEMISTRY

The majority of the leukemic infiltrate shows strong reactivity for lysozyme, myelo-peroxidase, CD45, CD43, CD68, and CD74 (Fig. 6). Staining for chloroacetate esterase may be positive in some cases of AMoL and AMMoL. CD3, CD20, CD30 and S-100 are not expressed on leukemic cells (3,20).

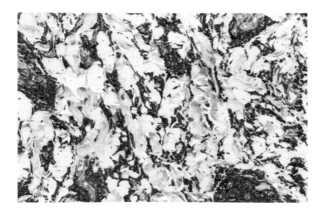

Figure 6 Acute monocytic leukemia (AMoL, M5). Immunohistochemical stain shows strong positivity of neoplastic cells for CD68.

REFERENCES

1. Lukens JN. Classification and differentiation of the acute leukemias. In: Lee GR, Bithell TC, Foerster J, Athens JW, Lukens JN, eds. Wintrobe's Clinical Hematology. Philadelphia, London: Lea & Febiger, 1993:1873.
2. Burg G, Schmoeckel C, Braun Falco O, Wolff HH. Monocytic leukemia. Clinically appearing as 'malignant reticulosis of the skin'. Arch Dermatol 1978; 114:418–420.
3. Ratnam KV, Khor CJL, Su WPD. Leukemia cutis. Dermatol Clin 1994; 12:419–431.
4. Su WPD. Clinical, histopathologic, and immunohistochemical correlations in leukemia cutis. Sem Dermatol 1994; 13:223–230.
5. Buechner SA, Su WPD. Leukemia cutis. In: Arndt KA, Robinson JK, Leboit PE, Wintroub BU, eds. Cutaneous Medicine and Surgery. Philadelphia: W.B. Saunders Company, 1996:1670.
6. Dreizen S, McCredie KB, Keating MJ, Luna MA. Malignant gingival and skin "infiltrates" in adult leukemia. Oral Surg 1983; 55:572–579.
7. Agis H, Weltermann A, Fonatsch C, Haas O, Mitterbauer G, Müllauer L, Schreiber S, Schwarzinger I, Juretzka W, Valent P, Jäger U, Lechner K, Geissler K. A comparative study on demographic, hematological, and cytogenetic findings and prognosis in acute myeloid leukemia with and without leukemia cutis. Ann Hematol 2002; 81:90–95.
8. Su WPD, Buechner SA, Li CY. Clinicopathologic correlations in leukemia cutis. J Am Acad Dermatol 1984; 11:121–128.
9. Baden TJ, Gammon WR. Leukemia cutis in acute myelomonocytic leukemia. Arch Dermatol 1987; 123:88–90.
10. Eubanks SW, Patterson JW. Subacute myelomonocytic leukemia—an unusual skin manifestation. J Am Acad Dermatol 1983; 9:581–584.
11. Lee DA, Su WPD. Acute myelomonocytic leukemia cutis presenting as a conjunctival lesion. Int J Dermatol 1985; 24:369–370.
12. Hoen B, Neidhardt AC, Aghassian C, Dorvaux V, Witz F, Canton P. Acute myelomonocytic leukemia revealed by a chickenpox-like rash. J Eur Acad Dermatol Venereol 1996; 6:76–79.
13. Metzler G, Cerroni L, Schmidt H, Soyer H, Sill H, Kerl H. Leukemic cells within skin lesions of psoriasis in a patient with acute myelogenous leukemia. J Cutan Pathol 1997; 24:445–448.
14. Török L, Lueff S, Garay G, Tapai M. Monocytic aleukemic leukemia cutis. J Eur Acad Dermatol Venereol 1999; 13:54–58.
15. Daoud MS, Snow JL, Gibson LE, Daoud S. Aleukemic monocytic leukemia cutis. Mayo Clin Proc 1996; 71:166–168.
16. Benez A, Metzger S, Metzler G, Fierlbeck G. Aleukemic leukemia cutis presenting as benign-appearing exanthema. Acta Derm Venereol 2001; 81:45–47.
17. Okun MM, Fitzgibbon J, Nahass GT, Forsman K. Aleukemic leukemia cutis, myeloid subtype. Eur J Dermatol 1995; 5:290–293.
18. Hansen RM, Barnett J, Hanson G, Klehm D, Schneider T, Ash R. Aleukemic leukemia cutis. Arch Dermatol 1986; 122:812–814.
19. Ohno S, Yokoo T, Ohta M, Yamamoto M, Danno K, Hamato N, Tomii K, Ohno Y, Kobashi Y. Aleukemic leukemia cutis. J Am Acad Dermatol 1990; 22:374–377.
20. Kaddu S, Zenahlik P, Beham-Schmid C, Kerl H, Cerroni L. Specific cutaneous infiltrates in patients with myelogenous leukemia: a clinicopathologic study of 26 patients with assessment of diagnostic criteria. J Am Acad Dermatol 1999; 40:966–978.
21. Baer MR, Barcos M, Farrell H, Raza A, Preisler HD. Acute myelogenous leukemia with leukemia cutis. Cancer 1989; 63:2192–2200.
22. Gambichler T, Herde M, Hoffmann K, Altmeyer P, Jansen T. Poor prognosis of acute myeloid leukaemia associated with leukaemia cutis. J Eur Acad Dermatol Venereol 2002; 16:177–178.

23. Buechner SA, Li CY, Su WPD. Leukemia cutis. A histopathologic study of 42 cases. Am J Dermatopathol 1985; 7:109–119.

24. Horiuchi Y, Masuzawa M, Nozaki O, Shibahara N, Shiga T, Yoshida M. Unusual cutaneous lesions associated with chronic myelomonocytic leukaemia. Clin Exp Dermatol 1992; 17:121–124.

25. Tomasini C, Quaglino P, Novelli M, Fierro M. "Aleukemic" granulomatous leukemia cutis. Am J Dermatopathol 1998; 20:417–421.

43.7. Acute Granulocytic (Myeloid) Leukemia (AML)

Stanislaw Buechner
Department of Dermatology, University of Basel, Basel, Switzerland

Daniel W.P. Su
Department of Dermatology, Mayo Clinic, Rochester, Minnesota, U.S.A.

Acute granulocytic (myeloid) leukemia (AML) (M0–M3) accounts approximately for 40–50% of all acute leukemias with the incidence of the different FAB types reported as M1 18%, M2 28%, M3 8% (1). The AML types differ with respect to cell line and degree of differentiation. In AML with minimal evidence of myeloid differentiation (M0) or without maturation (M1), the predominant cell is undifferentiated by light microscopy, peroxidase negative and expresses CD34+, CD33+ but lacks CD15. Acute granulocytic (myeloid) leukemia with maturation (M2) is distinguished from M1 by clear evidence of maturation. Myeloblasts with granules and promyelocytes accounts for more than 50% of nucleated cells. Acute promyelocytic leukemia (APL, M3) is recognized by a predominance of promyelocytes, many of which contain large azurophilic granules. In the M2 and M3 variants, the majority of blasts usually are peroxidase positive. The blasts express CD15 and are usually negative for CD34. Patients with AML M2 may present with splenomegaly and frequently anemia and thrombocytopenia at diagnosis. Acute granulocytic (myeloid) leukemia M3 occurs at a median age of 30–35 years (2). The most common complaint is nonspecific fatigue or malaise that usually has been present for several months. Patients often have relatively low leukocyte counts, and usually have thrombocytopenia with disseminated intravascular coagulation (DIC). The disease typically presents with a bleeding diathesis, leading to a relatively high early mortality rate. Virtually, all patients have a characteristic chromosome abnormality involving a balanced translocation between chromosomes 15 and 17 [t(15;17)] (1). The molecular basis of the t(15;17) is the fusion of the retinoic acid receptor rara gene on chromosome 17 with the pml gene on chromosome 15 forming a chimeric pml/rara gene. Systemic retinoids can induce complete remissions in APL with the use of all-trans retinoic acid (ATRA) (3).

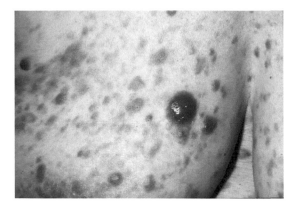

Figure 1   Acute granulocytic (myeloid) leukemia: erythematous papules and nodules on the trunk.

CLINICAL FEATURES

Specific skin lesions have been reported to occur in up to 10% of patients with AML subtypes M0–M3 (4,5). These lesions can be single or multiple. They are flesh-colored, pink, erythematous or red-brown papules, plaques or nodules, occurring primarily on the trunk, and extremities (6–9) (Fig. 1). The distribution is occasionally generalized. Hemorrhagic lesions may be present, and nodules may be ulcerated, especially as they enlarge. Some affected patients have bullous and hemorrhagic lesions (9). Generalized eruptions with purpuric nodules on the face, back, and extremities also occur in AML subtype M0 (10), as does transient acantholytic dermatosis (11). Oral involvement has been found in 3.7% of patients and may be the initial presentation of the disorder (Fig. 2) (12).

HISTOLOGY

Specific skin lesions in AML show dense infiltrates in the dermis and subcutaneous tissue with epidermal sparing. The infiltrates typically surround the dermal blood

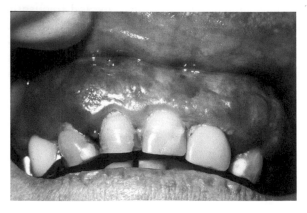

Figure 2   Acute granulocytic (myeloid) leukemia: oral manifestation with gingival involvement.

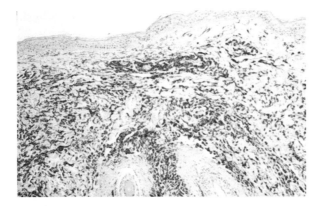

Figure 3 Acute granulocytic (myeloid) leukemia (AML, M2). Dermal infiltrate of neoplastic cells showing strong positivity for lysozyme.

vessels, hair follicles, muscle bundles, and sweat glands (13,14). Transmural infiltration of dermal blood vessels and intravascular clusters of atypical myeloid cells may be found. In some instances, vascular injury and even frank vasculitis may be observed (leukemic vasculitis). Typically, the leukemic myeloid cells spread between the collagen bundles and permeate the lobules of subcutaneous tissue. The predominant cell types in AML are medium-sized or large atypical myeloblasts and myelocytes with round or oval basophilic nuclei and prominent nucleoli. Immature myeloid cells with large bizarre nuclei can be identified within the dermal infiltrate (14). Occasionally, small lymphocytes and eosinophils can be admixed. Leukemic myeloblasts can be found intermingled with mature neutrophils in inflammatory reactions such as suppurative folliculitis associated with AML subtype M1 (15). In immature AML subtype M0, the infiltrate consists of a monomorphous population of medium-sized blasts with round or folded vesicular nuclei and prominent nucleoli (11). There are usually many mitotic figures.

IMMUNOHISTOCHEMISTRY

Staining for lysozyme and myeloperoxidase usually shows positivity in skin lesions of differentiated AML subtypes but is often negative in AML without maturation (Fig. 3) (14). Staining for naphthol AS-D chloroacetate-esterase is variable. In some cases, it is seen in most cells, while other cases show only a week or negative staining. The neoplastic cells usually express CD43, CD45, HLA-DR, and CD45RO. Staining for CD68 and CD74 shows positive reaction in up to 10% of neoplastic cells (14).

REFERENCES

1. Walker H, Smith FJ, Betts DR. Cytogenetics in acute myeloid leukaemia. Blood Rev 1994; 8:30–36.
2. Lukens JN. Classification and differentiation of the acute leukemias. In: Lee GR, Bithell TC, Foerster J, Athens JW, Lukens JN, eds. Wintrobe's Clinical Hematology. Philadelphia, London: Lea & Febiger, 1993:1873.

3. Warrell RP, de Thé H, Wang ZY, Degos L. Acute promyelocytic leukemia. N Engl J Med 1993; 329:177–189.
4. Ratnam KV, Khor CJL, Su WPD. Leukemia cutis. Dermatol Clin 1994; 12:419–431.
5. Baer MR, Barcos M, Farrell H, Raza A, Preisler HD. Acute myelogenous leukemia with leukemia cutis. Cancer 1989; 63:2192–2200.
6. Su WPD, Buechner SA, Li CY. Clinicopathologic correlations in leukemia cutis. J Am Acad Dermatol 1984; 11:121–128.
7. Su WPD. Clinical, histopathologic, and immunohistochemical correlations in leukemia cutis. Sem Dermatol 1994; 13:223–230.
8. Buechner SA, Su WPD. Leukemia cutis. In: Arndt KA, Robinson JK, LeBoit PE, Wintroub BU, eds. Cutaneous Medicine and Surgery. Philadelphia: W.B. Saunders Company, 1996:1670.
9. Ochonisky S, Aractingi S, Dombret H, Daniel MT, Verola O, Degos L, Dubertret L. Acute undifferentiated myeloblastic leukemia revealed by specific hemorrhagic bullous lesions. Arch Dermatol 1993; 129:512–513.
10. Benucci R, Annessi G, Signoretti S, Simoni R. Minimally differentiated acute myeloid leukaemia revealed by specific cutaneous lesions. Br J Dermatol 1996; 135:119–123.
11. Sakalosky P, Fenske N, Morgan M. A case of acantholytic dermatosis and leukemia cutis. Am J Dermatopathol 2002; 24:257–259.
12. Dreizen S, McCredie KB, Keating MJ, Luna MA. Malignant gingival and skin "infiltrates" in adult leukemia. Oral Surg 1983; 55:572–579.
13. Buechner SA, Li CY, Su WPD. Leukemia cutis. A histopathologic study of 42 cases. Am J Dermatopathol 1985; 7:109–119.
14. Kaddu S, Zenahlik P, Beham-Schmid C, Kerl H, Cerroni L. Specific cutaneous infiltrates in patients with myelogenous leukemia: a clinicopathologic study of 26 patients with assessment of diagnostic criteria. J Am Acad Dermatol 1999; 40:966–978.
15. Inuzuka M, Tokura Y. Sterile suppurative folliculitis associated with acute myeloblastic leukaemia. Br J Dermatol 2002; 146:904–907.

Granulocytic Sarcoma (Chloroma)

Stanislaw Buechner
Department of Dermatology, University of Basel, Basel, Switzerland

Daniel W.P. Su
Department of Dermatology, Mayo Clinic, Rochester, Minnesota, U.S.A.

CLINICAL FEATURES

Granulocytic sarcoma (GS) is a rare manifestation of acute myelogenous leukemia that may be present concurrent with or may precede the onset of acute leukemia M0–M5 FAB subtypes (1–3). It has been defined as a localized tumor mass composed of immature cells of myeloid series or the cells of each maturation step in extramedullary sites. The disease has been reported to occur in 2–8% of patients with acute nonlymphoblastic leukemia. Of the 102 tumor nodules of 74 patients with GS in the literature, 14 (14%) involved the skin (2). Recently, GS was observed in 34 out of 744 (4.6%) children prior to bone marrow manifestation of leukemia (3). Fourteen of these lesions were located in the skin. Seventeen patients had AMoL M5, seven

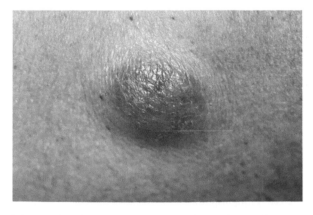

Figure 1 Violaceous raised nodule on the trunk.

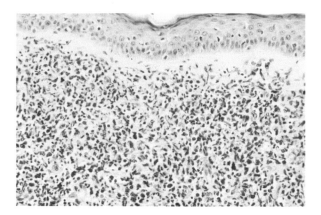

Figure 2   Dense diffuse dermal infiltrate of pleomorphic mononuclear cells.

had AMMoL M4, and nine had AML M0–M2. The lesions vary in size and usually present as erythematous or violaceous nodules (Fig. 1). The nodules, when cut, may also have a diagnostic yellow-green coloration, which is caused by the high concentration of myeloperoxidase, which changes color on exposure to air. Sites of mucocutaneous involvement include the trunk, head, extremities, oral mucosa (4), and conjunctiva (5). In adults and children, the prognosis of GS is poor.

HISTOLOGY

There is a dense, diffuse, confluent dermal infiltrate extending to the subcutaneous tissue. The infiltrate is pleomorphic, consisting of abnormal myeloid cells with oval to angulated nuclei and small nucleoli (Fig. 2). The infiltrates tend to be centered about blood vessels and adnexal structures and either grow as cellular sheets or track along individual collagen bundles (4). The lesions are occasionally associated with an inflammatory infiltrate, which includes eosinophils, neutrophils, and small lymphocytes.

IMMUNOHISTOCHEMISTRY

In most cases of GS, positive strong staining for lysozyme and myeloperoxidase can be observed. The staining with myeloperoxidase is variable. Granulocytic sarcoma cells also label with CD45 and CD43, and CD15 is also variably expressed (4).

REFERENCES

1. Sun NCJ, Ellis R. Granulocytic sarcoma of the skin. Arch Dermatol 1980; 116:800–802.
2. Yamauchi K, Yasuda M. Comparison in treatments of nonleukemic granulocytic sarcoma. Cancer 2002; 94:1739–1746.
3. Reinhardt D, Pekrun A, Lakomek M, Zimmermann M, Ritter J, Creutzig U. Primary myelosarcomas are associated with a high rate of relapse: report on 34 children from the acute myeloid leukaemia—Berlin–Frankfurt–Münster studies. Br J Haematol 2000; 110:836–866.

4. Ritter JH, Goldstein NS, Argenyi Z, Wick MR. Granulocytic sarcoma: an immunohisto-logic comparison with peripheral T-cell lymphoma in paraffin sections. J Cutan Pathol 1994; 21:207–216.
5. Hon C, Shek T, Liang R. Conjunctival chloroma (granulocytic sarcoma). Lancet 2002; 359:2247.

Large Granular Lymphocyte Leukemia

Dmitry V. Kazakov, Günter Burg, and Werner Kempf
Department of Dermatology, University Hospital, Zürich, Switzerland

Large granular lymphocyte leukemia (LGL) encompasses a group of disorders characterized by a clonal or reactive proliferation of large granular lymphocytes in the peripheral blood with or without systemic involvement. In the peripheral blood and bone marrow films, abnormal large granular lymphocytes have slightly eccentric, round to oval (sometimes irregular, hyperchromatic) nuclei, which are slightly larger than those of normal large granular lymphocytes. Nucleoli may be inconspicuous or distinct. The abundant pale or slightly basophilic cytoplasm contains characteristic fine or coarse azurophilic granules (Wright–Giemsa staining). In tissue sections, the granules may no longer be visible. Three forms of LGL can be delineated on the basis of clinicopathological features, immunophenotype, and course (1).

1. T-cell large granular lymphocyte leukemia (T-LGL) (T-cell chronic lymphocytic leukemia, Tγ-lymphoproliferative disorder, proliferation of large granular lymphocytes, large granular lymphocyte leukemia)
2. Aggressive NK-cell leukemia (large granular lymphocyte leukemia, NK-type; aggressive NK-cell leukemia/lymphoma)
3. NK-cell large granular lymphocyte lymphocytosis (chronic NK-cell lymphocytosis, indolent NK-cell lymphoproliferative disorder)

While T-LGL is a heterogeneous disorder of mature T-cells, the other two entities represent NK-cell neoplasms. Aggressive NK-cell leukemia may show a considerable overlap with nasal-type NK/T-cell lymphoma with multiorgan involvement and might represent its leukemic counterpart. It is not clear yet whether NK-cell large granular lymphocyte lymphocytosis is a clonal or reactive process. The main features of large granular lymphocyte leukemias are summarized in Table 1.

Cutaneous involvement in LGL is rare. Clinically, LGL patients may present with multiple nodules, erythematous plaques, ulcerated lesions, leg edema, telangiectases, and recurrent pyogenic infections (2–4). A subset of Asian patients (mostly children, median age 6.7 years) with otherwise typical features of *aggressive NK-cell leukemia* have a

Table 1 Clinicopathological Features of Large Granular Lymphocyte Leukemias

	T-cell large granular lymphocyte leukemia	Aggressive NK-cell leukemia	NK-cell large granular lymphocyte lymphocytosis
Epidemiology	Adults (median age 55 years), M~F	Asians > whites, teenagers and young adults, M=F	Adults
Main sites of involvement	PB, LN, spleen, liver	PB, LN, spleen, liver	PB
Clinical features	Asymptomatic in 60%, splenomegaly, rheumatoid arthritis	Fever, lymphadenopathy, hepatospleno-megaly	Mostly asympto-matic, vasculitis or nephrotic syndrome rare
Laboratory findings	Lymphocytosis (2–20 × 10^9/L, lymphocytes < 50%, CIC, hyper-gamma-globulinemia, anemia	Lymphocytosis, anemia, neutropenia, thrombocytopenia, soluble FAS ligand	Lymphocytosis
Phenotype	CD3+, TCRαβ+, CD4–, CD8+[a]	CD2+, sCD3–, CD3ε+, CD8+, CD56+, CD57–/+	CD2+, sCD3–, CD16+, CD56+, CD57+
TCR	TCRβ≫TCRγ	Germline	Germline
EBV	–	+	–
Course	Indolent, progression to aggressive disease rare	Aggressive to fulminant	Indolent, transformation to aggressive phase extremely rare
Prognosis	Good	Poor[b]	Good

PB, peripheral blood; LN, lymph nodes; TCR, T-cell receptor rearrangements; EBV, Epstein–Barr virus; CIC, circulating immune complexes.

[a] This is the phenotype seen in 80% of cases (common variant). Other forms include: (1) CD3+, TCRαβ+, CD4–, CD8–, (2) CD3+, TCRαβ+, CD4+, CD8+, (3) CD3+, TCRγδ+. Expression of CD56 and CD57 is variable, with the latter more often expressed in the common variant.

[b] Death is usually caused by multiorgan failure. Many patients die within days to weeks of initial presentation. In other patients, the fatal outcome occurs within 2 years.

peculiar hypersensitivity to mosquito bites, a condition referred to as HMB–EBV–NK disease (HMB, hypersensitivity to mosquito bites; EBV, Epstein–Barr virus; NK, natural killers) (5). Clinically, they show indurated bullae with clear or hemorrhagic contents that appear at the bite sites, then undergo necrosis and ulceration and heal with scarring.

REFERENCES

1. Jaffe ES, Harris NL, Stein H, Vardiman JW, eds. World Health Organization Classification of Tumours. Pathology and Genetics of Tumours of Haematopoietic and Lymphoid Tissue. Lyon: IARC Press, 2001.

2. De Lord C, Mercieca J, Ashton-Key M, Singh L, Ryley S, Isaacson P, Catovsky D. Aggressive NK cell lymphoma preceded by a ten year history of neutropenia associated with large granular lymphocyte lymphocytosis. Leuk Lymphoma 1998; 31:417–421.
3. Shiozawa S, Ogawa R, Morimoto I, Tanaka Y, Kanda N, Tatsumi E, Yamaguchi N, Fujita T. Polyarthritis, mononeuritis multiplex and eczematous ulcerative skin rash in a patient with myelodysplastic syndrome and peripheral large granular lymphocytosis. Clin Exp Rheumatol 1991; 9:629–633.
4. Loughran TP Jr, Starkebaum G. Large granular lymphocyte leukemia. Report of 38 cases and review of the literature. Medicine (Baltimore) 1987; 66:397–405.
5. Tokura Y, Ishihara S, Tagawa S, Seo N, Ohshima K, Takigawa M. Hypersensitivity to mosquito bites as the primary clinical manifestation of a juvenile type of Epstein–Barr virus-associated natural killer cell leukemia/lymphoma. J Am Acad Dermatol 2001; 45:569–578.

43.10. Chronic Neutrophilic Leukemia

Dmitry V. Kazakov, Günter Burg, and Werner Kempf
Department of Dermatology, University Hospital, Zürich, Switzerland

DEFINITION

Chronic neutrophilic leukemia (CNL) is a very rare form of leukemia with sustained peripheral blood neutrophilia, proliferation of neutrophilic granulocytes in the bone marrow, and absence of the Philadelphia (Ph) chromosome or the BCR/ABL fusion gene. Diagnosis of CNL is achieved by the exclusion of other myeloproliferative/myelodysplastic disorders. Since the original description by Tuohy in 1920, only approximately 100 cases of CNL have been reported (1,2).

CLINICAL FEATURES

Chronic neutrophilic leukemia affects mainly adults older than 50 years and occurs with equal distribution among males and females. Specific skin involvement is exceedingly rare. Nonspecific changes such as pruritus, purpura, petechiae, and ecchymoses are seen in approximately 25–30% of cases (2). Specific cutaneous involvement occurs as pruritic, infiltrative plaques on the extremities accompanied by scaling erythematous on palms and soles. In addition, patients may show hepatosplenomegaly and fatigue (2).

HISTOLOGY

There is a superficial and deep perivascular infiltrate composed of mature (neutrophils and eosinophils) and immature (myelocytes and metamyelocytes) myeloid cells.

IMMUNOHISTOCHEMISTRY

The majority of the cells stain positively with chloroacetate esterase and lysozyme, as well as other myeloid cell markers (myeloperoxidase, CD68, and CD34).

LABORATORY FINDINGS

There is peripheral blood leukocytosis ($\geq 25 \times 10^9/L$) with presence of immature granulocytes, bone marrow hypercellularity due to an increase of neutrophils, an increased myeloid to erythroid ratio (10:1 or greater), an elevated vitamin B_{12} level and an increased leukocyte alkaline phosphatase (LAP) score.

CYTOGENETICS

There is no Ph chromosome or BCR/ABL fusion gene.

TREATMENT

Skin lesions may improve with systemic chemotherapy. Topical steroids appear not to be beneficial (2).

CLINICAL COURSE AND PROGNOSIS

Survival is variable and ranges from 5 months to 20 years. The impact of skin involvement on survival is not known.

DIFFERENTIAL DIAGNOSIS

Specific skin involvement should be distinguished from Sweet syndrome and reactive neutrophilic dermatosis in CNL (3). A clue to the diagnosis of specific cutaneous involvement in CNL is the presence of immature granulocytes in the dermal infiltrate.

REFERENCES

1. Jaffe ES, Harris NL, Stein H, Vardiman JW, eds. World Health Organization Classification of Tumours. Pathology and Genetics of Tumours of Haematopoietic and Lymphoid Tissue. Lyon: IARC Press, 2001.
2. Willard RJ, Turiansky GW, Genest GP, Davis BJ, Diehl LF. Leukemia cutis in a patient with chronic neutrophilic leukemia. J Am Acad Dermatol 2001; 44:365–369.
3. Castanet J, Lacour JP, Garnier G, Perrin C, Taillan B, Fuzibet JG, Ortonne JP. Neutrophilic dermatosis associated with chronic neutrophilic leukemia. J Am Acad Dermatol 1993; 29:290–292.

44

Paraneoplastic Cutaneous Reactions in Leukemia and Lymphomas

Werner Kempf, Reinhard Dummer, Dmitry V. Kazakov, and Günter Burg
Department of Dermatology, University Hospital, Zürich, Switzerland

DEFINITION

Paraneoplastic cutaneous syndromes are nonneoplastic skin disorders which occur in strict association with an underlying malignant neoplasm (1).

CLASSIC PARANEOPLASTIC DISEASES

The most common paraneoplastic skin disorders comprise acanthosis nigricans (2), acrokeratosis Bazex (3), erythema gyratum repens (4) (Fig. 1), necrolytic migratory erythema (5), acquired hypertrichosis lanuginosa (6), and the Leser–Trélat sign (7).

These paraneoplastic dermatoses are mostly associated with solid tumors, in particular those involving visceral organs such as the lung and gastrointestinal system. Only rarely, do these dermatoses indicate the presence of nodal or primary cutaneous lymphomas. The sudden appearance of seborrheic keratoses known as Leser–Trélat sign and acanthosis nigricans are so far the only ones reported to arise in primary cutaneous lymphomas such as MF and Sézary syndrome (SS). In contrast, acrokeratosis Bazex, erythema gyratum repens, and necrolytic migratory erythema have not yet been observed in patients with primary cutaneous lymphomas. Two cases have been described in which pityriasis lichenoides chronica (PLC) preceded the occurrence of a medium or large-cell pleomorphic CD30–negative T-cell lymphoma of the skin (8). Recently, we reported for the first time a patient with MF and PLEVA (Fig. 2) (23).

ACUTE FEBRILE NEUTROPHILIC DERMATOSIS

Acute febrile neutrophilic dermatosis (Sweet syndrome) occurs in close association with hematological and lymphoproliferative disorders (9,10). Paraneoplastic Sweet syndrome is most often associated with acute myeloid leukemia (11). However, some cases may be induced by retinoic acid used for treatment of leukemia (12). Clinically,

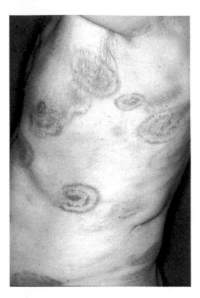

Figure 1 Erythema gyratum repens: concentric expanding rings on the trunk.

Sweet syndrome is characterized by painful erythematous plaques on the face, extremities and the trunk (Fig. 3). In addition, patients are febrile and suffer from malaise. Laboratory examination reveals an elevated neutrophil count. Histologically, a diffuse heavy infiltrate of neutrophils extending through the entire dermis is the hallmark of the lesion. Subepidermal edema can lead to blister formation. Additional findings may include erythrocyte extravasation, mild leukocytoklasia, and presence of lymphocytes and a few eosinophils. The differential diagnosis includes vasculitis secondary to leukemia as well as leukemia cutis in chronic neutrophilic leukemia (13,14).

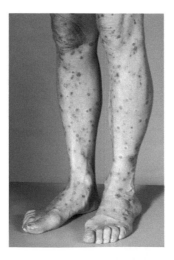

Figure 2 Paraneoplastic pityriasis lichenoides et varioliformis acuta (PLEVA): disseminated eroded scaly papules in a patient with MF.

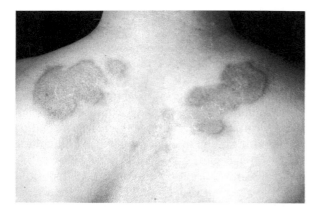

Figure 3 Sweet syndrome: infiltrated plaques on the back in patient with acute myeloid leukemia.

VASCULITIS

Vasculitis is most often seen in patients with leukemia, especially acute or chronic myeloid leukemia (15), and also rarely observed in patients with malignant lymphoma (16). Reactive vasculitis must be distinguished from vasculitis due to infiltration of vessel walls by neoplastic cells (so called leukemic vasculitis (17)), and drug-induced vasculitis in those patients with leukemia receiving multiagent chemotherapy and antibiotics (18). Vasculitic changes may represent the first marker for the underlying malignancy. Clinically, malignancy-associated vasculitis may present as maculopapular exanthems, purpura, and ulcers (19) (Fig. 4). Histologically, leukocytoclastic vasculitis is most often found. Recently, systemic vasculitis of medium-sized vessels associated with chronic myelomonocytic leukemia (CMML) has been reported (20). The prognosis of CMML-associated vasculitis seems to be poor with fatal outcome in some patients. Therefore, it is of clinical importance to recognize as early as possible paraneoplastic vasculitis.

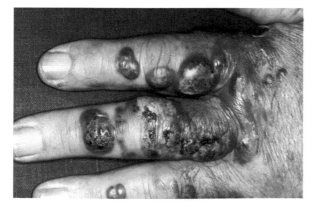

Figure 4 Paraneoplastic vasculitis: neutrophilic infiltrates with vascular damage producing nodules, bullae, and early erosions.

PATHOGENESIS

The pathogenetic mechanisms behind paraneoplastic reactions are still enigmatic. Immunologic mechanisms, either humoral or cell mediated, triggered by substances released by the tumor, may be the most important factors. This hypothesis is based on the observation that paraneoplastic dermatoses regress in almost all cases after remission of the underlying neoplasm. In many cases of primary cutaneous lymphomas such as MF and SS, the release of cytokines interacting with growth regulation of keratinocytes by the underlying neoplasm results in epidermal hyperproliferation as seen in acanthosis nigricans, Leser–Trelat sign, and acrokeratosis Bazex (21). Similar epidermal hyperplastic reactions have been observed in CD30–positive cutaneous T-cell lymphomas (22). In other disorders, inflammatory reactions like erythema gyratum repens and PLEVA may be triggered by proinflammatory cytokines. The vasculitis seen in PLEVA and associated with some leukemia may be induced by circulating immune complexes or cross-reacting antigens (19).

TREATMENT

By definition, paraneoplastic reactions resolve after removal of the underlying neoplasm. Symptomatic treatment includes systemically administered or topically applied corticosteroids. Keratolytics may be beneficial as adjunctive therapy in paraneoplastic disorders with hyperkeratosis.

COMMENT

It is of therapeutic and prognostic importance to recognize paraneoplastic skin diseases, since some of them such as leukemia-associated systemic vasculitis can be accompanied by life-threatening complications. Moreover, early recognition is of particular value in a patient with leukemia since prompt intervention may significantly affect survival.

REFERENCES

1. Poole S, Fenske NA. Cutaneous markers of internal malignancy. II. Paraneoplastic dermatoses and environmental carcinogens. J Am Acad Dermatol 1993; 28:147–164.
2. Safai B, Grant JM, Kurtz R, Lightdale CJ, Good RA. Cutaneous manifestation of internal malignancies (I) acanthosis nigricans. Int J Dermatol 1978; 17:312–315.
3. Bazex A. Paraneoplatische Akrokeratose. Hautarzt 1979; 30:119–123.
4. Boyd AS, Neldner KH, Menter A. Erythema gyratum repens: a paraneoplastic eruption. J Am Acad Dermatol 1992; 26:757–762.
5. Braverman I. Commentary: migratory necrolytic erythema. Arch Dermatol 1982; 118: 796–798.
6. Samson MK, Buroker TR, Henderson MD, Baker LH, Vaitkevicius VK. Acquired hypertrichosis languiginosa. Report of two new cases and a review of the literature. Cancer 1975; 36:1519–1521.
7. Safai B, Grant JM, Good RA. Cutaneous manifestation of internal malignancies (II): the sign of Leser–Trelat. Int J Dermatol 1978; 17:494–495.

8. Panizzon RG, Speich R, Dazzi H. Atypical manifestations of pityriasis lichenoides chronica: development into paraneoplasia and non-Hodgkin lymphomas of the skin. Dermatology 1992; 184:65–69.
9. Avivi I, Rosenbaum H, Levy Y, Rowe J. Myelodysplastic syndrome and associated skin lesions: a review of the literature. Leuk Res 1999; 23:323–330.
10. Callen JP. Neutrophilic dermatoses. Dermatol Clin 2002; 20:409–419.
11. Paydas S, Sahin B, Zorludemir S. Sweet's syndrome accompanying leukemia: seven cases and review of the literature. Leuk Res 2000; 24:83–86.
12. Astudillo L, Loche F, Reynish W, Rigal-Huguet F, Lamant L, Pris J. Sweet's syndrome associated with retinoic acid syndrome in a patient with promyelocytic leukemia. Ann Hematol 2002; 81:111–114.
13. Willard RJ, Turiansky GW, Genest GP, Davis BJ, Diehl LF. Leukemia cutis in a patient with chronic neutrophilic leukemia. J Am Acad Dermatol 2001; 44:365–369.
14. Malone JC, Slone SP, Wills-Frank LA, Fearneyhough PK, Lear SC, Goldsmith LJ, Hood AF, Callen JP. Vascular inflammation (vasculitis) in Sweet syndrome: a clinicopathologic study of 28 biopsy specimens from 21 patients. Arch Dermatol 2002; 138: 345–349.
15. Longley S, Caldwell JR, Panush RS. Paraneoplastic vasculitis: unique syndrome of cutaneous angiitis and arthritis associated with myeloproliferative disorder. Am J Med 1986; 80:1027–1030.
16. Greer JM, Longley S, Edwards NL, Elfenbein GJ, Panush RS. Vasculitis associated with malignancy. Experience with 13 patients and literature review. Medicine 1988; 67: 220–230.
17. Paydas S, Zorludemir S. Leukemia cutis and leukaemic vasculitis. Br J Dermatol 2000; 143:773–779.
18. Paydas S, Zorludemir S, Sahin B. Vasculitis and leukemia. Leuk Lymphoma 2000; 40: 105–112.
19. Mertz LE, Conn DL. Vasculitis associated with maligancy. Curr Opin Rheumatol 1992; 4:39–46.
20. Hamidou MA, El Kouri D, Audrain M, Grolleau JY. Systemic antineutrophil cytoplasmic antibody vasculitis associated with lymphoid neoplasia. Ann Rheum Dis 2001; 60: 293–295.
21. Horiuchi Y, Katsuoka K, Takezaki S, Nishiyama S. Study of epidermal growth activity in cultured human keratinocytes from peripheral-blood lymphocytes of a patient with Sezary syndrome associated with the Leser–Trelat sign. Arch Dermatol Res 1985; 278:74–76.
22. Scarisbrick JJ, Calonje E, Orchard G, Child FJ, Russell Jones R. Pseudocarcinomatous change in lymphomatoid papulosis and primary cutaneous CD30+ lymphoma: a clinicopathologic and immunohistochemical study of 6 patients. J Am Acad Dermatol 2001; 44:239–247.
23. Kempf W, Kutzuer H, Vetfelhack N, Palmedo G, Burg G. Paraveoplastic pityriasis liduenoides in cutaueous lymphoma—Case report and review of the literature on paraveoplastic reactions of the skin in lymphoma and leukenima. Br J Deermatol 2005 in press.

45

Histiocytic Disorders

Dmitry V. Kazakov, Günter Burg, and Werner Kempf
Department of Dermatology, University Hospital, Zürich, Switzerland

Histiocytoses are reactive or neoplastic disorders that arise from cells of the mono-nuclear phagocyte system (MPS). The cells constituting the MPS can be divided into two major groups based on their functional, cytological and ultrastructural features, namely *phagocytes* and *dendritic cells*. The main characteristics of these two categories are presented in Table 1. The *phagocytes* are derived from proliferating monoblasts and promonocytes, which give rise to nonproliferating monocytes, which in turn enter the blood and later migrate into the peripheral tissues to differentiate into macrophages. Tissue macrophages include short-living phagocytes appearing as a part of an inflammatory response and long-living residents in perivascular and interstitial spaces such as Kupffer cells in the liver and alveolar macrophages in the lungs. The *dendritic cell compartment* includes: (1) follicular dendritic cells, (2) Langerhans cells, (3) interstitial dendritic cells (the counterpart of Langerhans cells in parenchymal organs), (4) indeterminate (veiled) cells, (5) interdigitating dendritic cells and (6) dermal dendritic cells (dermal dendrocytes). The origin, distribution, immunophenotype

Table 1 Main Properties of Phagocytes and Dendritic Cells

	Phagocytes	Dendritic cells
Ultrastructural features	Numerous vacuoles, lysosomes, mitochondria, residual bodies	Dendrites, veils, lamellipodia
Endocytic activity	High (pinocytosis, phagocytosis)	Weak
Secretory activity	Cytokines (IL-1, IL-6, TNF), H_2O_2, Proteases	Few known secretory products
Receptors	Immune complexes FcR (CD16, 32, 64) and C3R (CDIIb) Lipopolysaccharide serum protein complexes (CD14)	HLA-DR, MHC class I and class II molecules, CD45, FcIgG
Response to M-CSF	Yes	No
Main function	Antigen processing (phagocytosis)	Antigen presentation

IL-interleukin; TNF-tumor necrosis factor; MHC-major histocompatibility complex; M-CSF-macro-phage-colony-stimulating factor.

and main ultrastructural features of dendritic cells (and also of macrophages for comparison) are summarized in Table 2. In addition, there are two types of cells with hybrid cell function and phenotype between phagocytes and dendritic cells (transitional cells), namely plasmacytoid monocytes and sinus-lining cells. A detailed description of the structure and functions of the MPS has been provided elsewhere (1–9) and is beyond the scope of this book.

The classification of the histiocytoses is still a matter of discussion. In 1987, the Writing Group of the Histiocyte Society (10) classified the histiocytoses into three classes:

Class 1. Langerhans cell histiocytosis
Class 2. Non-Langerhans cell histiocytosis
Class 3. Malignant histiocytoses

Table 2 Origin, Distribution, Immunophenotype and Key Ultrastructural Features of Dendritic Cells and Macrophages

Cell types	Distribution	Origin	Immunophenotype	Key ultrastructural features
Follicular dendritic cells	Germinal centers of lymph nodes	Controversial	**CD21+, CD35+,** CD45+, S-100– CD1a– Factor XIIIa–	Desmosomes
Langerhans cells	Skin (epidermis), cervix, vagina, stomach and esophagus	Bone marrow	**CD1a+, S-100+** CD45+ CD21–, CD35–, CD86– Factor XIIIa–	Birbeck granules
Interstitial dendritic cells	Parenchymal organs with exception of brain and cornea	Bone marrow	=Langerhans cells	Birbeck granules
Indeterminate cells	Migrating cells to local lymphoid tissue	Langerhans cells or interstitial dendritic cells	=Langerhans cells	No Birbeck granules
Interdigitating dendritic cells	T-zones of lymph nodes	Bone marrow	**S-100+, CD86+** CD45+ **CD1a–** CD21–, CD35– factor XIIIa–	Complex interdigitating cellular junctions
Dermal dendrocytes	Skin (papillary dermis, around vessels and adnexae)	Controversial	**Factor XIIIa+** CD45+, CD68+ CD21–, CD35– S-100, CD1a–	
Macrophages	Peripheral tissues	Bone marrow	**Lysozyme+,** S-100[b], CD1a– Factor XIIIa– CD21–, CD35–	Lysosomes (see Table 1)

Expression of factor XIIIa by neoplastic cells in cutaneous lesions of indeterminate cell histiocytosis has been detected.
Other markers expressed by macrophages include CD64, CD68, Mac387, alpha1-antitrypsin, CD11b, CD11c, CD14, CD32.

Table 3 Classification of Histiocytoses Applied to Dermatology and Dermatopathology

---

1. Langerhans cell histiocytoses (Class 1)
Letterer–Siwe disease
Hand-Schüller–Christian disease
Eosinophilic granuloma
Congenital self-healing Langerhans cell
    histiocytosis (Hashimoto–Pritzker disease)
2. Non-Langerhans cell histiocytoses (Class 2)
Proliferative non-Langerhans cell histiocytoses
Generalized eruptive histiocytosis
Progressive nodular histiocytosis
Benign cephalic histiocytosis
Multicentric reticulohistiocytosis
Solitary reticulohistiocytoma
Indeterminate cell histiocytosis
Granulomatous and storage non-Langerhans cell
    histiocytoses (including histiocytic reactions to
    exogenous and endogenous material)
Xanthomas (eruptive, tuberous, tendinous, xanthelasma, plane)
Verruciform xanthoma
Xanthoma disseminatum (Montgomery syndrome)
Plexiform xanthomatous tumor
Juvenile and adult xanthogranuloma
Necrobiotic xanthogranuloma
Progressive mucinous histiocytosis (hereditary and sporadic)
Crystal-storing histiocytosis
Disseminated lipogranulomatosis (Farber disease)
Niemann–Pick disease
Erdheim–Chester disease
Reactions to silica, zirconium, beryllium, polyvinylpyrrolidone, etc
Miscellaneous histiocytic reactions (including infections)
    histologically resembling neoplasm
Sinus histiocytosis with massive lymphadenopathy
Histioid leprosy
Malakoplakia
Hemophagocytic disorders
Hemophagocytic lymphohistiocytoses (familial and sporadic)
Histiocytic cytophagic panniculitis
3. **Malignant histiocytoses (including malignant tumors**
   of dendritic cells) (Class 3)
Histiocytic sarcoma
Langerhans cell sarcoma
Interdigitating cell tumor/sarcoma
Follicular dendritic cell tumor/sarcoma

While the class 1 disorders are well-defined and not a subject of debate, great confusion exists concerning class 2, in which there is a number of clinically distinct entities sharing the same or very similar histo- and immunopathological features. A range of hypotheses and proposals regarding the reclassification of class 2 histiocytoses have been set forward and we believe that future observations will bring about consensus on the topic. Recently, a reclassification of histiocytic disorders primarily affecting children has been proposed by the World Health Organization's Committee on histiocytic/reticulum cell proliferations and the Reclassification Working Group of the Histiocyte Society (8). This classification takes into account the ontogeny of histiocytes (macrophages or dendritic cells), lineage of lesional cells and biologic behavior of a correspondent entity. Finally and most recently, the International Lymphoma Study Group has offered a classification of tumors of histiocytes and accessory dendritic cells based on an immunohistochemical approach (11). Table 3 lists a classification which can be used in clinical dermatological and dermatopathological practice.

REFERENCES

1. Foucar K, Foucar E. The mononuclear phagocyte and immnuregulatory effector (M-PIRE) system: evolving concepts. Sem Diagn Pathol 1990; 7:4–18.
2. Lieberman PH, Jones CR, Steinman RM, Erlandson RA, Smith J, Gee T, Huvos A, Garin-Chesa P, Filippa DA, Urmacher C, Gangi MD, Sperber M. Langerhans cell (eosinophilic) granulomatosis. A clinicopathological study encompassing 50 years. Am J Surg Pathol 1995; 20:519–552.
3. Murphy GF, Liu V. The dermal immune system. In: Skin Immune System. Bos JD, ed. Boca Raton: CRC Press, 1997:347.
4. Caputo R. Text Atlas of Histiocytic Syndromes. London: Martin Dunitz Ltd, 1998.
5. Jaffe ES. Histiocytic and dendritic cell neoplasm: introduction. In: Pathology and Genetics of Tumours of Haemotapoietic and Lymphoid Tissues. World Health Organization Classification of Tumours. Lyon: IARC Press, 2001:275–277.
6. Headington JT. The dermal dendrocyte. Adv Dermatol 1986; 1:159–171.
7. Balogh P, Aydar Y, Tew JG, Szakal AK. Ontogeny of the follicular dendritic cell phenotype and function in the postnatal murine spleen. Cell Immunol 2001; 214:45–53.
8. Favara BE, Feller AC, Pauli M, Jaffe ES, Weiss LM, Arico M, Bucsky P, Egeler RM, Elinder G, Gadner H, Gresik M, Henter JI, Imashuku S, Janka-Schaub G, Jaffe R, Ladisch S, Nezelof C, Pritchard J. Contemporary classification of histiocytic disorders. The WHO committee on histiocytic/reticulum cell proliferations. reclassification working group of the histiocyte society. Med Pediatr Oncol 1997; 29:157–166.
9. Imal Y, Yamakawa M. Morphology, function and pathology of follicular dendritic cells. Pathol Int 1996; 46:807–833.
10. Writing group of the Histiocytic Society. Histiocytic syndromes in children. Lancet 1987; 1:208–209.
11. Pileri SA, Grogan TM, Harris NL, Banks P, Campo E, Chan JK, Favera RD, Delsol G, De Wolf-Peeters C, Falini B, Gascoyne RD, Gaulard P, Gatter KC, Isaacson PG, Jaffe ES, Kluin P, Knowles DM, Mason DY, Mori S, Muller-Hermelink HK, Piris MA, Ralfkiaer E, Stein H, Su IJ, Warnke RA, Weiss LM. Tumours of histiocytes and accessory dendritic cells: an immunohistochemical approach to classification from the international lymphoma study group based on 61 cases. Histopathology 2002; 41:1–29.

45.1. Langerhans Cell Histiocytosis (Histiocytosis X)

Dmitry V. Kazakov, Günter Burg, and Werner Kempf
Department of Dermatology, University Hospital, Zürich, Switzerland

DEFINITION

Langerhans cell histiocytosis (LCH) (also known as histiocytosis-X) is a proliferative disorder of Langerhans cells with a wide spectrum of cutaneous and extracutaneous manifestations.

CLINICAL FEATURES

The clinical presentation of LCH is very diverse. Four forms of LCH have been delineated, taking into account the clinical setting, course, and prognosis (Table 1). This classification has certain limitations because of the highly variable manifestations of the disease with many overlapping features. The skin may be involved in LCH either as single organ involvement or as part of a multiorgan systemic disease. Skin lesions may be the first manifestation of LCH (50% of cases). They may occur simultaneously with extracutaneous involvement or follow the latter. Both generalized lesions or solitary lesions can be seen. Any anatomic site can be involved including scalp, nails, palms, and soles as well as mucous membranes.

The simplest classification divides LCH into localized disease (skin lesions, solitary or limited bone disease) and disseminated disease (multifocal bone disease or multiorgan involvement). In the latter case, the most crucial organs are the hematopoietic system, spleen, liver, and lungs. Dysfunction of these organs and age of the patient (<1 year and >60 years) are the most important factors.

The unifying feature is the histological findings. For this reason, the clinical features and differential diagnoses of each variant are discussed separately, followed by a common discussion of histology, immunohistochemistry, electron microscopy, and therapy.

Table 1 Langerhans Cell Histiocytoses and Their Characteristics

Disease	Age	Skin involvement	Clinical features	Course	Prognosis
Letterer–Siwe	First years of life	~90–100%	Fever, weight loss, lymphadenopathy, hepatosplenomegaly, pancytopenia, bone lesions	Acute	Mortality rate: 50–66%
Hand–Schüller–Christian	Children, adults	~30%	Osteolytic bone lesions, diabetes insipidus, exophthalmus, otitis	Subacute to chronic	Mortality rate: <50%
Eosinophilic granuloma	Mainly adults	<10%	Solitary bone or skin lesions	Chronic	Favorable
Congenital self-healing reticulohistiocytosis	Congenital	100%	Skin lesions only	Self-healing[a]	Excellent

[a] Both relapses and conversion to systemic disease can occur, so long-term follow-up is needed.

Letterer–Siwe Disease

The disease usually manifests during the first year of life. There is little epidemiologic information (1), but the incidence has been estimated as 0.1–0.5 per 100,000 inhabitants per year. There have been reports on familial cases with autosomal recessive inheritance.

Symptoms include fever, weight loss, rash, lymphadenopathy, hepatosplenomegaly, pancytopenia and purpura. The most common sites of involvement are the scalp and diaper area. Other seborrhoeic sites such as the postauricular area, nasolabial folds, perioral region, and upper trunk are often involved. There are tiny (0.5 mm in diameter) rose-yellow or brownish-red, translucent papules and patches (Fig. 1). In time, the papules become scaly and crusted and may coalesce into plaques. Petechial and purpuric lesions, pustules, and vesicles as well as small erosions can also be seen. Nodules are uncommon, but may be found on the trunk and tend to ulcerate.

Clinical Course and Prognosis

Without treatment, the disease was frequently fatal in the past. Today, the mortality rate is 50–66% assuming major organ dysfunction.

Differential Diagnosis

Seborrhoeic dermatitis, other eczematous lesions and other forms of LCH.

Hand–Schüller–Christian Disease

The typical triad includes osteolytic skull lesions (100%), diabetes insipidus (50%), and exophthalmus (10%). Otitis media, generalized lymphoadenopathy, hepatosplenomegaly, and pulmonary disease may be additional findings.

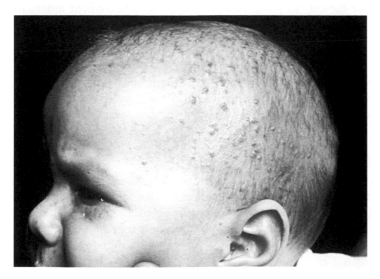

Figure 1   Letterer–Siwe disease: Multiple small papules on the scalp in an infant. (Kindly provided by R. Caputo.)

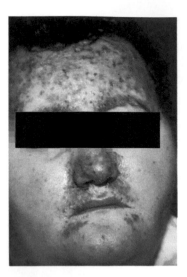

Figure 2 Hand–Schüller–Christian disease: Scaly and crusted papules and plaques in the seborrhoeic areas of the face.

Skin lesions occur in about 30% of cases, usually in the intertriginous areas, most often as papules and nodules which may be ulcerated or superinfected. Typical intertriginous and perinasal lesions as seen in Letterer–Siwe disease may also occur (Fig. 2).

Clinical Course and Prognosis

The disease shows a prolonged course and has a relatively good prognosis with a mortality rate of less than 50%, but detailed data are not available. The biggest problems in survivors are (i) permanent major organ dysfunction due to "internal scarring" (i.e., persistent liver dysfunction), (ii) endocrine defects, mainly diabetes insipidus, and (iii) bone defects. In patients with cutaneous involvement alone, no matter what age or type of lesions, survival is 100% (age-matched).

Differential Diagnosis

The nodules may be confused with juvenile xanthogranuloma, Spitz's nevus, mastocytoma, or lymphoma. The intertriginous lesions simulate eczema, psoriasis, Hailey–Hailey disease, or tinea corporis.

Eosinophilic Granuloma

Patients have one or a few localized lesions. The most common site of involvement is the bone. A clinically distinct form is the involvement of the maxilla or mandible with loss of teeth (floating teeth). The uncommon cutaneous lesions are deep dermal or subcutaneous nodules which are not clinically distinct (2,3). In rare cases, only the skin is involved.

Clinical Course and Prognosis

Most lesions can be easily treated, but may locally recur. On rare occasions, the disease may spread to multiple organs (4).

Differential Diagnosis

The spectrum of skin lesions with predominant eosinophilic infiltration is wide and includes granuloma faciale, insect bite reaction, and Wells syndrome.

Congenital Self-healing Reticulohistiocytosis

Multiple papules and nodules on the trunk, head, palms, and soles are found, sometimes showing central ulceration. They occur in otherwise healthy infants with no or mild systemic symptoms (5–8). As the lesions involute, they leave behind hypo- or hyperpigmented macules or patches. Due to the spontaneous regression within a few weeks or months of lesions, no therapy is needed.

Clinical Course and Prognosis

The prognosis is excellent, but on rare occasions, the young patients may develop LS disease with the corresponding worse outlook.

HISTOPATHOLOGY

In 1868, Langerhans described the cell that bears his name (9). In 1961, Birbeck et al. discovered the organelle that became the "condition sine qua non" of the Langer-

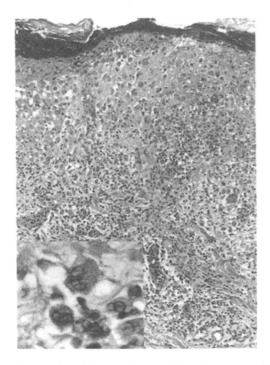

Figure 3 Diffuse infiltrate of lymphocytes, epithelioid histiocytes, eosinophils, neutrophils, plasma cells, and tumor cells with large, pale, reniform nucleus, and abundant, slightly eosinophilic cytoplasm (insert).

hans cell (LC). The hallmark of LCH is a cell with a large, pale, reniform, vesicular nucleus, and abundant, slightly eosinophilic or amphophilic cytoplasm (Fig. 3). These cells were described by Lichtenstein (10) in 1953 in his classical paper unifying the many variants of histiocytosis X. Histological variations mainly concern the architecture of the infiltrate and its cellular composition and correlate with the clinical appearance of the lesions. Fully developed papules and plaques show a dense band-like infiltrate obscuring the dermo-epidermal junction. Epidermotropism of LCs with Pautrier-like microabscess formation can be found. In addition, erosion or ulceration is frequently found. Nodular lesions demonstrate larger, more deeply located circumscribed or diffuse infiltrates often accompanied by eosinophils (eosinophilic granuloma). In addition to LCs and eosinophils, the infiltrate may contain variable numbers of lymphocytes, epithelioid histiocytes, neutrophils, plasma cells, giant cells, foam cells, and extravasated erythrocytes (Fig. 3). Xanthomatous lesions with foamy histiocytes are common in bones, but extremely rare in the skin.

IMMUNOHISTOCHEMISTRY

The phenotypic hallmarks in LCH are expression of CD1a and S-100 by the tumor cells (11,12). Macrophage markers are almost always negative and have no diagnostic significance.

ELECTRON MICROSCOPY

Rod-shaped or rocket-shaped granules measuring 200–400 nm (Birbeck granules, Langerhans cell granules) are the ultrastructural hallmark of LCs. The number of cells with demonstrable granules is variable in a given lesion. Early lesions usually contain a greater number of Birbeck granules. In addition, the cytoplasm of LCs contains high numbers of lysosomes. The coexistence of laminated dense bodies and Birbeck granules may be more common in congenital self-healing reticulohistiocytosis (12–15).

TREATMENT

The significant differences in prognosis depending on major organ dysfunction mean that the treatment of LCH must be carefully tailored to the individual patient.

Solitary skin lesions can be treated with intralesional corticosteroids or even excision. Multiple lesions can be approached with topical corticosteroids; if these fail, then in adults, topical nitrogen mustard is an effective alternative. We do not employ it in children. Superficial radiation therapy is also effective, but is rarely used in children.

Patients with multiorgan involvement generally require systemic therapy. Those who are older than 2 years and do not have involvement of the liver, lungs, spleen, or hematopoietic system tend to do very well and can generally be treated with systemic corticosteroids and vinblastine. Others have a much higher risk and a much lower response to therapy. They should be treated in cooperation with oncologists, ideally as part of a study protocol, as the ideal approach to this group remains to be determined.

REFERENCES

1. Nicholson HS, Egeler RM, Nesbit ME. The epidemiology of Langerhans cell histiocytosis. Hematol Oncol Clin North Am 1998; 12:379–384.
2. Gerbig AW, Zala L, Hunziker T. Tumorlike eosinophilic granuloma of the skin. Am J Dermatopathol 2000; 22:75–78.
3. Mahzoon S, Wood MG. Multifocal eosinophilic granuloma with skin ulceration. Histiocytosis X of the Hand–Schüller–Christian type. Arch Dermatol 1980; 116:218–220.
4. Rodman OG, Cooper PH. Multifocal eosinophilic granuloma of skin and bone. Thirteen year surveillance of a patient. Cutis 1980; 26:487–488, 495–498.
5. Hashimoto K, Pritzker MS . Electron microscopic study of reticulohistiocytoma: an unusual case of congenital, self-healing reticulohistiocytosis. Arch Dermatol 1973; 107:263–270.
6. Laugier P, Hunziker N, Laut J, Orusco M, Osmos LP. Reticulohistiocytosis of benign evolution (Hashimoto–Pritzker type). Ann Dermatol Syphiligr Paris 1975; 102:21–31.
7. Rufli T, Fricker HS. Congenital, self-healing reticulohistiocytosis. Z Hautkr 1979; 54: 554–558.
8. Larralde M, Rositto A, Giardelli M, Gatti CF, Santos Munoz A. Congenital self-healing histiocytosis (Hashimoto–Pritzker). Int J Dermatol 1999; 38:693–696.
9. Langerhans P. Über die Nerven der menschlichen Haut. Virchow Arch B 1868; 44:325.
10. Lichtenstein L, Histiocytosis X. Integration of eosinophilic granuloma of bone, Letterer–Siwe disease and Hand–Schüller–Christian disease as related manifestations of a single nosologic entity. Arch Path 1953; 56:84–102.
11. Emile JF, Wechsler J, Brousse N, Boulland ML, Cologon R, Fraitag S, Voisin MC, Gaulard P, Boumsell L, Zafrani ES. Langerhans' cell histiocytosis. Definitive diagnosis with the use of monoclonal antibody O10 on routinely paraffin-embedded samples. Am J Surg Pathol 1995; 19:636–641.
12. Hashimoto K, Kagetsu N, Taniguchi Y, Weintraub R, Chapman-Winokur RL, Kasiborski A. Immunohistochemistry and electron microscopy in Langerhans cell histiocytosis confined to the skin. J Am Acad Dermatol 1991; 25:1044–1053.
13. Gianotti F, Caputo R, Ranzi T. Ultrastructural study of giant cells and "Langerhans cell granules" in cutaneous lesions and lymph-node and liver biopsies from four cases of subacute disseminated histiocytosis of Letterer–Siwe. Arch Klin Exp Dermatol 1968; 233:238–252.
14. Gianotti F, Caputo R. Skin ultrastructure in Hand–Schüller–Christian disease. Report on abnormal Langerhans' cells. Arch Dermatol 1969; 100:342–349.
15. Gianotti F. Cutaneous benign histiocytoses of childhood. Mod Probl Paediatr 1975; 17:193–203.

45.2. Indeterminate Cell Histiocytosis

Dmitry V. Kazakov, Günter Burg, and Werner Kempf
Department of Dermatology, University Hospital, Zürich, Switzerland

DEFINITION

Indeterminate cell histiocytosis (ICH) is a rare neoplastic disorder typified by the proliferation of indeterminate histiocytic cells first described by Wood and colleagues in 1985 (1). These cells are morphologically and immunophenotypically (CD1a+, S100+) related to Langerhans cells but lack Birbeck granules on electron microscopy.

CLINICAL FEATURES

The disease usually affects otherwise healthy adults without predilection for age and gender and commonly manifests itself as multiple (in some cases more than 100), asymptomatic, non-confluent papules and nodules, varying from 1 to 10 mm in size (Fig. 1). The trunk and limbs are the most common sites (2). In the beginning, the lesions are reddish-brown and may be dome-shaped, but in the course of the disease some lesions may develop a yellow discoloration while others regress leaving atrophy, wrinkling of the overlying epidermis, or hyperpigmented macules.

HISTOLOGY

There is a non-epidermotropic infiltrate composed of mononuclear cells intermingled with some giant cells and foamy cells. On occasion, a whorled and storiform arrangement of the infiltrative cells can be seen (3).

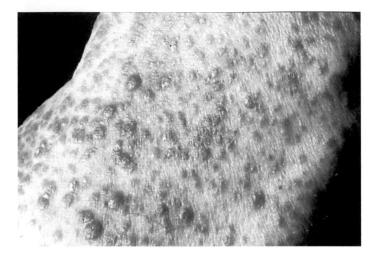

Figure 1 Multiple papules on the arm.

IMMUNOHISTOCHEMISTRY

The coexpression of CD1a (often focal) and S-100 is characteristic. In addition, the neoplastic cells are positive for histiocytic markers such as factor XIIIa, KiM1p, CD68, HAM 56, Mac387, lysozyme, alpha1-antitrypsin, CD11b, CD11c, CD14, CD32, and HLA-DR (4,5). Different patterns of staining in the superficial dermis vs. the deep dermis for some of these histiocytic markers have been noted (4).

ELECTRON MICROSCOPY

The histiocytes in ICH lack Birbeck granules and contain dense bodies and/or comma-shaped bodies/worm-like particles. These ultrastructural features may help in separating ICH from Langerhans cell histiocytosis.

Indeterminate cell histocytosis

Clinical features
  No gender or age predilection
  Multiple, asymptomatic, nonconfluent papules and nodules; size: 1–10 mm
  Mostly on the trunk and limbs
  Reddish-brown lesions, later yellow discoloration, regression with atrophy, wrinkling of the overlying epidermis or hyperpigmentation
Histological features
  Non-epidermotropic infiltrate
  Mononuclear histiocytic cells admixed with some vacuolated cells and multinucleated giant cells
Immunophenotype
  CD1a+ S-100+, macrophage markers+

Indeterminate cell histocytosis

Electron microscopy
  No Birbeck granules
  Dense bodies and/or comma-shaped bodies/worm-like particles
Clinical course and prognosis
  Usually benign with spontaneous regression

TREATMENT

Due to the spontaneous regression of the lesions, no treatment is usually required. In persistent lesions, successful treatment with vinblastine or 2-chlorodeoxyadenosine has been reported (6).

CLINICAL COURSE AND PROGNOSIS

The disease usually follows a benign course with spontaneous resolution. Recurrences may occur. One case with evolution to acute mast cell leukemia has been described (7).

COMMENTS

Several theories exist regarding the origin of indeterminate cells. Some authors believe that indeterminate cells may represent precursors of Langerhans cells that acquire Birbeck granules as they transit from dermal to epidermal sites as a result of the interaction of their receptors and epidermis-specific ligands (8). More recently it has been suggested that indeterminate cells represent members of the epidermal/dermal dendritic (antigen-presenting) cell system that are on their way from the skin to the regional lymph nodes (9). According to this concept, indeterminate cell histiocytosis can be regarded as a disorder of proliferating indeterminate cells that have been locally arrested before leaving the skin and traveling as veiled cells via the lymphatics to the T-cell-dependent paracortical areas of the regional lymph nodes (4).

REFERENCES

1. Wood GS, Hu CH, Beckstead JH, Turner RR, Winkelmann RK. The indeterminate cell proliferative disorder: report of a case manifesting as an unusual cutaneous histiocytosis. J Dermatol Surg Oncol 1985; 11:1111–1119.
2. Winkelmann RK. Cutaneous syndromes of non-X histiocytosis. A review of the macrophage–histiocyte diseases of the skin. Arch Dermatol 1981; 117:667–672.
3. Rosenberg AS, Morgan MB. Cutaneous indeterminate cell histiocytosis: a new spindle cell variant resembling dendritic cell sarcoma. J Cutan Pathol 2001; 28:531–537.
4. Sidoroff A, Zelger B, Steiner H, Smith N. Indeterminate cell histiocytosis—a clinicopathological entity with features of both X- and non-X histiocytosis. Br J Dermatol 1996; 134:525–532.

5. Burgdorf WHC, Zelger B. The histiocytoses. In: Elder D, ed. Lever's Histopathology of the Skin 9th ed. Philadelphia: Lippincott Williams & Wilkins, 2003.
6. Winkelmann RK, Hu CH, Kossard S. Response of nodular non-X histiocytosis to vinblastine. Arch Dermatol 1982; 118:913–917.
7. Kolde G, Brocker EB. Multiple skin tumors of indeterminate cells in an adult. J Am Acad Dermatol 1986; 15:591–597.
8. Murphy GF, Harrist TJ, Bhan AK, Mihm MC Jr. Distribution of cell surface antigens in histiocytosis X cells. Quantitative immunoelectron microscopy using monoclonal antibodies. Lab Invest 1983; 48:90–97.
9. Berti E, Gianotti R, Alessi E. Unusual cutaneous histiocytosis expressing an intermediate immunophenotype between Langerhans' cells and dermal macrophages. Arch Dermatol 1988; 124:1250–1253.

Sinus Histiocytosis with Massive Lymphadenopathy

Dmitry V. Kazakov, Günter Burg, and Werner Kempf
Department of Dermatology, University Hospital, Zürich, Switzerland

DEFINITION

Sinus histiocytosis with massive lymphadenopathy (SHML) or Rosai–Dorfman disease is a rare, benign, self-limiting, proliferative histiocytic disorder of unknown origin. It was first described by Rosai and Dorfman in 1969, although Destombes had previously described the disorder in Africa.

CLINICAL FEATURES

SHML mainly occurs in childhood and early adolescence (mean age 20 years) and demonstrates a slight male predominance of 1.5:1 (1). Patients typically present with painless, bilateral-, cervical lymphadenopathy, usually accompanied by fever. Other lymph nodes can also be involved. Laboratory findings include leukocytosis with neutrophilia, an elevated erythrocyte sedimentation rate and polyclonal hypergammaglobulinemia. An increased incidence of various autoimmune and rheumatological disorders in patients with SHML has been noted (1). Extranodal involvement occurs in approximately 40% of cases, with the skin and soft tissue being the most commonly affected organs. Most often firm red-brown papules or nodules are seen. Other sites of involvement are the nasal cavity, paranasal sinuses, eyelids, orbits, bones, upper respiratory tract, salivary glands, breasts, and central nervous system. Patients with purely extranodal disease have been reported and referred to as purely cutaneous SHML. In contrast to the systemic disease, purely cutaneous SHML occurs in older people with a predilection for women (2). The most common presentation of the disease is multiple (sometimes single), firm, indurated papules, and nodules ranging in color from red-brown to orange and yellow and ranging in size from 1 to 10 cm (3). At times, the lesions can exhibit ulceration or central atrophy (4). There is no predilection site. Other reported manifestations of cutaneous SHML

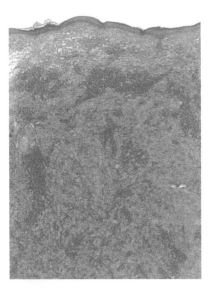

Figure 1 Sinus histiocytosis with massive lymphadenopathy: dermal infiltrate with sheets of pale sinusoidal histiocytes and dark small lymphocytes at the periphery.

include changes resembling vasculitis, eczema, psoriasis, exfoliative dermatitis, lupus vulgaris, acne, sarcoidosis, hidradenitis suppurativa, and pyogenic granuloma (5,6).

HISTOLOGY

The histologic features of primary cutaneous SHML and secondary skin involvement are similar. The hallmark of the conditions is the tendency of the infiltrate to recapitulate its architecture seen in the lymph nodes, i.e., aggregates of lymphocytes simulate the appearance of germinal centers with surrounding sheets of large histiocytes and dilated vessels (pseudosinuses) (Fig. 1). Within the infiltrate, the histiocytes are usually arranged in clusters of different size and shape (Fig. 2). They

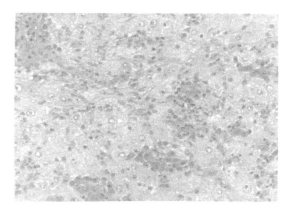

Figure 2 Sinus histiocytosis with massive lymphadenopathy: sheets of clear histiocytes some of which display emperipolesis.

possess large vesicular nuclei, centrally placed nucleoli, abundant eosinophilic cytoplasm, and indistinct cellular margins. The lymphoid aggregates are usually located at the periphery of the infiltrate. In addition, variable numbers of plasma cells, small well-differentiated lymphocytes, and neutrophils are dispersed between the aggregates of histiocytes. Emperipolesis (phagocytosis of lymphocytes and/or granulocytes) is frequently seen. The lymphatic vessels are dilated and contain sinus histiocytes. Histological variations include the presence of foamy histiocytes, occasional Touton cells, and fibrosis, which is seen in late stages.

IMMUNOHISTOCHEMISTRY

The histiocytes express S-100 protein and stain positively for monocyte-macrophage-associated antigens (CD68, Mac387, CD11b, CD11c, CD13, and lysozyme) and variably for activation markers such as CD38, CD69, CD71, and HLA-DR (Fig. 3). CD1a is not expressed. The lymphoid infiltrate represents a mixture of mature T cells and polyclonal B cells.

TREATMENT

Since the disorder is self-limiting, no treatment is usually required. Treatment may be required in the patients with systemic disease showing life-threatening organ involvement or progression. Systemic corticosteroids, multiagent chemotherapy, antiviral drugs, interferon, radiotherapy, and surgical interventions have been used with variable success. If needed, cutaneous lesions can be treated with topical steroids or cryotherapy or can be excised.

CLINICAL COURSE AND PROGNOSIS

Most patients with both the systemic disease and the purely cutaneous form have a favorable prognosis. Usually, the disease runs a benign although protracted course

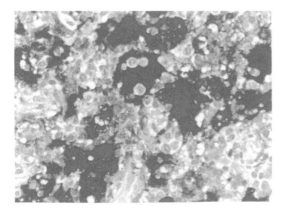

Figure 3 Sinus histiocytosis with massive lymphadenopathy: histiocytic cells express S-100 as shown here, but fail to express CD1a.

with spontaneous regression. However, death due to immune dysfunction can occur in the patients with systemic disease in approximately 10% of cases (7).

Sinus histiocytosis with massive lymphadenopathy

Clinical features
  Systemic disease
    Young patients
    Marked lymphadenopathy (bilateral, cervical), systemic features
    Extranodal involvement in 40%
  Purely cutaneous disease
    Nodules in older patients
Histological features
  Clusters of histiocytes with large vesicular nuclei, centrally placed nucleoli, abundant eosinophilic cytoplasm, and indistinct margins.
  Emperipolesis
Immunophenotype
  Histiocytes: S-100+, CDla−
Treatment
  Excision of solitary lesions. No standardized approach for systemic disease
Clinical course and prognosis
  Favorable, spontaneous remission in most cases

DIFFERENTIAL DIAGNOSIS

The differential diagnosis of SHML includes other benign and malignant histiocytoses as well as lymphomas. The unique constellation of histological and immunohistochemical features make the diagnosis of SHML straightforward in most cases.

COMMENTS

The cause of the disease is unknown. It has been suggested that SHML may represent an abnormal reactive response of histiocytes to an infectious agent. EBV and HHV-6 have been considered as possible causative infection agents since elevated titers of HHV-6 and EBV antibodies have been detected in blood, and HHV-6 has been demonstrated in the involved lymph nodes. PCR studies from the lesional skin have been negative. Clonality studies have given evidence of a polyclonal nature of the histiocytes in SHML (8–10).

REFERENCES

1. Foucar E, Rosai J, Dorfman R. Sinus histiocytosis with massive lymphadenopathy (Rosai–Dorfman disease): review of the entity. Semin Diagn Pathol 1990; 7:19–73.
2. Skiljo M, Garcia-Lora E, Tercedor J, Massare E, Esquivias J, Garcia-Mellado V. Purely cutaneous Rosai–Dorfman disease. Dermatology 1995; 191:49–51.

3. Perrin C, Michiels JF, Lacour JP, Chagnon A, Fuzibet JG. Sinus histiocytosis (Rosai–Dorfman disease) clinically limited to the skin. An immunohistochemical and ultrastructural study. J Cutan Pathol 1993; 20:368–374.
4. Quaglino P, Tomasini C, Novelli M, Colonna S, Bernengo MG. Immunohistologic findings and adhesion molecule pattern in primary pure cutaneous Rosai–Dorfman disease with xanthomatous features. Am J Dermatopathol 1998; 20:393–398.
5. Thawerani H, Sanchez RL, Rosai J, Dorfman RF. The cutaneous manifestations of sinus histiocytosis with massive lymphadenopathy. Arch Dermatol 1978; 114:191–197.
6. Ang P, Tan SH, Ong BH. Cutaneous Rosai–Dorfman disease presenting as pustular and acneiform lesions. J Am Acad Dermatol 1999; 41:335–337.
7. Grabczynska SA, Toh CT, Francis N, Costello C, Bunker CB. Rosai–Dorfman disease complicated by autoimmune haemolytic anaemia: case report and review of a multisystem disease with cutaneous infiltrates. Br J Dermatol 2001; 145:323–326.
8. Perez A, Rodriguez M, Febrer I, Aliaga A. Sinus histiocytosis confined to the skin. Case report and review of the literature. Am J Dermatopathol 1995; 17:384–388.
9. Middel P, Hemmerlein B, Fayyazi A, Kaboth U, Radzun HJ. Sinus histiocytosis with massive lymphadenopathy: evidence for its relationship to macrophages and for a cytokine-related disorder. Histopathology 1999; 35:525–533.
10. Levine PH, Jahan N, Murari P, Manak M, Jafee ES. Detection of human herpesvirus 6 in tissues involved by sinus histiocytosis with massive lymphadenopathy (Rosai–Dorfman disease). J Infect Dis 1992; 166:291–295.

Multicentric Reticulohistiocytosis (Lipoid Dermatoarthritis)

Dmitry V. Kazakov, Günter Burg, and Werner Kempf
Department of Dermatology, University Hospital, Zürich, Switzerland

DEFINITION

Multicentric reticulohistiocytosis (MR) is a rare histiocytic proliferative disease of unknown cause affecting mainly skin, joints, and mucous membranes. It was first described by Weber and Freundenthal in 1937. Since then, approximately 200 cases have been published; other names used for MR include lipoid dermatoarthritis, giant cell histiocytoma, reticulohistiocytic granuloma, and reticulohistiocytoma (RH).

CLINICAL FEATURES

The disease typically affects women in their fourth or fifth decade of life with a male:female ratio of 1:2–3. Children and adolescents are rarely involved. In 40–60% of cases, the joint disease precedes skin and mucosal involvement. Patients tend to present with polyarthritis, which most commonly affects the distal interphalangeal joints of the hands. Other joints may also be involved. Whatever the anatomic location, the arthritis in MR is symmetrical, chronic, and destructive. Radiological examination shows well-circumscribed periarticular "punched out" erosions and reabsorption of the juxtarticular zone corresponding to a secondary osteoarthritis (1).

The skin lesions in most cases are firm, reddish, brown or yellow papules, nodules, or plaques ranging in diameter from a few millimeters to centimeters located in a somewhat symmetrical fashion predominantly on the extensor surfaces of the hands and forearms (Fig. 1). The face, scalp, and hands are also commonly involved. Multiple confluent lesions of the face may result in leonine facies. Very typical if not pathognomonic are the rings of papules along the nail folds (coral

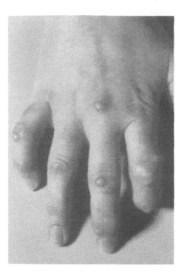

Figure 1   Multicentric reticulohistiocytosis: multiple papules and nodules in typical acral locations.

bead-like lesions) seen in a third of patients. They sometimes produce nail dystrophy. Although observed less frequently, vermicular erythematous lesions bordering the nostrils are also quite characteristic of MR (2). Involvement of the lower trunk and the legs is rarely seen. The skin lesions, which rarely ulcerate, are often in proximity to the affected joints. Pruritus is reported in about 25% of cases.

About half of the patients have mucosal involvement affecting the oral mucosa, lips, tongue, nasal mucosa, pharynx, larynx, and sclera (3). Cystic swellings of tendon sheaths may also develop. Constitutional symptoms include fever, malaise, and weight loss. Lymphadenopathy is present in 3% of cases (2). Laboratory findings are usually normal.

An associated internal malignancy including carcinomas of internal organs, multiple myeloma, melanoma, and lymphomas is found in about 15–25% of patients (4–6). In most cases, the diagnosis of MR precedes that of the neoplasm. In approximately 15% of cases, MR is accompanied by an autoimmune disease such as Sjögren syndrome or systemic lupus erythematosus (7,8).

HISTOLOGY

The hallmarks of the disease are diffuse infiltrates of oncocytic histiocytes with ample eosinophilic, finely granular ("ground-glass") cytoplasm, and small round nuclei (Figs. 2 and 3). Along with these mononuclear histiocytes, large (50–100 μm) multinucleated cells (up to 20 nuclei) are observed. In addition, the infiltrate contains a few small lymphocytes, neutrophils, plasma cells, and eosinophils. The cytoplasm of the histiocytic cells is PAS-positive and diastase resistant. In addition, in most cases, the cells stain strongly with Sudan black B fat stain and oil red O. The infiltrate usually displays an interstitial pattern. An increase in reticular fibers (Gomori stain) can be seen. In older lesions, fibrosis may develop (9,10).

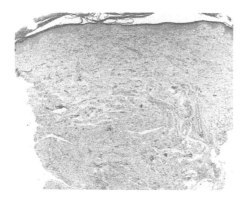

Figure 2 Multicentric reticulohistiocytosis: diffuse infiltrate of histiocytes throughout the entire dermis. (Specimen courtesy of W. Burgdorf, Germany.)

IMMUNOHISTOCHEMISTRY

The histiocytes of MR exhibit positivity for CD68, KiM1P, HAM56, lysozyme, alpha 1-antitrypsin, and vimentin, but are negative for Mac 387, CD34, CD1a, S-100, factor XIIIa, desmin, and smooth muscle actin (HHF35) (9–11).

TREATMENT

No consistently successful treatment approach has been delineated. Systemic corticosteroids alone or in combination with azathioprine, immunosuppressive drugs (methotrexate and cyclophosphamide), and nonsteroid anti-inflammatory agents have been used with variable success (12,13).

ELECTRON MICROSCOPY

The histiocytes contain dense bodies, coated vesicles, myeloid bodies, fat droplets, and dilated rough endoplasmic reticulum filled with granular material. Intra- and

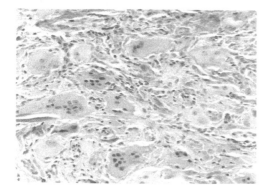

Figure 3 Multicentric reticulohistiocytosis: histiocytes with ground-glass cytoplasm and multiple irregularly distributed nuclei in giant cells. (Specimen courtesy of W. Burgdorf.)

extracytoplasmic type IV collagen inclusions similar to those seen in lymphohistiocytic neoplasms have been detected.

Multicentric reticulohistiocytosis

Clinical features
   Adults, mainly women
   Symmetrical, chronic, destructive polyarthritis
   Acral red-brown or yellow papules or nodules
   Associated internal malignancy or connective tissue disease possible
Histological features
   Mono- and multinucleated histiocytes with "ground-glass" cytoplasm,
      lymphocytes, neutrophils, plasma cells, and eosinophils
Immunophenotype
   CD68+, CDla−, S-100−
Treatment
   No standardized therapy
Clinical course and prognosis
   Gradual loss of activity in 7–8 years
   Depends on systemic findings

CLINICAL COURSE AND PROGNOSIS

In most cases, the disease gradually burns out over a period of 7–8 years. The deforming polyarthritis produces permanent damage, including shortening of the fingers and other mutilating changes resulting in significant disability. Involvement of internal organs, bone marrow, skeletal muscle, and lymph nodes may occur. Deaths have been reported in cases with cardiac or pulmonary involvement. In cases where MR is associated with malignancy, the disease may relapse with recurrence of the tumor.

COMMENTS

Recent studies have provided evidence that MR and solitary reticulohistiocytoma (SRH) appear to be different entities, considering their clinical setting, histological features, and immunophenotype (10). The histopathological features distinguishing between the two disorders are discussed in detail under the latter entity.

REFERENCES

1. Friedman PD, Kalisher L. Multicentric reticulohistiocytosis in a child: radiologic findings and clinical correlation. Can Assoc Radiol J 1998; 49:378–380.
2. Luz FB, Gaspar TAP, Kalil-Gaspar N, Ramos-e-Silva M. Multicentric reticulohistiocytosis. J Eur Acad Dermatol Venereol 2001; 15:524–531.
3. Eagle RC Jr, Penne RA, Hneleski IS Jr. Eyelid involvement in multicentric reticulohistiocytosis. Ophthalmology 1995; 102:426–430.
4. Gibson G, Cassidy M, O'Connell P, Murphy GM. Multicentric reticulohistiocytosis associated with recurrence of malignant melanoma. J Am Acad Dermatol 1995; 32: 134–136.

5. Kenik JG, Fok F, Huerter CJ, Hurley JA, Stanosheck JF. Multicentric reticulohistiocytosis in a patient with malignant melanoma: a response to cyclophosphamide and a unique cutaneous feature. Arthritis Rheum 1990; 33:1047–1051.

6. Valencia IC, Colsky A, Berman B. Multicentric reticulohistiocytosis associated with recurrent breast carcinoma. J Am Acad Dermatol 1998; 39:864–866.

7. Shiokawa S, Shingu M, Nishimura M, Yasuda M, Yamamoto M, Tawara T, Wada T, Nobunaga M. Multicentric reticulohistiocytosis associated with subclinical Sjogren's syndrome. Clin Rheumatol 1991; 10:201–205.

8. Takahashi M, Mizutani H, Nakamura Y, Shimizu M. A case of multicentric reticulohistiocytosis, systemic sclerosis and Sjogren syndrome. J Dermatol 1997; 24:530–534.

9. Perrin C, Lacour JP, Michiels JF, Flory P, Ziegler G, Ortonne JP. Multicentric reticulohistiocytosis. Immunohistological and ultrastructural study: a pathology of dendritic cell lineage. Am J Dermatopathol 1992; 14:418–425.

10. Zelger B, Cerio R, Soyer HP, Misch K, Orchard G, Wilson-Jones E. Reticulohistiocytoma and multicentric reticulohistiocytosis. Histopathologic and immunophenotypic distinct entities. Am J Dermatopathol 1994; 16:577–584.

11. Gorman JD, Danning C, Schumacher HR, Klippel JH, Davis JC Jr. Multicentric reticulohistiocytosis: case report with immunohistochemical analysis and literature review. Arthritis Rheum 2000; 43:930–938.

12. Franck N, Amor B, Ayral X, Lessana-Leibowitch M, Monsarrat C, Kahan A, Escande JP. Multicentric reticulohistiocytosis and methotrexate. J Am Acad Dermatol 1995; 33:524–525.

13. Pandhi RK, Vaswani N, Ramam M, Singh MK, Bhutani LK. Multicentric reticulohistiocytosis: response to dexamethasone pulse therapy. Arch Dermatol 1990; 126: 251–252.

45.5. Juvenile Xanthogranuloma

Dmitry V. Kazakov, Günter Burg, and Werner Kempf
Deparment of Dermatology, University Hospital, Zürich, Switzerland

DEFINITION

Juvenile xanthogranuloma (JXG) is a benign, self-limiting histiocytic disorder of unknown cause predominantly affecting infants and children. The following synonyms have been used in the literature for JXG: nevoxanthoendothelioma, xanthoma multiplex, juvenile xanthoma, multiple eruptive xanthoma in infancy, congenital xanthoma tuberosum, xanthoma neviforme, and juvenile giant-cell granuloma. Since not all JXG occur in children, the designation xanthogranuloma might be preferable but it has been applied to a variety of cutaneous and systemic lesions and thus lacks specificity.

CLINICAL FEATURES

In nearly half of the cases, the disease affects infants under 6 months of age. There is no gender predilection. Occurrence of JXG is reported to be 10 times more frequent in whites than in blacks. Juvenile xanthogranuloma typically presents as a single or several asymptomatic, small (1–2 cm in diameter), flat or dome-shaped, firm, shiny, yellow-red papules (Fig. 1). Rarely do the lesions exceed the size of 2–3 cm. Ulceration and satellite lesions have been described. Spontaneous regression occurs over a period of months or years, leaving small atrophic scars. Many different clinical variants have been described including eruptive, plaque-like, lichenoid, giant, and disfiguring forms. Attempts to correlate the number and size of the lesions with the risk of systemic involvement have not been helpful.

Extracutaneous involvement may occur in visceral organs, lymph nodes, soft tissue, and skeletal muscles. Eye involvement occurs in up to 10% of cases and may lead to secondary glaucoma due to hemorrhage into the anterior chamber (1–3). The association of JXG with neurofibromatosis I and chronic juvenile myelogenous leukemia is well-established. Many other perhaps coincidence associations have also been reported such as with Niemann–Pick disease and urticaria pigmentosa (4–6).

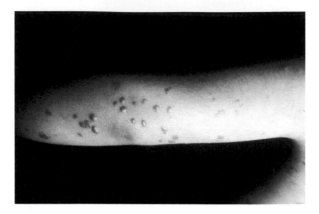

Figure 1 Small yellow nodules. (Kindly provided by R. Caputo.)

HISTOLOGY

Early lesions are characterized by a moderately dense perivascular and interstitial infiltrate composed mainly of medium-sized histiocytes with oval or irregular nuclei and eosinophilic, granular cytoplasm. As the lesions evolve, circumscribed infiltrates surrounded by an epidermal collarette at the margins are present (Fig. 2). In addition, Touton cells and foamy cells appear and increase in numbers (Fig. 3). The infiltrate acquires a diffuse or large nodular, sheet-like appearance. Admixture of small lymphocytes and eosinophils is found. Fibrosis signals the regression of the lesions.

IMMUNOHISTOCHEMISTRY

The most common immunophenotype of the histiocytic cells is CD68+, factor XIIIa+, fascin+, CD64+ (HAM56), HLA-DR+, LCA+, vimentin+, CD1a– (7,8) A positive reaction for S-100 is found in 30%. In around 80% of cases, expression of CD4 is observed (9).

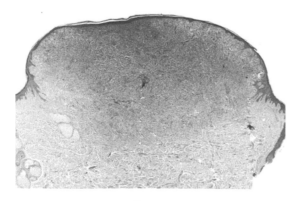

Figure 2 Nodular infiltrate with epidermal collarette.

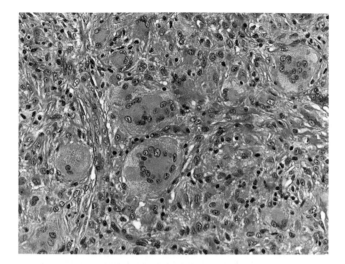

Figure 3 Touton giant cells admixed with histiocytes and lymphocytes.

TREATMENT

No treatment is necessary, since the lesions usually resolve spontaneously. Disturbing JXG can be excised. Surgery or radiotherapy give good results in cases with ocular involvement.

CLINICAL COURSE AND PROGNOSIS

The outlook is excellent; typically, childhood lesions resolve spontaneously in 1–6 years.

Juvenile xanthogranuloma

Clinical features
　Mainly infants, rarely adults
　Single or multiple, asymptomatic, papules and nodules. Rarely extracutaneous
　　involvement, especially ocular
Histological features
　Moderately dense perivascular and interstitial infiltrate of medium-sized histiocytes.
　Touton cells and foamy cells in later stages
Immunophenotype
　CD68+, factor XIIIa+, fascin+, CD1a–
　S-100+ in 30%, CD4+ in 80%
Treatment
　Excision or observation
Clinical course and prognosis
　Childhood lesions resolve spontaneously in 1–6 years; adult lesions tend to be
　　persistent

COMMENTS

In 15–30% of cases, JXG occur in adults, producing a misnomer. While the lesions are histologically identical, those in adults tend to be more often solitary, larger, and less likely to resolve spontaneously (10).

The origin of JXG remains unclear. Some consider it a macrophage disorder (histologic picture with giant cells, foam cells, etc.), while others favor the concept of a tumor of dermal dendrocytes due to factor XIIIa positivity (11–13). Recently, it has been suggested that the mononuclear cells of JXG represent bone marrow-derived cells with a morphology and phenotype consistent with the plasmacytoid monocyte (9).

REFERENCES

1. Chang MW, Frieden IJ, Good W. The risk intraocular juvenile xanthogranuloma: survey of current practices and assessment of risk. J Am Acad Dermatol 1996; 34:445–449.
2. Labalette P, Guilbert F, Jourdel D, Nelken B, Cuvellier JC, Maurage CA. Bilateral multifocal uveal juvenile xanthogranuloma in a young boy with systemic disease. Graefes Arch Clin Exp Ophthalmol 2002; 240:506–509.
3. Hamdani M, El Kettani A, Rais L, El Belhadji M, Rachid R, Laouissi N, Zaghloul K, Amraoui A. Juvenile xanthogranuloma with intraocular involvement. A case report. J Fr Ophtalmol 2000; 23:817–820.
4. Deb G, Habetswallner D, Helson L, De Sio L, Caniglia M, Donfrancesco A. Sporadic acute lymphocytic leukemia arising in a patient with neurofibromatosis and xanthogranulomatosis. Cancer Invest 1996; 14:109–111.
5. Burgdorf WH, Zelger B. The non-Langerhans' cell histiocytoses in childhood. Cutis 1996; 58:201–207.
6. Okubo T, Okabe H, Kato G. Juvenile xanthogranuloma with cutaneous and cerebral manifestations in a young infant. Acta Neuropathol (Berl) 1995; 90:87–92.
7. Jaffe R, DeVaughn D, Langhoff E. Fascin and the differential diagnosis of childhood histiocytic lesions. Pediatr Dev Pathol 1998; 1:216–221.
8. Zelger B, Cerio R, Soyer HP, Misch K, Orchard G, Wilson-Jones E. Reticulohistiocytoma and multicentric reticulohistiocytosis. Histopathologic and immunophenotypic distinct entities. Am J Dermatopathol 1994; 16:577–584.
9. Kraus MD, Haley JC, Ruiz R, Essary L, Moran CA, Fletcher CD. "Juvenile" xanthogranuloma: an immunophenotypic study with a reappraisal of histogenesis. Am J Dermatopathol 2001; 23:104–111.
10. Chang SE, Cho S, Choi JC, Choi JH, Sung KJ, Moon KC, Koh JK. Clinicohistopathologic comparison of adult type and juvenile type xanthogranulomas in Korea. J Dermatol 2001; 28:413–418.
11. Burgdorf WHC, Zelger B. The histiocytoses. In: Elder D, ed. Lever's Histopathology of the Skin. 9th ed. Philadelphia: Lippincott Williams & Wilkins, 2003.
12. Freyer DR, Kennedy R, Bostrom BC, Kohut G, Dehner LP. Juvenile xanthogranuloma: forms of systemic disease and their clinical implications. J Pediatr 1996; 129:227–237.
13. Misery L, Boucheron S, Claudy AL. Factor XIIIa expression in juvenile xanthogranuloma. Acta Derm Venereol 1994; 74:43–44.

Benign Cephalic Histiocytosis

Dmitry V. Kazakov, Günter Burg, and Werner Kempf
Department of Dermatology, University Hospital, Zürich, Switzerland

DEFINITION

Benign cephalic histiocytosis (BCH) is a benign, self-healing, non-Langerhans cell proliferation of unknown cause affecting infants and children. It was first described by Gianotti in 1968 (1).

CLINICAL FEATURES

The disease affects infants and children under the age of 3 years without gender predisposition and presents with multiple, asymptomatic, red-brown, or brown-yellow papules confined to the head and neck area (Fig. 1). Mucous membranes and viscera are not usually involved. The lesions persist for several months to years and show spontaneous regression (2–4).

HISTOLOGY

The histological features are very similar if not identical to those seen in juvenile xanthogranuloma, generalized eruptive histiocytoma, and xanthoma disseminatum. The cellular composition of the infiltrate may vary somewhat depending on its architecture (diffuse vs. perivascular and lichenoid vs. superficial confined to the papillary dermis) (Fig. 2). The infiltrative cells are histiocytes with round nuclei and sparse cytoplasm (Fig. 3). No reniform cells are seen (4,5).

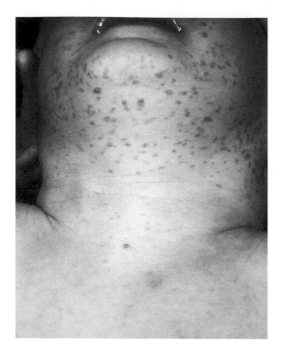

Figure 1 Multiple small papules in typical facial location. (Courtesy of R. Caputo.)

IMMUNOHISTOCHEMISTRY

The histiocytes in BCH express CD68, CD64, and factor XIIIa. They are negative for CD1a and S-100. Rare cases are S-100 positive representing a diagnostic pitfall.

ELECTRON MICROSCOPY

Ultrastructural features are not specific. The histiocytes in BCH contain intracytoplasmic comma-like (worm-like) bodies and membrane-bound vesicles. Desmosome-like junctions between histiocytes have also been detected (6).

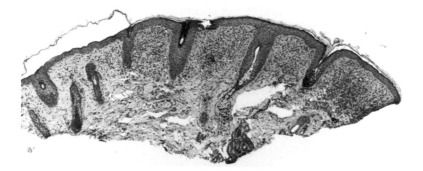

Figure 2 Lichenoid infiltrate in the upper dermis. (Specimen courtesy of W. Burgdorf M.D., Germany.)

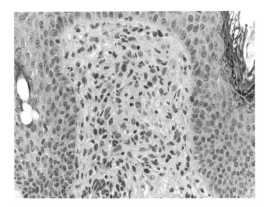

Figure 3 Infiltrate composed of histiocytes with round nuclei and sparse cytoplasm, and admixed eosinophils. (Specimen courtesy of W. Burgdorf, Germany.)

TREATMENT

Usually, no treatment is necessary due to the self-healing nature of the disease (7).

CLINICAL COURSE AND PROGNOSIS

The disease follows a benign course with spontaneous regression of the lesions at the mean age of 9 years (1).

Benign cephalic histiocytosis

Clinical features
　　Children under 3 years of age
　　Multiple, asymptomatic, papules with facial involvement
Histological features
　　Medium-sized histiocytes with oval or irregular nuclei and eosinophilic cytoplasm
Immunophenotype
　　Factor XIIIa+, CD68+, CD1a−, S-100−
Treatment
　　Not required
Clinical course and prognosis
　　Benign with spontaneous regression

COMMENTS

Considering the similarity of histological features of BCH, juvenile xanthogranuloma, generalized eruptive histiocytoma, and xanthoma disseminatum, some authors believe that these conditions are not separate entities but represent a spectrum within the family of non-Langerhans histiocytoses (8).

REFERENCES

1. Gianotti F, Caputo R, Ermacora E. Singular "infantile histiocytosis with cells with intra-cytoplasmic vermiform particles". Bull Soc Fr Dermatol Syphiligr 1971; 78:232–233.
2. Gianotti F, Caputo R, Ermacora E, Gianni E. Benign cephalic histiocytosis. Arch Dermatol 1986; 122:1038–1043.
3. de Luna ML, Glikin I, Golberg J, Stringa S, Schroh R, Casas J. Benign cephalic histiocytosis: report of four cases. Pediatr Dermatol 1989; 6:198–201.
4. Gianotti R, Alessi E, Caputo R. Benign cephalic histiocytosis: a distinct entity or a part of a wide spectrum of histiocytic proliferative disorders of children? A histopathological study. Am J Dermatopathol 1993; 15:315–319.
5. Khoo BP, Tay YK. Benign cephalic histiocytosis in Singapore—a review of 8 cases. Singapore Med J 1999; 40:697–699.
6. Eisenberg EL, Bronson DM, Barsky S. Benign cephalic histiocytosis. A case report and ultrastructural study. J Am Acad Dermatol 1985; 12:328–331.
7. Weston WL, Travers SH, Mierau GW, Heasley D, Fitzpatrick J. Benign cephalic histiocytosis with diabetes insipidus. Pediatr Dermatol 2000; 17:296–298.
8. Zelger BW, Sidoroff A, Orchard G, Cerio R. Non-Langerhans cell histiocytoses. A new unifying concept. Am J Dermatopathol 1996; 18:490–504.

45.7. Solitary Reticulohistiocytoma

Dmitry V. Kazakov, Günter Burg, and Werner Kempf
Department of Dermatology, University Hospital, Zürich, Switzerland

DEFINITION

Solitary reticulohistiocytoma (SRH) is a rare histiocytic proliferative disease of unknown cause affecting exclusively the skin.

CLINICAL FEATURES

This disease is most often seen in young adult men. The typical lesion is a solitary yellow-brown papule or nodule. There is no predilection site. In less than 20% of cases, multiple lesions are found but the criteria for multicentric reticulohistiocytosis (MR) including extracutaneous involvement are lacking.

HISTOLOGY

The infiltrate in SRH is usually circumscribed, dense, and sheet-like. It is composed of oncocytic histiocytes with ample eosinophilic, finely granular ("ground-glass") cytoplasm similar to those seen in MR. The nuclei are round to oval, occasionally reniform, with one to two prominent nucleoli. Multinucleated oncocytic histiocytes are very large (>200 µm), have numerous (>25) nuclei, and frequently possess scalloped or bizarre cellular outlines. Their cytoplasm demonstrates no or only weak granular reactivity with PAS. In addition, an admixture of Touton cells, vacuolated/xanthomatized and spindle-shaped histiocytes, and lymphocytes is seen. Mitotic figures are rare or absent (1,2).

Table 1 Main Discriminative Histological and Immunophenotypical Features of SRH and MR

Features	SRH	MR
Infiltrate: architecture	Well-circumscribed	More interstitial
Infiltrate: composition	Admixture of Touton cells, vacuolated/xanthomatized and spindled histiocytes	No admixture of Touton cells, vacuolated/xanthomatized and spindled histiocytes
Giant cells	>200 μm	50–100 μm
	>25 nuclei	<20 nuclei
	PAS-negative	PAS-positive
	Scalloped cell borders	Regular cell borders
Immunophenotype	Factor XIIIa+	Factor XIIIa–
	SMA (HHF35)+	SMA (HHF35)–

IMMUNOHISTOCHEMISTRY

The oncocytic histiocytes consistently express CD68, KiM1P, HAM56, factor XIIIa, smooth muscle actin (SMA) (HHF35), and vimentin. Expression of lysozyme and alpha 1-antitrypsin is variable. The cells are negative for Mac 387, CD34, CD1a, S-100, and desmin (1,3).

ELECTRON MICROSCOPY

Ultrastructurally, the cells show lipid droplets, lysosomes, and coarse, electron-dense endoplasmic reticulum (3).

Solitary reticulohistiocytoma

Clinical features
  Adult men
  Solitary yellow-brown papule or nodule
  No extracutaneous involvement
Histological features
  Well-circumscribed sheet-like infiltrate of mono- and multinucleated histiocytes
    with "ground-glass" cytoplasm
  Admixture of Touton cells, lymphocytes, vacuolated or spindle histiocytes
Immunophenotype
  CD68+, CD1a–, S-100–, SMA+, KiM1p+
Treatment
  Excision
Clinical course and prognosis
  Excellent

CLINICAL COURSE AND PROGNOSIS

The lesions are entirely benign. If disturbing, they may be excised.

COMMENTS

Some have attempted to group together SRH, multiple reticulohistiocytomas without extracutaneous involvement and MR as part of a disease spectrum under the rubric reticulohistiocytoma cutis (4). Recent studies have provided evidence that at least the very ends of the spectrum, SRH and MR, show different clinical, histopathological as well as immunophenotypical features and therefore might better be considered different entities (1,4). The principal distinguishing histological and immunophenotypical features of SRH and MR are summarized in Table 1.

REFERENCES

1. Zelger B, Cerio R, Soyer HP, Misch K, Orchard G, Wilson Jones E. Reticulohistiocytoma and multicentric reticulohistiocytosis. Histopathologic and immunophenotypic distinct entities. Am J Dermatopathol 1994; 16:577–584.
2. Perrin C, Lacour JP, Michiels JF, Ortonne JP. Reticulohistiocytomas versus multicentric reticulohistiocytosis. Am J Dermatopathol 1995; 17:625–626.
3. Hunt SJ, Shin SS. Solitary reticulohistiocytoma in pregnancy: immunohistochemical and ultrastructural study of a case with unusual immunophenotype. J Cutan Pathol 1995; 22:177–181.
4. Oliver GF, Umbert I, Winkelmann RK, Muller SA. Reticulohistiocytoma cutis—review of 15 cases and an association with systemic vasculitis in two cases. Clin Exp Dermatol 1990; 15:1–6.

45.8. Malignant Histiocytic Tumors

Dmitry V. Kazakov, Günter Burg, and Werner Kempf
Department of Dermatology, University Hospital, Zürich, Switzerland

INTRODUCTION

The topic of true histiocytic malignancies is complex and controversial for many reasons. First, these disorders are very rare. Second, the criteria applied in the past to categorize a neoplasm as a "malignant histiocytic tumor" differ from those used today. Many previously published cases that were reassessed after the introduction of immunohistochemistry lacked convincing evidence for a histiocytic origin of the neoplastic cells and most turned out to be lymphoproliferative disorders. In addition, the older literature is replete with terms such as "histiocytic medullary reticulosis," "malignant histiocytosis," "true histiocytic lymphoma," "true histiocytic lymphoma/sarcoma," and "monocytic sarcoma." This terminology makes the comparison of various entities very difficult (1,2).

MALIGNANT HISTIOCYTIC TUMORS OF THE SKIN

The dermatopathologic aspects of malignant histiocytic tumors are even more perplexing because of the extreme scarcity of observations. No typical clinical pattern or course has been identified. In those cases where the histiocytic nature of a malignant neoplasm of the skin has been unequivocally proven, the malignant histiocytic tumors (histiocytic sarcomas) of the skin have occurred as single or multiple tumors and have been either confined to the skin (no extracutaneous involvement) or a part of multisystemic involvement ("malignant histiocytosis"). The prognosis in the latter case is poor. Histologically, these tumors demonstrate a proliferation of large, pleomorphic, round to oval or polygonal cells with slightly eccentric nuclei, small distinct nucleoli, and abundant eosinophilic (H&E staining) or grayish (Giemsa staining) cytoplasm. Spindle cells, giant cells, and emperipolesis can be seen. The immunophenotype is decisive for the categorization of a neoplasm as histiocytic sarcoma and for its differential diagnosis from lymphomas and malignant tumors of accessory den-

Table 1 Immunohistochemistry in Differential Diagnosis of Malignant Histiocytic and Dendritic Cell Neoplasm

Neoplasm	CD68, LYS	CD1a, S-100	CD21/CD35
Histiocytic sarcoma	CD68+, LYS+	CD1a−, S-100−/+	−
Langerhans cell tumor/sarcoma	CD68+, LYS−/+	CD1a+, S-100+	−
Interdigitating cell tumor/sarcoma	CD68+/−, LYS−	CD1a−, S-100−/+	−
Follicular dendritic cell tumor/sarcoma	CD68+/−, LYS−	CD1a−, S-100−/+	+

LYS, lysozyme.
Source: From Ref. 2.

dritic cells (Table 1). Expression of histiocytic markers (CD68+, lysozyme+) with the simultaneous absence of follicular dendritic cell markers (CD21, CD35), lymphoid markers (B- and T-associated antigens and CD30), and myeloid-specific markers (myeloperoxidase, CD33) is required for the diagnosis of histiocytic sarcoma. S-100 and CD4 may be expressed. Diagnostic ultrastructural findings include the presence of cytoplasmic lysosomes and the lack of Birbeck granules, desmosomes, and interdigitating junctions (2).

REFERENCES

1. Jaffe ES, Harris NL, Stein H, Vardiman JW, eds. World Health Organization Classification of Tumours. Pathology and Genetics of Tumours of Haematopoietic and Lymphoid Tissue. Lyon: IARC Press, 2001.
2. Pileri SA, Grogan TM, Harris NL, Banks P, Campo E, Chan JK, Favera RD, Delsol G, de Wolf-Peeters C, Falini B, Gascoyne RD, Gaulard P, Gatter KC, Isaacson PG, Jaffe ES, Kluin P, Knowles DM, Mason DY, Mori S, Muller-Hermelink HK, Piris MA, Ralfkiaer E, Stein H, Su IJ, Warnke RA, Weiss LM. Tumours of histiocytes and accessory dendritic cells: an immunohistochemical approach to classification from the International Lymphoma Study Group based on 61 cases. Histopathology 2002; 41:1–29.

46

Etiology and Pathogenesis of Cutaneous Lymphomas

Günter Burg, Werner Kempf, Reinherd Dummer, Dmitry V. Kazakov, Frank O. Nestle, Antonio Cozzio, Sonja Michaelis, and Udo Döbbeling
Department of Dermatology, University Hospital, Zürich, Switzerland

46.1. Introduction

The etiology and the exact steps in the pathogenesis of cutaneous lymphomas are only partially understood. Most probably, lymphomagenesis of CL represents a *multifactorial and multistep process* due to the impact of various etiologic factors over a long period of time. The disease most probably starts as a (hyper-)reactive, inflammatory process. Deficits in cell proliferation regulation and defective oncogene and/or suppressor gene expression later promotes transition from preneoplastic conditions to neoplasia.

Among the many potential initiating factors to be considered, genetic, environmental, infectious, and immunologic ones will be briefly discussed, before presenting a multifactorial concept of the pathogenesis of cutaneous lymphomas.

46.2. Genetic Factors

A limited genetic diathesis is suggested by the enhanced risk of CTCL in first degree relatives of CTCL patients. An association to certain histocompatibility antigens has been described (1). Familial occurrence of cutaneous T-cell lymphoma has been rarely reported. Shelley (2) in 1980 reviewed familial MF, and after examining several cases in detail, concluded it was a rare phenomenon. Only a few documented examples have been reported (3–5) including occurrence in twins (6,7) or siblings (4).

There are congenital diseases with chromosomal abnormalities such as familial hemophagocytic reticulosis (8). Down syndrome or Bloom syndrome that have an increased risk to develop lymphoma/leukemia.

In contrast to nodal lymphomas, the large cell transformation in cutaneous T-cell lymphoma is not associated with t(2;5) (p23;q35) chromosomal translocation (9,10). Nodal follicular B-cell lymphomas are associated with the t14;18 translocation and subsequent bcl-2 expression (11), while in CBCL, this translocation is rare (12,13).

The most frequent chromosomal breakpoints in malignant lymphoma, including cutaneous T-cell lymphoma and adult T-cell leukemia-lymphoma, involve chromosomes 1 and 6q, 14q11, 7p15p21, and 7q32q35, 14q32, 2p11–p14, 2p23–p25, 17cen, 9p21p23, and 10p13p15 (14). In G-banding studies, numerical raberrations of chromosomes 6, 13, 15, and 17, marker chromosomes, and structural aberrations of chromosomes 3, 9, and 13 were increased in mycosis fungoides (MF) compared with healthy controls (15). Studies should be concentrated on these chromosomal regions in order to identify the underlying molecular mechanisms that may be involved in T-cell malignancies. Increased expression of C-myc p62, p53 and PCNA proteins has been found in pleomorphic medium–large CTCL and advanced stages of MF as compared to early stages of MF suggesting a relationship between levels of these proteins and aggressiveness of the cutaneous T-cell lymphomas. Furthermore, C-myc p62 and bcl-2 proteins, both important for lymphomagenesis, have been found to be frequently coexpressed (16).

46.3. Environmental Factors

Three case control studies have investigated the possibility of an environmental etiology for MF. The first recorded a high incidence of allergies, of fungal, and viral infections and found a higher than expected proportion of patients in the petrochemical, textile, metal, and machine industries in the United States (17). A second study from Scotland failed to confirm these observations, but recorded a higher incidence than expected of atopic diathesis in MF patients (18). The third study from the United States failed to confirm any differences in occupational environmental exposure but noticed an increased rate of other malignancies including skin cancers (19).

Close contacts with fertilizers and insecticides have been suggested to play a possible role as environmental hazards in the development of parakeratosis variegata (20) which may be related to MF. Plant-derived diterpene esters have an Epstein–Barr virus (EBV)-activating/tumor-promoting potency. Many active diterpene ester-containing plants are widely used as herbal medicaments in geographic areas, in which the EBV-associated diseases—Burkitt lymphoma, nasopharyngeal carcinoma—and adult T-cell leukemia/lymphoma—are endemic (21).

46.4. Infectious Factors

Several studies have investigated the possible involvement of viral agents, particularly herpes and retroviruses, in primary CL.

HUMAN T-CELL LYMPHOTROPIC VIRUSES

The impact of human T-cell lymphotropic virus type I (HTLV-I) in the pathogenesis of CTCL has been illuminated by numerous studies. The Tax sequence of HTLV-I has been found in the peripheral blood mononuclear cells of patients with CTCL (22). By in situ PCR, Tax has been demonstrated in the lymphocytes infiltrating the skin as well as in the keratinocytes of CTCL patients (23). Although it is well established that the HTLV-I causes adult T-cell leukemia/lymphoma (ATLL) in regions of the world where this virus is endemic, CTCL in the Western world usually are negative for antibodies to the structural proteins of HTLV-I, which does not appear to be a primary etiologic agent in CTCL (24–27). HTLV-II pol and tax gene sequences can be detected in a minority of CTCL patients, but this does not necessarily imply an etiologic role (25). They have also been found in Japanese patients with cutaneous T-cell lymphoma different from ATLL. There never has been further confirmation for the finding that a new human retrovirus (HTLV-V) is associated with cutaneous T-cell lymphoma or mycosis fungoides (28). Recently, detection of endogenous retroviral particles has been described in CD30+ lymphoproliferative disorders of the skin (29).

EPSTEIN–BARR VIRUS AND OTHER HERPESVIRUSES

Epstein–Barr virus is unequivocally involved in the etiology of endemic African Burkitt lymphoma (30). EBV is also implicated in some types of extranodal lymphomas such as T/NK- and NK-cell lymphomas, CTCL with an angiocentric growth pattern (31) or hydroa vacciniformia-like lymphoproliferative disorders, which are prevalent in Asia (32) and less frequent in Western countries. Search for the presence of DNA, RNA, and EBV proteins in cutaneous lesions of primary cutaneous CD30+ ALCL by PCR, in situ hybridization and immunohistochemistry does not support a role of EBV in these lymphomas (33,34). The pathogenic role of the virus in such cases remains obscure as the virus frequently infects only a minority of the cells (35).

Other herpesviruses like human herpesviruses 7 (HHV-7) and 8 (HHV-8) seem not to be involved in the pathogenesis of primary cutaneous lymphomas (36,37).

BORRELIA BURGDORFERI

Some cases of low-grade malignant CBCL in Europe seem to be associated with *Borrelia burgdorferi* infection (38–41), whereas *Borrelia burgdorferi* DNA has not been detected in CBCL from the United States (42). Borrelial escape from immunosurveillance mechanisms, persistence of both their mitogenic and antigenic stimuli for B-cells, and activation of the skin associated lymphoid tissue (SALT) may be involved in the pathogenesis of Borrelia-associated CBCL (43).

SUPERANTIGENS

Superantigens are microbial proteins produced by bacteria as well as by viruses, yeasts, and parasites. Superantigens are able to stimulate up to 20% of the naive T-cell population in a nonspecific way (44). Superantigens induce inflammation by extensive cytokine release after T-cell stimulation and/or T-cell-mediated cytotoxicity. They are considered to play an important role in the pathogenesis of many diseases including autoimmune disorders and T-cell lymphoma (45). They may be able to induce autoimmune processes by stimulation of autoreactive T-cells as well as autoantibody production by stimulation of B-cells (46). These processes may also exhibit an adjuvant effect in the pathogenesis of chronic lymphoproliferative disorders. Sézary T-cell activating factor (SAF) has been identified as a Chlamydia-associated protein that possibly plays a pathogenetic role in the pathogenesis of CTCL, specifically in erythrodermic forms (47).

46.5. Immunological Factors

Disturbances of immune surveillance by autoimmune diseases, chronic infections, or immunosuppression increase the risk for lymphoma development. There are many immunologic phenomena found especially in CTCL, which may be mere epiphenomena or may be involved in lymphomagenesis. On the basis of clinical observations that chronic immune stimulation may lead to tumor formation, the hypothesis was advanced that MF is an "immunoma" (48).

Stimulation of the T-cell receptor (TCR)/CD3 complex using anti-CD3 monoclonal antibodies induces Sézary-like morphology (nuclear contour indices >6.5) in a significant portion (9–28%) of T-cells from normal donors (49). There is strong morphologic evidence for a functional relationship between lymphocytes and dendritic cells in the dermal infiltrate of CTCL which is in favor of the hypothesis that the disease is a consequence of chronic immune stimulation (50).

Two basic functional types of T helper (Th) cells can be distinguished. Th1 clones secrete mainly IL-2 and IFN-gamma. They are involved in cell-mediated inflammatory functions, e.g., the induction of delayed type hypersensitivity. Th2 clones produce IL-4, IL-5, IL-6, IL-10, and IL-13 (51,52) and stimulate IgE antibody by IL-4 and IL-13, activate eosinophils by IL-5 (53). In addition, they inhibit macrophages, antigen presenting cells, and T helper 1 (Th1) T-cells by IL-10 (54). The phenotype of the malignant T-cell clone patients with Sézary syndrome is consistent with peripheral T memory cells. Their cytokine transcription and secretion is comparable to human T helper 2 (Th2) cells with IL-5, IL-10, and IL-13. Attempts to reveal Th1 and 2 profiles in skin biopsies of CTCL patients revealed conflicting results. Saed et al. (55) demonstrated the presence of IL-2 and IFN-gamma, but no IL-4, IL-5, or IL-10 in the epidermis of MF by RT-PCR and concluded that MF exhibits a Th1 cytokine profile. Other groups disagree and interpret MF and SS as Th2 lymphomas since they found IL-2 as well as IFN-gamma in normal skin (56,57).

When functional properties of peripheral blood mononuclear cells (PBMC) of nonleukemic CTCL patients, primed with phytohemagglutinin (PHA) for three days are compared with those of normal age-matched donors, a diminished number of PBMC from CTCL patients are capable of proliferating after IL-2, but not after IL-4 stimulation. PHA induces a significantly higher release of IL-4 and a significantly lower secretion of IFN-gamma in CTCL-derived PBMC compared to PBMC of healthy donors (58). This discrepancy (59,60) reflects one of the problems, which is the discrimination between the clonal T-cell population and the nonclonal reactive CD8+ or CD4+ lymphocytes, as well as between the cytokines produced by these different cell populations.

One of the cytokines, which plays a significant role and exhibits pleiotropic effects on tumor-defense and escape mechanisms, is IL-10. Its original name was cytokine synthesis inhibitory factor (CSIF), since it reduces the production and secretion of IL-2, IFN-gamma, IL-1β, TNF-alpha, and granulocyte monocyte-colony stimulating factor (GM-CSF), as well as downregulates the proliferation of mitogen-activated peripheral blood lymphocytes. While IL-10 limits T-cell expansion by directly inhibiting IL-2 production by these cells (54,61a,61b), it is a growth factor for human B-lymphocytes. IL-10 indirectly prevents antigen-specific T-cell activation by downregulation of antigen presentation and accessory cell functions of monocytes, macrophages, Langerhans' cells, and dendritic cells. Asadullah et al. (62) have used a quantitative RT-PCR to evaluate the IL-10 mRNA in lesional skin of MF patients and found that the IL-10 mRNA levels increase with the stage of the disease.

Since Th1 cells are the principle effectors for cell-mediated immunity against tumor cells and delayed type hypersensitivity reaction, it seems to be an advantage for the malignant cells to switch the immune response of the host to a Th2 type. The dominance of the Th2 cells explains many clinical phenomena seen in CTCL patients, such as pruritus, edema of the skin, reduced cutaneous delayed type hypersensitivity reactions, hypereosinophilia, alterations in serum immunoglobulin levels (IgE, IgA), an increased risk of infections and second malignancies and immunological abnormalities of PBMC such as reduced natural killer cell activity and decreased mitogen-induced proliferation (58,63).

Other cytokines that are important for the development of CTCL are IL-15 (64) and IL-7 (65). IL-15 is a growth factor for the IL-2 dependent CTCL cell line SeAx, which is 10–20 times more potent than IL-2 and can replace IL-2. It prolongs the in vitro survival of CTCL cells isolated from Sézary syndrome patients. The expression of IL-15 by basal layer keratinocytes and skin dendritic cells (66) might explain the observation that CTCL cells are found in close vicinity to the basal layer in the earliest stages of the disease. During the course of the disease, CTCL cells acquire the ability to express IL-15 and they become IL-15 independent, when they have "learned" to produce IL-15 themselves leading to an autocrine cell stimulation loop.

Insights into reasons for homing of neoplastic T-cells into skin are important for the understanding of disease pathogenesis. Chemokines are small molecules of about 8 kDa which are involved in leukocyte migration to specific tissue sites and are essential for the host immune response. Epidermal IFN-gamma inducible protein-10 (IP-10) and monokine induced by gamma-interferon (Mig) expression is associated with epidermotropism in cutaneous CD30– T-cell lymphomas (67). In CD30+ CTCL, it was recently shown that expression of CCR3 and its ligand eotaxin/CCL11 play a role in the recruitment and retention of CD30+ malignant T-cells to the skin. Understanding and modulating factors which attract neoplastic T-cells to skin will most likely impact future therapeutic approaches to CTCL.

46.6. Pathogenetic Models of Cutaneous Lymphomagenesis

THE THYMUS BYPASS MODEL

This interesting model (68) proposes that some cases of CTCL are due not to malignant clonal proliferation of thymus-derived T-lymphocytes but rather to an error of histogenesis in which bone marrow-derived precursors of T-cells go directly to the skin where an aberrant proliferation occurs representing an abortive attempt at thymocyte differentiation. This aberrant proliferation may be promoted by selfantigens present in the skin or possibly by influences due to viral infection or to incomplete viral DNA sequences present in cutaneous cells, to foreign or autoantigens or to some combination of endogenous or exogenous pathogenetic factors.

A MULTIFACTORIAL CONCEPT OF THE PATHOGENESIS OF CUTANEOUS LYMPHOMAS (69,70)

There is increasing evidence that cancerogenesis is not a big bang event but a step-wise evolutionary process due to the accumulation of mutations in DNA repair genes, oncogenes, or tumor suppressor genes (71).

Chromosomal Alterations

Analyses of the karyotype and genome of CTCL cells have revealed chromosomal abnormalities (15,72) containing chromosome breaks and translocations. The sequence analyses of DNA breakpoints found in different kinds of leukemias suggested that the observed translocations have been caused by illegitimate V(D)J recombination. However, expression of the RAG-1 or the RAG-2 genes, which are essential for V(D)J recombination could not be detected in samples of CTCL, indicating that illegitimate V(D)J recombination may not be the reason for the increased number of chromosomal aberrations and translocations in CTCL cells (73).

NFκB

As a result of chromosomal breaks, the translocation of the NFκB2 (lyt-10) gene is found in malignant cells of 5–10% of all CTCL patients (74,75). The NFκB2 (lyt-10) gene codes for a transcription factor which is a member of the NFκB/Rel/IkB gene family comprising at least 10 different genes regulating gene expression (see for review Ref. 76). Proteins of the members of the NFκB and Rel subfamilies occur in the nuclei of cells only after stimulation by an external inducer which can be a growth factor (e.g., IL-1) or a stress signal (e.g., oxygen radicals, hypoxia). The inducers activate tyrosine and serine/threonine kinases which in turn activate proteases which process the transcriptionally inactive NFκB1 and NFκB2 gene products p105 and p100 to their active forms p50 and p52 by degradation of the carboxy-terminus which retains these proteins in the cytoplasm. The processed p50 and p52 proteins can form heterodimers with members of the Rel subfamily. These heterodimers translocate to the nucleus where they activate the transcription of their target genes. Beside the NFκB/Rel heterodimers, the p50/p50 homodimers and p52/bcl-3 heterodimers can also be found in the nuclei of stimulated cells. An alternative NFκB activation pathway is the recruitment of p50/Rel heterodimers from cytoplasmic transcriptionally inactive p50/rel/IkB trimeric complexes by the proteolytic degradation of the IkB component (76).

   The observed NFκB2 translocations result in NFκB2 gene products which lack parts of their carboxy-termini which retain them in the cytoplasm. These proteins can translocate to the nucleus where they may disturb the "normal" pattern of gene transcription (77–82).

   Electrophoretic mobility shift assays (EMSA) and western blotting demonstrate that other family members of the NFκB/Rel/IkB gene family also are constitutively active in the nucleus (own unpublished data). In nucleic extracts from the three CTCL cell lines (HUT78, MyLa and SeAx), p50 (NFκB1), p52 (NFκB2), p65 (RelA), RelB, and bcl-3 could be detected. The truncated NFκB2 protein (79,82) also could be demonstrated in the HUT78 cell line. In the nuclei, this protein was less abundant than the properly processed p52 protein. These proteins bind as p50/p50 homodimers, p50/p65 and p50/RelB heterodimers to an NFκB consensus sequence. P52/Bcl-3 heterodimers may also occur, but probably bind to another sequence. Western blots showed that the p50 and p52 proteins were of correct size and it is therefore unlikely that these proteins derive from translocated genes. The processed p50 and p52 proteins must therefore be the products of a constitutive protease activity that may be triggered by constitutive tyrosine or serine/threonine kinase activities, since the tyrosine kinase inhibitor herbimycin suppresses the DNA binding of NFκB proteins in CTCL cell lines (own unpublished data). This protease activity is also present in the malignant cells of CTCL patients since p50/p50 homodimers are also found in these cells. The appearance of this constitutive protease activity seems to be an early step in the development of cutaneous T-cell lymphoma. This activity has been found in 10 of 11 (91%) patients tested so far. Whether the appearance of gene products of the Rel family in CTCL cell lines is a late step in CTCL tumorigenesis or an adaptation to in vitro cell culture, has to be established.

Microenvironment

The proliferation of T-cells in the skin significantly relies on interaction with other cellular and humoral components (83). Clinical as well as histological features suggest that CTCL clones, in most cases, need the presence of epidermal cells to survive, and thus depend on the epidermal cytokine network (84). Paracrine loops between epidermal cells and lymphocytes create a microenvironment which allows the growth of malignant T-cell clones, but suppresses reactive cells like macrophages, natural killer cells or cytotoxic T-cells. In addition, fibrobasts also may be essential microenvironmental components by preventing IL-2-deprived T-cells from going into apoptosis without inducing proliferation due to a selective effect on Bcl-X$_L$ expression (85,86). If the conditions are changed and lymphocytes isolated from a skin biopsy are cultured in the presence of IL-2 and IL-4, only the reactive, not tumor-clone derived, cells expand (87), unless the growth of tumor cells is stimulated by immature dendritic cells (88).

Hypothesis for CTCL Lymphomagenesis

For CTCL lymphomagenesis, we propose the following hypothesis. Abnormal but not primarily neoplastic lymphocytes showing genomic instability ("genotraumatic lymphocytes") (89,90) are driven into activation and reactive cell proliferation by antigenic stimulation. The risk of the occurrence of mutations in the susceptible "genotraumatic" cell clone increases with every new cell division. The accumulation of mutations is usually limited by controlling mechanisms leading to cell death in order to prevent cells with chromosomal aberrations from unlimited, neoplastic expansion. Such controlling mechanisms are programmed cell death (apoptosis) which can be blocked by increased bcl-2 protein expression (91) due to bcl-2 gene mutation or translocation.

Normal cells in culture have a limited proliferative capacity of 50–70 cell cycles. Thereafter, they die due to cutting off *telomeres* which are repetitive base sequences (TTAGGG) at the end of each chromosome, responsible for the maintenance of chromosomal structure and function (92,93). Immortal cells overcome this regulation and proliferate indefinitely by reactivation of telomerase activity, a ribonucleoprotein complex, which can prevent shortening of the telomeres. Telomerase is believed to be induced upon proliferation and inhibited when cells differentiate. Thus, regulation of telomerase activity may be an important mechanism to limit growth of normal and cancer cells. The enzyme telomerase, present especially in highly replicating cell systems, such as keratinocytes (94) or lymphocytes, shows a significant increase of activity in CTCL (95) and in CTCL cell lines. The unlimited proliferation leads to accumulation of mutations finally resulting in a highly abnormal cell clone which grows independently from external stimuli due to autocrine or paracrine stimulation. In this pathogenetic model, tumor formation results from multiple independent genetic changes accumulated in the same cell and a series of clonal expansions after > 100 doublings, provided a frequency of spontaneous mutations of 10 to the 6.

The transformation from "normal" lymphocytes in preneoplastic stages to highly atypical neoplastic cells in the tumor stage of CTCL is a stepwise process with clear-cut breakpoints in the clinical and histological features as well as immunophenotypic profile of the skin infiltrates (Fig. 1). Four possible steps in lymphomagenesis of CL can be delineated.

Step One

Chronic activation of lymphocytes with genetic instability leads to the development of preneoplastic lymphoproliferative condition. This step represents a *potentially reversible process* caused by increased activities of some transcription factors (c-myb, bcl-3, STAT5)—which in turn increase the expression of survival genes (bcl-2, bcl-xL, mcl-1)—and the endogenous production of cell growth factors (IL-15) (64,96–98).

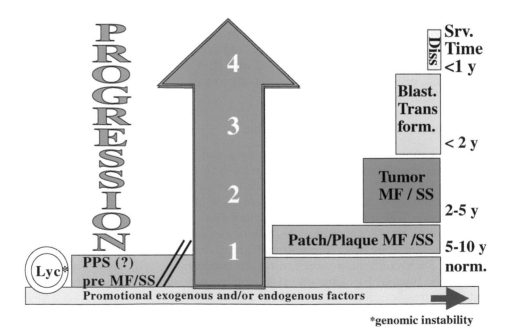

Figure 1 Stepwise progression of CTCL from cutaneous patches to plaque stage (Step One), to tumor stage (Step Two), to blastic transformation (Step Three), and to dissemination (Step Four).

Step Two

Endogenous tyrosine kinases are activated and can then mimic and augment the effects of persistent antigen stimulation. This results in activation of further transcription factors (NFκB p50, p65, p52, STAT2, STAT3) and their target genes and initiates the *transition into definitive low-grade lymphoma* such as plaque-stage mycosis fungoides. Lesional T-cells which accumulate in the dermis and epidermis in psoriasis and in mycosis fungoides express B7-1. Such expression may permit self-co-stimulation involving the CD28-mediated activation pathway, and thereby contribute to the ongoing T-cell proliferation present in these chronic, benign, and malignant skin diseases (83). The hypothesis that CTCL cell growth may be driven through TCR recognition of class II-presented selfpeptides (88). Cell to cell contacts, dendritic cells (83,88), CD40/CD40L, FAS are of utmost importance in the promotion of lymphoproliferation in this early stage of the disease.

Step Three

Further activation of endogenous tyrosine kinases, of ras genes and of transcription factors (RelB, c-Rel, STAT6, c-myc) replaces the pathogenetic effects of persistent antigen stimulation which in conjunction with inactivation of apoptosis promoting proteins (Bad, Bax), inactivation of Rb and p53, and downregulation of cell cycle regulating genes (p15, p16) leads to *proliferation of neoplastic lymphoid cells, independent from microenvironmental factors*, i.e., cytokines. At this stage, tumor formation and transformation into large cell blastic lymphoma of high-grade malignancy evolves.

Step Four

Extracutaneous dissemination with involvement of lymph nodes, peripheral blood, bone marrow, and visceral organs is a result of change in homing receptors which are responsible for the settling of the cells in distinct microenvironments and organs (99–103).

REFERENCES

1. MacKie R, Dick HM, deSousa MB. Letter: HLA and mycosis fungoides. Lancet 1976; 1:1179.
2. Shelley WB. Familial mycosis fungoides revisited. Arch Dermatol 1980; 116:1177–1178.
3. Cameron OJ. Mycosis fungoides in mother and in daughter. Arch Dermatol Syphilol 1933; 27:232–236.
4. Sandbank M, Katzenellenbogen I. Mycosis fungoides of prolonged duration in siblings. Arch Dermatol 1968; 98:620–627.
5. Matutes E, Spittle MF, Smith NP, Eady RA, Catovsky D. The first report of familial adult T-cell leukaemia lymphoma in the United Kingdom. Br J Haematol 1995; 89:615–619.
6. Naji AA, Waiz MM, Sharquie KE. Mycosis fungoides in identical twins. J Am Acad Dermatol 2001; 44:532–533.
7. Schneider BF, Christian M, Hess CE, Williams ME. Familial occurrence of cutaneous T cell lymphoma: a case report of monozygotic twin sisters. Leukemia 1995; 9:1979–1981.
8. Farquhar JC. Familial haemophagocytic reticulosis. Arch Dis Child 1952; 529:519–525.
9. Li G, Salhany KE, Rook AH, Lessin SR. The pathogenesis of large cell transformation in cutaneous T-cell lymphoma is not associated with t(2;5)(p23;q35) chromosomal translocation. J Cutan Pathol 1997; 24:403–408.

10. DeCoteau JF, Butmarc JR, Kinney MC, Kadin ME. The t(2;5) chromosomal translocation is not a common feature of primary cutaneous CD30+ lymphoproliferative disorders: comparison with anaplastic large-cell lymphoma of nodal origin. Blood 1996; 87:3437–3441.

11. Tycko B, Sklar J. Chromosomal translocations in lymphoid neoplasia: a reappraisal of the recombinase model. Cancer Cells 1990; 2:1–8.

12. Volkenandt M, Cerroni L, Rieger E, Soyer HP, Koch O, Wienecke R, Atzpodien J, Bertino JR, Kerl H. Analysis of the 14;18 translocation in cutaneous lymphomas using the polymerase chain reaction. J Cutan Pathol 1992; 19:353–356.

13. Child FJ, Russell-Jones R, Woolford AJ, Calonje E, Photiou A, Orchard G, Whittaker SJ. Absence of the t(14;18) chromosomal translocation in primary cutaneous B-cell lymphoma. Br J Dermatol 2001; 144:735–744.

14. Berger R, Baranger L, Bernheim A, Valensi F, Flandrin G, Berheimm A. Cytogenetics of T-cell malignant lymphoma. Report of 17 cases and review of the chromosomal breakpoints. Cancer Genet Cytogenet 1988; 36:123–130.

15. Karenko L, Hyytinen E, Sarna S, Ranki A. Chromosomal abnormalities in cutaneous T-cell lymphoma and in its premalignant conditions as detected by G-banding and interphase cytogenetic methods. J Invest Dermatol 1997; 108:22–29.

16. Kanavaros P, Ioannidou D, Tzardi M, Datseris G, Katsantonis J, Delidis G, Tosca A. Mycosis fungoides: expression of C-myc p62 p53, bcl-2 and PCNA proteins and absence of association with Epstein–Barr virus. Pathol Res Pract 1994; 190:767–774.

17. Greene MH, Dalager NA, Lamberg SI, Argyropoulos CE, Fraumeni JF. Mycosis fungoides: epidemiologic observations. Cancer Treat Rep 1979; 63:597–606.

18. Tuyp E, Burgoyne A, Aitchison T, MacKie R. A case-control study of possible causative factors in mycosis fungoides. Arch Dermatol 1987; 123:196–200.

19. Whittemore AS, Holly EA, Lee IM, Abel EA, Adams RM, Nickoloff BJ, Bley L, Peters JM, Gibney C. Mycosis fungoides in relation to environmental exposures and immune response: a case-control study. J Natl Cancer Inst 1989; 81:1560–1567.

20. Rogozinski TT, Zekanowski C, Kaldan L, Blaszczyk M, Majewski S, Jablonska S. Parakeratosis variegata: a possible role of environmental hazards?. Dermatology 2000; 201:54–57.

21. Ito Y, Tokuda H, Ohigashi H, Koshimizu K. Distribution and characterization of environmental promoter substances as assayed by synergistic Epstein–Barr virusactivating system. Princess Takamatsu Symp 1983; 14:125–137.

22. Pancake BA, Wassef EH, Zucker-Franklin D. Demonstration of antibodies to human T-cell lymphotropic virus-I tax in patients with the cutaneous T-cell lymphoma, mycosis fungoides, who are seronegative for antibodies to the structural proteins of the virus. Blood 1996; 88:3004–3009.

23. Zucker-Franklin D. The role of human T cell lymphotropic virus type I tax in the development of cutaneous T cell lymphoma. Ann N Y Acad Sci 2001; 941:86–96.

24. Whittaker SJ, Luzzatto L. HTLV-1 provirus and mycosis fungoides [letter]. Science 1993; 259:1470–1471.

25. Li G, Vowels BR, Benoit BM, Rook AH, Lessin SR. Failure to detect human T-lymphotropic virus type-I proviral DNA in cell lines and tissues from patients with cutaneous T-cell lymphoma. J Invest Dermatol 1996; 107:308–313.

26. Wood GS, Salvekar A, Schaffer J, Crooks CF, Henghold W, Fivenson DP, Kim YH, Smoller BR. Evidence against a role for human T-cell lymphotrophic virus type I (HTLV-I) in the pathogenesis of American cutaneous T-cell lymphoma. J Invest Dermatol 1996; 107:301–307.

27. Kikuchi A, Nishikawa T, Ikeda Y, Yamaguchi K. Absence of human T-lymphotropic virus type I in Japanese patients with cutaneous T-cell lymphoma. Blood 1997; 89: 1529–1532.

28. Fine RM. HTLV-V: a new human retrovirus associated with cutaneous T-cell lymphoma (mycosis fungoides). Int J Dermatol 1988; 27:473–474.

29. Kempf W, Kadin ME, Dvorak AM, Lord CC, Burg G, Letvin NL, Koralnik IJ. Endogenous retroviral elements, but not exogenous retroviruses, are detected in CD30-positive lymphoproliferative disorders of the skin. Carcinogenesis 2003; 24: 301–306.

30. Ziegler JL. Burkitt's lymphoma. N Engl J Med 1981; 305:735–745.

31. Misago N, Ohshima K, Aiura S, Kikuchi M, Kohda H. Primary cutaneous T-cell lymphoma with an angiocentric growth pattern: association with Epstein–Barr virus. Br J Dermatol 1996; 135:638–643.

32. Jung DY, Kim JW, Lee SK, Lee WW. Epstein–Barr virus-associated lymphoproliferative skin lesion with recurrent necrotic papulovesicles of the face. J Dermatol 1999; 26:448–451.

33. Hellier I, Dereure O, Segondy M, Guillot B, Baldet P, Guilhou JJ. Unlikely role of Epstein–Barr virus in the pathogenesis of primary cutaneous CD30+ anaplastic large cell lymphoma. Eur J Dermatol 2001; 11:203–208.

34. Peris K, Niedermeyer H, Cerroni L, Radaskiewicz T, Chimenti S, Höfler H. Detection of Epstein–Barr virus genome in primary cutaneous T and B cell lymphomas and pseudolymphomas. Arch Derm Res 1994; 286:364–368.

35. Anagnostopoulos I, Hummel M, Kaudewitz P, Korbjuhn P, Leoncini L, Stein H. Low incidence of Epstein–Barr virus presence in primary cutaneous T-cell lymphoproliferations. Br J Dermatol 1996; 134:276–281.

36. Nagore E, Ledesma E, Collado C, Oliver V, Perez-Perez A, Aliaga A. Detection of Epstein–Barr virus and human herpesvirus 7 and 8 genomes in primary cutaneous T- and B-cell lymphomas. Br J Dermatol 2000; 143:320–323.

37. Kempf W, Kadin ME, Kutzner H, Lord CL, Burg G, Letvin NL, Koralnik IJ. Lymphomatoid papulosis and human herpesviruses—a PCR-based evaluation for the presence of human herpesvirus 6, 7 and 8 related herpesviruses. J Cutan Pathol 2001; 28:29–33.

38. Braun-Falco O, Guggenberger K, Burg G, Fateh-Moghadam A. Immunozytom unter dem bild einer acrodermatitis chronica atrophicans. Hautarzt 1978; 29:644–647.

39. Garbe C, Stein H, Dienemann D, Orfanos CE. Borrelia burgdorferi-associated cutaneous B cell lymphoma: clinical immunohistologic characterization of four cases. J Am Acad Dermatol 1991; 24:584–590.

40. Cerroni L, Zochling N, Putz B, Kerl H. Infection by Borrelia burgdorferi and cutaneous B-cell lymphoma. J Cutan Pathol 1997; 24:457–461, ISSN: 0303–6987.

41. Roggero E, Zucca E, Mainetti C, Bertoni F, Valsangiacomo C, Pedrinis E, Borisch B, Piffaretti JC, Cavalli F, Isaacson PG. Eradication of Borrelia burgdorferi infection in primary marginal zone B-cell lymphoma of the skin. Hum Pathol 2000; 31:263–268.

42. Wood GS, Kamath NV, Guitart J, Heald P, Kohler S, Smoller BR, Cerroni L. Absence of Borrelia burgdorferi DNA in cutaneous B-cell lymphomas from the United States. J Cutan Pathol 2001; 28:502–507.

43. Jelic S, Filipovic-Ljeskovic I. Positive serology for Lyme disease borrelias in primary cutaneous B-cell lymphoma: a study in 22 patients; is it a fortuitous finding?. Hematol Oncol 1999; 17:107–116.

44. Haffner AC, Zepter K, Elmets CA. Major histocompatibility complex class I molecule serves as a ligand for presentation of the superantigen staphylococcal enterotoxin B to T cells. Proc Natl Acad Sci USA 1996; 93:3037–3042.

45. Tokura Y, Heald PW, Yan SL, Edelson RL. Stimulation of cutaneous T-cell lymphoma cells with superantigenic staphylococcal toxins. J Invest Dermatol 1992; 98:33–37.

46. Jappe U. Superantigens and their association with dermatological inflammatory diseases: facts and hypotheses. Acta Derm Venereol 2000; 80:321–328.

47. Abrams JT, Vonderheid EC, Kolbe S, Appelt DM, Arking EJ, Balin BJ. Sezary T-cell activating factor is a Chlamydia pneumoniae-associated protein. Clin Diagn Lab Immunol 1999; 6:895–905.

48. Schuppli R. Is mycosis fungoides an "immunoma"? Dermatologica 1976; 153:1–6.

49. Reinhold U, Herpertz M, Kukel S, Oltermann I, Uerlich M, Kreysel HW. Induction of nuclear contour irregularity during T-cell activation via the T-cell receptor/CD3 complex and CD2 antigens in the presence of phorbol esters. Blood 1994; 83:703–706.

50. Romagnoli P, Moretti S, Fattorossi A, Giannotti B. Dendritic cells in the dermal infiltrate of Sezary syndrome. Histopathology 1986; 10:25–36.

51. Mosmann TR, Sad S. The expanding universe of T-cell subsets—TH1, TH2 and more. Immunol Today 1996; 17:138–146.

52. Mosmann TR, Cherwinski H, Bond MW, Giedlin MA, Coffman RL. Two types of murine helper T cell clone. I. Definition according to profiles of lymphokine activities and secreted proteins. J Immunol 1986; 136:2348–2357.

53. Romagnani S. Human TH1 and TH2 subsets: regulation of differentiation and role in protection and immunopathology. Int Arch Allergy Immunol 1992; 98:279–285.

54. de Vries JE. Immunosuppressive and anti-inflammatory properties of interleukin 10. Ann Med 1995; 27:537–541.

55. Saed G, Fivenson DP, Naidu Y, Nickoloff BJ. Mycosis fungoides exhibits a Th1-type cell-mediated cytokine profile whereas Sezary syndrome expresses a Th2-type profile. J Invest Dermatol 1994; 103:29–33.

56. Vowels B, Cassin M, Vonderheid E, Rook A. Aberrant cytokine production by Sezary syndrome patients: cytokine secretion pattern resembles murine Th2 cells. J Invest Dermatol 1992; 99:90–94.

57. Dummer R, Heald PW, Nestle FO, Ludwig E, Laine E, Hemmi S, Burg G. Sézary syndrome's T-cell clones display T helper 2 cytokines and express the accessory factor-1 (interferon gamma receptor beta chain). Blood 1996; 88:1383–1389.

58. Dummer R, Kohl O, Gillessen J, Kagi M, Burg G. Peripheral blood mononuclear cells in patients with nonleukemic cutaneous T-cell lymphoma. Reduced proliferation and preferential secretion of a T helper-2-like cytokine pattern on stimulation. Arch Dermatol 1993; 129:433–436.

59. Saed G, Fivenson D, Nickoloff B. Th2 cytokine profile in cutaneous T-cell lymphoma [reply]. J Invest Dermatol 1995; 105:856.

60. Lessin SR, Vowels BR, Rook AH. Th2 cytokine profile in cutaneous T-cell lymphoma [letter]. J Invest Dermatol 1995; 105:855–856.

61a. Moore KW, O'Garra A, de Waal Malefyt R, Vieira P, Mosmann TR. Interleukin-10. Annu Rev Immunol 1993; 11:165–90

61b. Moore KW, O'Garra A, de Waal Malefyt R, Vieira P, Mosmann TR. Interleukin-10. Annu Rev Immunol 1996; 135:572–575.

62. Asadullah K, Döcke W-D, Haeussler A, Sterry W, Volk H-D. Progression of mycosis fungoides is associated with increasing cutaneous expression of interleukin-10 (IL-10) mRNA. J Invest Dermatol 1996; 107:833–837.

63. Liebe V, Burg G. Lymphozytentransformationstest bei kutanen lymphomen. Hautarzt 1977; 28:S200–S203.

64. Qin JZ, Dummer R, Burg G, Dobbeling U. Constitutive and interleukin-7/interleukin-15 stimulated DNA binding of Myc, Jun, and novel Myc-like proteins in cutaneous T-cell lymphoma cells. Blood 1999; 93:260–267.

65. Dalloul A, Laroche L, Bagot M, Mossalayi MD, Fourcade C, Thacker DJ, Hogge DE, Merle-Beral H, Debre P, Schmitt C. Interleukin-7 is a growth factor for Sezary lymphoma cells. J Clin Invest 1992; 90:1054–1060.

66. Blauvelt A, Asada H, Klaus-Kovtun V, Altman DJ, Lucey DR, Katz SI. Interleukin-15 mRNA is expressed by human keratinocytes Langerhans cells, and blood-derived dendritic cells and is downregulated by ultraviolet B radiation. J Invest Dermatol 1996; 106:1047–1052.

67. Tensen CP, Vermeer MH, van der Stoop PM, van Beek P, Scheper RJ, Boorsma DM, Willemze R. Epidermal interferon-gamma inducible protein-10 (IP-10) and monokine induced by gamma-interferon (Mig) but not IL-8 mRNA expression is associated

with epidermotropism in cutaneous T cell lymphomas. J Invest Dermatol 1998; 111: 222–226.

68. Lambert WC. The thymus bypass model. A new hypothesis for the etiopathogenesis of mycosis fungoides and related disorders. Dermatol Clin 1994; 12:305–310.

69. Burg G, Dummer R, Haeffner A, Kempf W, Kadin M. From inflammation to neoplasia: mycosis fungoides evolves from reactive inflammatory conditions (lymphoid infiltrates) transforming into neoplastic plaques and tumors. Arch Dermatol 2001; 137:949–952.

70. Burg G, Kempf W, Haeffner A, Dobbeling U, Nestle FO, Boni R, Kadin M, Dummer R. From inflammation to neoplasia: new concepts in the pathogenesis of cutaneous lymphomas. Recent Results Cancer Res 2002; 160:271–280.

71. Fearon ER, Vogelstein B. A genetic model for colorectal tumorigenesis. Cell 1990; 61:759–767.

72. Karenko L, Kahkonen M, Hyytinen ER, Lindlof M, Ranki A. Notable losses at specific regions of chromosomes 10q and 13q in the Sezary syndrome detected by comparative genomic hybridization [letter]. J Invest Dermatol 1999; 112:392–395.

73. Dobbeling U, Dummer R, Hess Schmid M, Burg G. Lack of expression of the recombination activating genes RAG-1 and RAG-2 in cutaneous T-cell lymphoma: pathogenic implications. Clin Exp Dermatol 1997; 22:230–233.

74. Schmid RM, Perkins ND, Duckett CS, Andrews PC, Nabel GJ. Cloning of an NF-kappa B subunit which stimulates HIV transcription in synergy with p65. Nature 1991; 352:733–736.

75. Neri A, Chang CC, Lombardi L, Salina M, Corradini P, Maiolo AT, Chaganti RS, Dalla-Favera R. B cell lymphoma-associated chromosomal translocation involves candidate oncogene lyt-10, homologous to NF-kappa B p50. Cell 1991; 67:1075–1087.

76. Baeuerle PA, Baltimore D. NF-kappa B: ten years after. Cell 1996; 87:13–20.

77. Fracchiolla NS, Lombardi L, Salina M, Migliazza A, Baldini L, Berti E, Cro L, Polli E, Maiolo AT, Neri A. Structural alterations of the NF-kappa B transcription factor lyt-10 in lymphoid malignancies. Oncogene 1993; 8:2839–2845.

78. Chang CC, Zhang J, Lombardi L, Neri A, Dalla-Favera R. Rearranged NFKB-2 genes in lymphoid neoplasms code for constitutively active nuclear transactivators. Mol Cell Biol 1995; 15:5180–5187.

79. Zhang J, Chang CC, Lombardi L, Dalla-Favera R. Rearranged NFKB2 gene in the HUT78 T-lymphoma cell line codes for a constitutively nuclear factor lacking transcriptional repressor functions. Oncogene 1994; 9:1931–1937.

80. Migliazza A, Lombardi L, Rocchi M, Trecca D, Chang CC, Antonacci R, Fracchiolla NS, Ciana P, Maiolo AT, Neri A. Heterogeneous chromosomal aberrations generate 3′ truncations of the NFKB2/lyt-10 gene in lymphoid malignancies. Blood 1994; 84:3850–3860.

81. Kim KE, Gu C, Thakur S, Vieira E, Lin JC, Rabson AB. Transcriptional regulatory effects of lymphoma-associated NFKB2/lyt10 protooncogenes. Oncogene 2000; 19:1334–1345.

82. Thakur S, Lin HC, Tseng WT, Kumar S, Bravo R, Foss F, Gelinas C, Rabson AB. Rearrangement and altered expression of the NFKB-2 gene in human cutaneous T-lymphoma cells. Oncogene 1994; 9:2335–2344.

83. Nickoloff BJ, Nestle FO, Zheng XG, Turka LA. T lymphocytes in skin lesions of psoriasis and mycosis fungoides express B7-1: a ligand for CD28. Blood 1994; 83:2580–2586.

84. Dummer R, Schwarz T. Cytokines as regulatory proteins in lymphoproliferative skin infiltrates. Dermatol Clin 1994; 12:283–294.

85. Pilling D, Akbar AN, Girdlestone J, Orteu CH, Borthwick NJ, Amft N, Scheel-Toellner D, Buckley CD, Salmon M. Interferon-beta mediates stromal cell rescue of T cells from apoptosis. Eur J Immunol 1999; 29:1041–1050.

86. Gombert W, Borthwick NJ, Wallace DL, Hyde H, Bofill M, Pilling D, Beverley PC, Janossy G, Salmon M, Akbar AN. Fibroblasts prevent apoptosis of IL-2-deprived T

cells without inducing proliferation: a selective effect on Bcl-XL expression. Immunology 1996; 89:397–404.

87. Reinhold U, Abken H, Kukel S, Goeden B, Uerlich M, Neumann U, Kreysel HW. Tumor-infiltrating lymphocytes isolated from a Ki-1-positive large cell lymphoma of the skin. Phenotypic characterization and analysis of cytokine secretion. Cancer 1991; 68:2155–2160.

88. Berger CL, Hanlon D, Kanada D, Dhodapkar M, Lombillo V, Wang N, Christensen I, Howe G, Crouch J, El-Fishawy P, Edelson R. The growth of cutaneous T-cell lymphoma is stimulated by immature dendritic cells. Blood 2002; 99:2929–2939.

89. Thestrup PK, Kaltoft K. Genotraumatic T cells and cutaneous T-cell lymphoma. A causal relationship?. Arch Dermatol Res 1994; 287:97–101.

90. Kaltoft K, Hansen BH, Thestrup PK. Cytogenetic findings in cell lines from cutaneous T-cell lymphoma. Dermatol Clin 1994; 12:295–304.

91. Dummer R, Michie S, Kell D, Gould J, Haeffner A, Smoller B, Warnke R, Wood G. Expression of BCL-2 protein and Ki-67 nuclear proliferation antigen in benign and malignant cutaneous T-cell infiltrates. J Cutan Pathol 1995; 22:11–17.

92. Harley CB, Sherwood SW. Telomerase, checkpoints and cancer. Cancer Surv 1997; 29:263–284.

93. Chiu CP, Harley CB. Replicative senescence and cell immortality: the role of telomeres and telomerase. Proc Soc Exp Biol Med 1997; 214:99–106.

94. Harle-Bachor C, Boukamp P. Telomerase activity in the regenerative basal layer of the epidermis inhuman skin and in immortal and carcinoma-derived skin keratinocytes. Proc Natl Acad Sci USA 1996; 93:6476–6481.

95. Taylor RS, Ramirez RD, Ogoshi M, Chaffins M, Piatyszek MA, Shay JW. Detection of telomerase activity in malignant and nonmalignant skin conditions. J Invest Dermatol 1996; 106:759–765.

96. Dobbeling U, Dummer R, Laine E, Potoczna N, Qin JZ, Burg G. Interleukin-15 is an autocrine/paracrine viability factor for cutaneous T-cell lymphoma cells. Blood 1998; 92:252–258.

97. Qin JZ, Kamarashev J, Zhang CL, Dummer R, Burg G, Dobbeling U. Constitutive and interleukin-7- and interleukin-15-stimulated DNA binding of STAT and novel factors in cutaneous T cell lymphoma cells. J Invest Dermatol 2001; 117:583–589.

98. Qin JZ, Zhang CL, Kamarashev J, Dummer R, Burg G, Dobbeling U. Interleukin-7 and interleukin-15 regulate the expression of the bcl-2 and c-myb genes in cutaneous T-cell lymphoma cells. Blood 2001; 98:2778–2783.

99. Heald PW, Yan SL, Edelson RL, Tigelaar R, Picker LJ. Skin-selective lymphocyte homing mechanisms in the pathogenesis of leukemic cutaneous T-cell lymphoma. J Invest Dermatol 1993; 101:222–226.

100. Rossiter H, van Reijsen F, Mudde GC, Kalthoff F, Bruijnzeel-Koomen CA, Picker LJ, Kupper TS. Skin disease-related T cells bind to endothelial selectins: expression of cutaneous lymphocyte antigen (CLA) predicts E-selectin but not P-selectin binding. Eur J Immunol 1994; 24:205–210.

101. Fritz TM, Kleinhans M, Nestle FO, Burg G, Dummer R. Combination treatment with extracorporeal photopheresis, interferon alfa and interleukin-2 in a patient with the Sézary syndrome. Br J Dermatol 1999; 140:1144–1147.

102. Armerding D, Kupper TS. Functional cutaneous lymphocyte antigen can be induced in essentially all peripheral blood T lymphocytes. Int Arch Allergy Immunol 1999; 119:212–222.

103. Ferenczi K, Fuhlbrigge RC, Pinkus J, Pinkus GS, Kupper TS. Increased CCR4 expression in cutaneous T cell lymphoma. J Invest Dermatol 2002; 119:1405–1410.

47

Therapy of Cutaneous Lymphomas

47.1. Introduction

Günter Burg, Werner Kempf, Reinhard Dummer, Antonio Cozzio, Sonja Michaelis, and Frank O. Nestle
Department of Dermatology, University Hospital, Zürich, Switzerland

Cutaneous lymphomas comprise a heterogeneous group of diseases, which differ not only in terms of cytogenetic phenotype (T- or B-cell lymphomas) but also with respect to type of skin lesions (patches, plaques, tumors, erythroderma), to the localization, number, and distribution of skin lesions, and to the grade and type of extra-

Table 1 Therapeutic Modalities in Cutaneous Lymphomas

Category of treatment	Topical treatment	Systemic treatment
Nonaggressive modalities	Heliotherapy	Glucocorticosteroids
	UVA	Low dose chemotherapy: chlorambucil, methotrexate
	UVB	Extracorporeal photopheresis
	Psoralen and UVA (PUVA)	Interferon alpha
	Glucocorticosteroids	Retinoids such as bexarotene
Aggressive modalities	Surgery	Low dose monochemotherapy: other agents
	Ionizing radiation (X-rays)	High dose polychemotherapy
	Total skin electron beam therapy (TSEB)	Bone marrow transplantation
	Nitrogen mustard (HN2)	
	Carmustin (BCNU)	
Experimental modalities	Imiquimod	Monoclonal antibodies (rituximab fusion proteins)
	Hexadecylphosphocholine	Acyclovir
	Photodynamic therapy	Interleukin-2
		Interleukin-12
		Vaccination therapy
		Gene therapy

Table 2 Therapeutic Agents Employed and Proposed for the Treatment of Cutaneous Lymphomas

Treatment	Stage[a] Early	Stage[a] Late	N[b]	OR[c]	Duration of response	Safety	Comments
Unimodal approach							
Topical therapies							
Corticosteroids	X		79	82–94		Skin atrophy, transient serum cortisol level depression	
Mechlorethamin (nitrogen mustard)	X		331	63–75		Allergic dermatitis (aqueous-based drug), non-melanoma skin cancer	DFS = 7.3 years. Useful in maintenance therapy
Bischlorethylnitrosurea (carmustin)	X		172	64–92		Residual telangectasias, myelosuppression	64 in T1; 92 in T2
Retinoids	X		167	44–86		Local irritation	Bexarotene
Phototherapy							
Ultraviolet B	X		68	71–74	22–51	Burning, non-melanoma skin cancer	
Ultraviolet A + psoralen	X		244	95		Burning, nausea, accelerated photoaging, non-melanoma skin cancer	DFS = 43 months
Extracorporeal photopheresis	X		116	20–88		Sepsis, fever, transient hypotension	Controversial data
Total surface electron beam therapy	X			70			
Biological response modifiers							
Interferons							
Interferon alpha	X	X		54	4–28	Flulike syndrome, asthenia, leukopenia, depression, thyroid dysfunction	
Interferon gamma	X	X	23	31–48	3–13	Flulike syndrome, asthenia, leukopenia	

						Toxicity
Retinoids						
Isotretinoin, etretinate, Acitretin	×	×	68	44–50		Transient hypertriglyceridemia, dry skin, cheilosis, asthenia, arthralgia
Oral bexarotene		×	84	48		Hypertriglyceridemia, hypercholesterolemia, hypothyroidism, leukopenia
Cytokines						
Interleukin-2		×	7	72		Flulike syndrome, hypotension, nausea, diarrhea, weight gain, anemia
Interleukin-12		×	34	56		Headache, depression
Chemotherapy						
Single agent	×					
Methotrexate		×		62		Hepatic toxicity, pulmonary fibrosis
Gemcitabine		×	44	20–70	15	Hematologic toxicity, nausea/vomiting
Pentostatin		×	94	20–70	1.3–8.3	Hematologic toxicity, renal insufficiency
Fludarabine		×	30	20		Hematologic toxicity, immunosuppression, sepsis, neurotoxicity
Cladribine		×	21	14–28	4.5	Myelosuppression, sepsis
Pegylated liposomal Doxorubicin		×	10	80	15	
Combined chemotherapy		×		85		Immunosuppression, leukopenia, sepsis

(Continued)

Table 2 Therapeutic Agents Employed and Proposed for the Treatment of Cutaneous Lymphomas (*Continued*)

Treatment	Stage[a]		N^b	OR^c	Duration of response	Safety	Comments
	Early	Late					
Monoclonal antibodies							
T 101 Y 90 conjugate		X	8	38		Bone marrow suppression	
Denileukin		X	71	30	4.3	Vascular leak syndrome, flulike syndrome, hypoalbuminemia	
Alentuzumab		X	8	50		Lymphopenia, neutropenia, sepsis, cardiac dysfunction	
Bone marrow transplantation							
Autologous		X	6	83		Sepsis	
Allogenic		X	8			Graft-vs.-host disease	
Multimodal approach							
PUVA + oral retinoid	X	X	69	95		Burning, non-melanoma skin cancer	
PUVA + interferon A	X	X	90	90–92	28	Fever, malaise, leukopenia, depression, photosensitivity	
PUVA + TSEB		X	53	NA			DFS > TSEB alone
Interferon A + oral retinoid		X	NA	71			
TSEB + ECP		X	44	73			DFS > TSEB alone
TSEB + chemotherapy		X	138	60–100	5–26		

DFS, disease free survival (months); PUVA, phototherapy with ultraviolet A; TSEB, total surface electron beam therapy; ECP, extracorporeal photopheresis.
[a] Early stage: stage IA–IIA; late stage: stage IIB–IVB.
[b] Number of patients included for OR estimation.
[c] Overall response rate.

cutaneous spread. Moreover since complete healing and eradication of the disease is usually not possible, control rather than cure is the best approach for treatment in most cases. Complete healing in this context means complete clearing of skin lesions without recurrence over a follow-up time of at least one year.

THERAPEUTIC MODALITIES

There is a broad spectrum of "classical" therapeutic modalities available, which can be classified into topical or systemic on one side and aggressive, nonaggressive, and experimental on the other side, as well as several possible combinations (Tables 1 and 2). *Nonaggressive* in this context means the absence of severe side effects during long-term use. *Aggressive* treatment modalities are intended to cure. Side effects may be moderate (WHO grade 2), severe (WHO grade 3), or even life threatening (WHO grade 4) after short-term or long-term use. *Experimental* treatment modalities mean therapeutic procedures with low empirical or evidence-based background.

The placing of treatment modalities into these three classes is not fixed and is debatable. A nonaggressive treatment modality may produce side effects, while aggressive modalities may be well tolerated. Treatment of cutaneous lymphoma has been extensively reviewed (1–9). In all cases, the treatment must be adjusted to the lymphoma type and stage (Chapter 47.5).

REFERENCES

1. Vonderheid EC, Micaily B. Treatment of cutaneous T-cell lymphoma. Dermatol Clin 1985; 3:673–687.
2. Jorg B, Kerl H, Thiers BH, Brocker EB, Burg G. Therapeutic approaches in cutaneous lymphoma. Dermatol Clin 1994; 12:433–441.
3. Foss FM, Kuzel TM. Experimental therapies in the treatment of cutaneous T-cell lymphoma. Hematol Oncol Clin North Am 1995; 9:1127–1137.
4. Herrmann JJ, Roenigk HJ, Honigsmann H. Ultraviolet radiation for treatment of cutaneous T-cell lymphoma. Hematol Oncol Clin North Am 1995; 9:1077–1088.
5. Jones GW, Hoppe RT, Glatstein E. Electron beam treatment for cutaneous T-cell lymphoma. Hematol Oncol Clin North Am 1995; 9:1057–1076.
6. Lim HW, Edelson RL. Photopheresis for the treatment of cutaneous T-cell lymphoma. Hematol Oncol Clin North Am 1995; 9:1117–1126.
7. Olsen EA, Bunn PA. Interferon in the treatment of cutaneous T-cell lymphoma. Hematol Oncol Clin North Am 1995; 9:1089–1107.
8. Ramsay DL, Meller JA, Zackheim HS. Topical treatment of early cutaneous T-cell lymphoma. Hematol Oncol Clin North Am 1995; 9:1031–1056.
9. Rosen ST, Foss FM. Chemotherapy for mycosis fungoides and the Sezary syndrome. Hematol Oncol Clin North Am 1995; 9:1109–1116.

Topical Therapies

Günter Burg, Reinhard Dummer, Werner Kempf, Sonja Michaelis, Philippa Golling, and Frank O. Nestle
Department of Dermatology, University Hospital, Zürich, Switzerland

NONAGGRESSIVE TOPICAL THERAPIES

Heliotherapy

Introduction

Heliotherapy as a natural source for UVB (280–320 nm) and UVA (320–400 nm) is a nonaggressive treatment modality, which has long been known to be beneficial for a variety of skin diseases. Phototherapy for CTCL was introduced by Karl Linser (1,2).

Mode of Action

The UV light exhibits multiple effects on lymphoproliferative infiltrates which are either due to direct effect on the lymphocytes or more likely to indirect effects through modulation of cellular and humoral (via cytokines) microenvironmental conditions. T-lymphocytes are very sensitive to UV light (3). Among several effects, apoptosis is induced and mediated via IL-10 and FasL (4,5). The UV light exhibits immunosuppressive effects. Altered antigen presentation and immune suppression are likely to derive from alterations induced in the antigen presenting cells (APC). There is compelling evidence that it is UV-induced DNA damage in cutaneous APC which leads to reduced immune function (6). Because almost all of the UV radiation is absorbed in the upper layers of the skin, it appears unlikely that the direct irradiation of APC can account for this effect. The UV-irradiated keratinocytes release IL-10, which in turn negatively affects antigen presentation (7). Also, UV exposure induces mast cell degranulation with subsequent vascular changes and inflammation.

Indication

The most important indication is early stages of CTCL.

Practical Application

The exposure to natural sun light especially at sea level or in the mountains is straightforward. Tan-Thru bathing suits allow patients to achieve full body exposure in a socially acceptable manner (8). The duration and frequency of exposure depends on the individual skin-type.

Combination with Other Modalities

Heliotherapy can be easily combined with other treatment modalities.

UVB, UVA, and Photochemotherapy (PUVA)

Introduction

The UV light includes the spectra of electromagnetic wavelengths between 280–400 nm, with the penetration depth through the epidermis and the energy delivered being inversely proportional. The use of psoralens (oral 8-methoxypsoralen, oxoralen, 5-methoxypsoralen) as amplifiers of UVA has brought a new dimension known as photochemotherapy or PUVA.

Mode of Action

The effects of UV light therapy are similar to those of heliotherapy. Photo(chemo)therapy primarily acts on the epidermis and to a lesser extent, depending on the wavelength administered, also on the dermis. There also is a systemic effect, inducing or suppressing cytokines and modulating directly or indirectly proliferation or differentiation of cells. Soluble keratinocyte-derived suppressive factors are involved in the induction of systemic immune suppression following UV radiation of epidermal cells (9). Broadband UV-B irradiation seems to be more efficient than narrowband UV-B at reducing the density and function of Langerhans cells, while UV-A irradiation is least effective (10).

Treatment with 8-methoxypsoralen (8-MOP) and ultraviolet A light (UVA) has been reported to modulate cytokine production in various cells. Synthesis of IL-6 and TNF alpha can be induced by UV-A irradiation (11). Also, 8-MOP/UV-A augments the expression of mRNAs for interferon-gamma (IFN-gamma) and interleukin (IL)-2 and reduces those for IL-4 and IL-10 in peripheral blood mononuclear cells (PBMCs) (12). The number of IFN-gamma-secreting lymphocytes was markedly increased in 8-MOP/UVA-treated PBMCs 20 hr after treatment, and its amount was elevated in culture supernatants. In addition, 8-MOP/UV-A-treated PBMCs produce enhanced amounts of IL-8 upon stimulation with anti-CD3/CD28 antibodies. Phototreated CD4+ but not CD8+ cells provided excellent T-cell help for monocytes to produce IL-8. Also, 8-MOP/UVA may exert a beneficial therapeutic effect on malignant Th2 neoplasms as a cytokine modifier and 8-MOP-phototreated CD4+ T cells allow monocytes to become effective tumor APCs for tumor-specific cytotoxic T cells (12).

Indication

Eczematous preneoplastic conditions of lymphoproliferative T-cell infiltrates are ideal indications for treatment with UV in the various modalities, since UV radiation—dependent on the wavelength used—reaches epidermal keratinocytes, Langerhans cells and the dermal infiltrate. Dermal edema, one of the features in CTCL, especially in Sézary syndrome, amplifies the depth of penetration for UV. Deep and dense dermal infiltrates, as seen in CBCL, are less susceptible to UV radiation. There are also reports on UVB therapy, most recently narrowband UVB, for patch stage CTCL cases (13–15).

Practical Application

The PUVA therapy has the advantages of widespread availability, ease of administration, relatively low cost and limited toxicity. For PUVA therapy, psoralens are given orally 1–3 hr before UV irradiation. Before initiating PUVA therapy, a phototoxicity assay is recommended in order to plan the precise dosage. Patients are treated three times twice weekly. In patients with normal skin type, UV dose can be increased by 10–20% every other treatment. Clear responses can be expected after 8–12 weeks of phototherapy. There are no convincing study results that indicate whether UV therapy should be stopped after the induction of remission or should be continued at a far-reduced frequency to maintain remission.

Results

Following the first report (16), several groups (17,18) confirmed high remission rates with PUVA, especially in limited plaque stage CTCL (T1/2). Remissions in this stage lasted for a median time of 13 months, in extensive plaques for 11 months.

Combination with Other Modalities

The UV or PUVA treatment can be combined with many other treatment modalities. Also, PUVA was initially combined with both nitrogen mustard topical therapy and with total skin electron beam (TSEB) therapy (19). In addition acitretin, interferon alpha and PUVA is a frequently used combination (20). The real question is which combinations produce the best results and reduce the total UV exposure.

UVA1

Introduction

Long-wave ultraviolet A radiation (UVA1R; 340–400 nm) is increasingly being used to treat patients with atopic dermatitis. Clinical improvement results from UVA-1R-induced apoptosis in skin-infiltrating helper T cells, indicating that helper T cells are sensitive targets for UVA1R and suggesting that UVA1 phototherapy may also be of benefit for other helper T cell-mediated skin diseases.

The UVA1 phototherapy represents a promising alternative to PUVA for the treatment of patients with CTCL because: (i) UVA1R reaches deeper layers of the dermis at higher intensities compared with PUVA; (ii) UVA1R is capable of inducing both protein-synthesis dependent and independent T-cell apoptosis (21), (iii) UVA1 phototherapy avoids the unwanted side effects resulting from the photosensitizer methoxsalen used with PUVA therapy, such as nausea, long-lasting skin photosensitivity, requirement for eye protection and possibly carcinogenesis.

Mode of Action

The precise mechanism of action underlying the effectiveness of UVA1 phototherapy for CTCL is currently unknown. Medium-dose UVA1 phototherapy (60 J/cm^2) induces apoptosis (programmed cell death) in skin infiltrating T-cells of CTCL in vivo (22). In vitro, UVA radiation-induced human T helper cell apoptosis is mediated through the FAS/FAS–ligand system, which is activated in irradiated T cells as a consequence of singlet oxygen generation which is a fundamental mechanism in phototherapy (23). Clinical improvement in UVA1-irradiated CTCL patients was associated with depletion of malignant T cells from lesional skin areas.

The type of apoptosis induced by UVA1R and PUVA differs qualitatively. UVA1R-induced apoptosis is mediated through the generation of singlet oxygen, which leads to the induction of both protein synthesis-independent and protein synthesis-dependent apoptosis (programmed cell death). This is in contrast to PUVA-induced apoptosis, which does not involve the generation of singlet oxygen and can only cause protein synthesis-dependent programmed cell death (21).

Indication

Patients with CTCL stages IA and IB can be treated effectively with UVA1 phototherapy (24).

Practical Application

Patients are treated 3–5 times per week with medium to high dose UVA1R.

Results

There is only limited experience with UVA1 in CTCL. It has been used in early stages IA and IB but also in advanced stages IIIB (25). Skin lesions began to resolve after only a few UVA1 radiation exposures. Complete clearance was observed between 16 and 20 exposures (24). Circulating CD4(+)/CD45RO(+) and CD4(+)/CD95(+) lymphocytes were significantly reduced by the therapy (25).

Combination with Other Modalities

The same guidelines and rules as for other UV treatment modalities.

Comments

The UVA1R is still an experimental therapy. Mechanisms of action of UVA1R predict positive results in CTCL. Larger randomized trials are necessary to get an insight into clinical efficacy.

Topical Glucocorticosteroids

Introduction

Topical glucocorticosteroids (GCS) play a crucial role in the treatment of a variety of inflammatory skin diseases. This nonaggressive therapy is most effective in flat lymphoproliferative infiltrates.

Mode of Action

Induction of peripheral blood T-cell apoptosis is an important mechanism contributing to the immunosuppression observed after high-dose GCS therapy (26). Peripheral blood T cells from normal subjects underwent DNA fragmentation after in vitro exposure to 2.5–10 µg/mL of methylprednisolone for 30 min (27).

There is a structure–function relationship between different types of GCS, for example dexamethasone and betamethasone (differences in position 16 of the molecules) with regard to two important aspects of GCS activity, namely the activation of transcription and induction of apoptosis in IL-2-dependent lymphoid cells. Dexamethasone induces a higher percentage of apoptotic cells compared to betamethasone. Two to four hours after high-dose steroid infusion (1 g methylprednisolone), apoptosis of peripheral blood T cells is seen, indicated by DNA fragmentation, which is more significant in CD4+ than CD8+ T cells. The susceptibility of CD4+ T cells to apoptosis is associated with a lower expression of Bcl-2 in these cells compared with that on CD8+ T cells.

Indication

Due to the limited penetration, topical GCS are indicated primarily in flat eczematous lymphoproliferative infiltrations.

Practical Application

Application of high strength GCS once or twice a day leads to clinical regression of lesions within 1–2 weeks. Maintenance therapy should be continued with low strength GCS, such as hydrocortisone, every second day for another 6–8 weeks.

Occlusion significantly increases percutaneous absorption of estradiol, testosterone, and progesterone, which are more lipophilic steroids, but does not effect the penetration of the more water-soluble hydrocortisone (28). Intralesional injection of GCS crystal suspension, diluted with lidocaine 1:2, may be beneficial especially in thick infiltrates.

Results

There are very few reports in the literature on the experience with topical GCS for the treatment of cutaneous lymphomas even though they probably are the most frequently used modality in early stages (29). Topical GCS of low to high potency twice daily resulted in complete remission in 63% of stage T1 patients and partial remission in 31% of patients, i.e., a total response rate of 94%. The comparable figures for stage T2 patients were 25, 57, and 82%, respectively. Reversible depression of serum cortisol levels occurred in 13% of patients (29).

Combination with Other Modalities

Topical GCS can be combined with all kinds of aggressive or nonaggressive topical or systemic treatment modalities.

AGGRESSIVE TOPICAL THERAPIES

Surgery
Introduction

Even though malignant lymphomas including cutaneous lymphomas basically are systemic neoplasms, excision of localized solitary or grouped tumors may be useful and even may lead to long lasting complete remission or even healing.

Mode of Action

Removal of the tumor bulk may allow other surveillance mechanisms to better handle or cure the systemically present, but clinically unapparent, tumor cells. Due to the systemic character of the disease, surgery certainly does not guarantee complete healing.

Indications

Cutaneous B-cell lymphomas and CD30-positive T-cell lymphomas are most often localized and thus best suited for surgery.

Practical Application

Excision can be done with local or general anesthesia. There is no need for a specific excision margin, although the lines of excision should be clinically free of disease.

Combination with Other Modalities

Surgery can be combined with adjuvant modalities to target minimal residual disease.

Soft X-ray (Orthovolt) Radiotherapy

Introduction

X-rays are electromagnetic radiations of high energy. When x-rays are used to treat superficial lesions, the energy spectrum of the x-ray beam is adjusted by selecting an appropriate combination of x-ray tube filtration and voltage, which is 30–100 kV (soft x-rays) in dermatology settings. Treatment of localized lesions and teleroentgen therapy with soft x-rays are two different approaches.

The first Nobel Prize in physics was awarded to Hans Conrad Röntgen in Würzburg, Germany, for his discovery of x-rays in 1896. Early reports on the use of orthovolt radiotherapy in cutaneous lymphoma were published by Scholtz in 1902 (30).

Mode of Action

Ionizing radiation induces free active radicals in the tissue and hits DNA by double-strand breaks. It has an impact on many functions such as enzyme activity, cell membrane permeability, and protein synthesis, finally resulting in the loss of reproductive integrity of the cells.

Indications

Early plaques and tumors in cutaneous lymphomas are highly radiosensitive and respond to low doses of ionizing radiation (31), provided that the half-value depth corresponds to the depth of infiltration, which in nontumoral stages of CTCL is usually a few millimeters in and beneath the epidermis.

Practical Application

For localized lesions, radiation therapy is given with D1/2 matching the depth of the lesion, in small doses of 2 Gy at weekly intervals or three times weekly until the lesion starts to involute. A total dose of 20–50 Gy is sufficient for most lesions (31).

Considering the malignant nature of the disease, additional radiation, perhaps even a second course, may be required despite side effects.

For widespread erythrodermic involvement, teleroentgen therapy with soft x-rays may be indicated. A distance of 2 m permits radiation of the entire body surface. When soft x-rays are used according to the technique described by Schirren in 1955, 50% of the surface dose is absorbed at a depth of only 2 mm (32,33). A high-output beryllium-window unit (50 kV) is used. Doses of 50–100 cGy are given daily or three times a week to the anterior, posterior, and lateral surfaces up to a total of 500–1000 cGy per course with the eyes and gonads shielded (31). There are some variations of the method in terms of distance (2 m in the technique described by Schirren in Munich (32) and 1.20 m in the Hamburg technique (34) and in terms of fractionation, which do not affect the basic principle of superficial total body "spray" irradiation.

Results

Irrespective of the technical differences, good long-term results have been reported from different centers (33,34) (Fig. 1).

Combination with Other Modalities

Topical agents especially topical cytostatic drugs (HN_2, BCNU) should be avoided during irradiation. Emollient creams or ointments may be useful to treat dryness and pruritus.

Comments

Soft x-ray therapy still is an excellent treatment modality for cutaneous T-cell and B-cell lymphomas. Erythrodermic patients may profit from teleroentgen therapy.

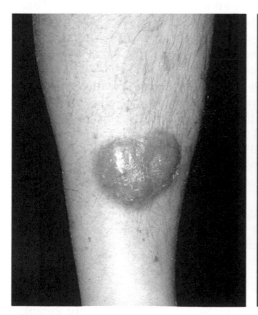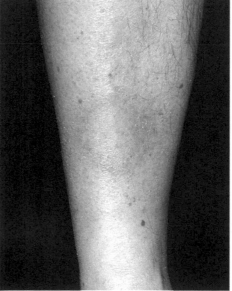

Figure 1 Follicle center lymphoma before (left) and after (right) soft X-ray therapy.

Total Skin Electron Beam (TSEB) Therapy

Introduction

Trump et al were the first to suggest using accelerated high energy electrons for the treatment of extensive superficial malignant lesions. A decade later modern linear accelerators came in use. Major contributions were made at Stanford, which included dual fixed-angle six-field beam arrangements with corresponding patient positions. Today TSEB therapy has become an important element in the management of patients with cutaneous lymphoma, especially in erythrodermic forms. Availability of TSEB depends on the willingness and ability of the radiation therapy facility to employ its electron beam facility for cutaneous therapy.

Mode of Action

A linear accelerator generates electrons at a point source. High energy electromagnetic waves induce DNA damage resulting in cell death. Tumor cells usually have an increased susceptibility to DNA damaging procedures.

Indications

Considering the radiobiological qualities of electrons and the dose gradient in the skin with a limited penetration depth on one side and the skin as a superficial widespread target, cutaneous T-cell lymphomas with disseminated or erythrodermic skin lesions are ideal indications for the use of TSEB therapy.

Practical Application

In a typical patient with mycosis fungoides, most of the disease lies superficially and—depending on the type of lesion—reaches 0.5–5 mm into the dermis.

If the source-to-skin distance is about 7 m, the intervening air between the source and the patient successfully spreads out the electrons in space and gives them incident trajectories that are fairly horizontal as they reach the target organ. A direct 4 MeV beam delivers a peak dose of 100% at 6 mm depth, and a 80% dose at 10 mm depth. In the TSEB technique used in most centers, a peak dose of 100% is reached on the surface and a 80% dose at a depth of 3.5 mm along the axis of each of the six fields. Increasing the nominal electron energy will increase the depth of treatment while the peak dose remains at the surface.

The dual fixed-angle, six fields method angles two complementary fields, each at 10–20° from the horizontal, to point over and under a standing patient. There are multiple fields and other alternatives to this technique. Six or more fields or rotational techniques reduce variation around the circumference of a patient's cylindrical mid-section to less then 10%. Dosimetric differences between six fields and rotational methods are minor. If treatment times are long or if the patient is ill, a rotating or lying position may be preferable. Most centers use 4–9 MeV electrons. Total dose is usually 2400–3600 cGy.

Besides acute toxicity, which depends on dose, nominal energy, degree of fractionation, and shielding, chronic toxicity may result in xerosis, telangiectases and diffuse fibrosis with itching and lack of sweating due to radiation-induced atrophy of sweat glands.

Results

The largest experience is from the Stanford group (35,36). The rates for complete clinical remission following TSEB therapy alone were 80% in patients with stage

IA disease, i.e., limited discrete (less than 10% skin involvement) patch or plaque disease, without tumors and without involvement of nodes, blood or viscera. In stages with more wide spread disease exceeding 10% of body surface or with tumors or erythroderma, remission rates were around 50 and 25%, respectively. Higher rates of complete remission were achieved with higher doses and energies in all stages of the disease.

About 40–60% of patients with stage IA disease remained relapse-free at 5 years and most of them were still without skin lesions after 20 years. In contrast to these encouraging results in stage IA, 5-year-relapse-free survivals for stages IB through III were about 10–20%. In erythrodermic forms of CTCL (stage III) radiation may be most efficacious in patients without blood involvement. When there is blood, lymph node, or visceral involvement, combined modality therapies should be explored (36).

Combination with Other Modalities

The TSEB can be combined with mechlorethamine (HN$_2$) (37,38), photon radiation, topical or systemic chemotherapy (39), oral etretinate (40), and biologic response modifiers.

Comments

Total skin electron beam is an efficient way to induce regression in cutaneous T-cell lymphomas, especially erythrodermic forms. The lasting side effects such as dryness of the skin and loss of sweating must be considered. The radiation process is complicated and expensive. There is no proven impact on overall survival (41). Therefore, this treatment approach is justified only in a minority of patients. Prospective randomized clinical trials are urgently needed to determine the relevance of this treatment modality.

Nitrogen Mustard (HN$_2$)

Introduction

Di (2-chloroethyl) sulfide, and less often HN$_2$, has been used as chemical weapons, with the skin being a principle target. The first reports on the use of topical HN$_2$ to treat CTCL were given by Sipos et al 1965 (42). Later on Van Scott and Kalmanson (43) reported on complete remissions of mycosis fungoides with topical HN$_2$, as well control of delayed hypersensitivity to HN$_2$ by desensitization and by induction of specific immunologic tolerance.

Mode of Action

Besides the DNA-damaging effect, HN$_2$ has a direct effect on the basement membrane zone. Pyknotic nuclei with or without dyskeratotic changes within epidermal keratinocytes can be seen (44), indicating that there is probably not only a direct cytostatic effect on the lymphocytes, but also epidermal changes possibly modulating the quality and the amount of cytokines released from keratinocytes.

Indications

Patches and thin plaques in CTCL are the main indications for the use of topical HN$_2$. One should be aware of the fact, that in the early premycotic stages of the dis-

ease, survival time is within normal range (45) and the results of early treatment have
to be assessed against this good outlook.

Practical Application

The therapy is generally initiated with a concentration of 10 mg of HN_2 in 60 mL of
water with 5 mL of propylene glycol and is increased only when no clinical response
is observed. Following preparation of the solution, patients should be instructed to
immediately paint the body surface excluding the genitalia and apply the drug spar-
ingly to intertriginous sites (46). The patient should wear protective plastic gloves
while applying HN_2. Treatment is applied daily until clearing which usually takes
3–4 months with the solution and 6–12 months when an ointment form is used.
Although treatment of the total skin surface is often recommended, the need to treat
clearly uninvolved areas is controversial (45).

Also, HN_2 can be applied as an aqueous solution for generalized treatment or
as an anhydrous ointment for localized treatment (47). The ointment may be simpler
to use because the patients do not need to dilute the mechlorethamine powder themselves. Additionally, the aqueous solution is drying. Many patients object to the
greasiness and resulting staining of clothing that occurs with ointment preparations
(46). Due to the vaporizing pressure of HN_2, nitrogen mustard evaporates into the
air during topical treatment of patients with mycosis fungoides (48). In order to estimate the risk for the nurse applying topical HN_2, the concentration of HN_2 in the air
during treatment was measured during a 20 min treatment period. The mean concentration of HN_2 in the air during treatment does not exceed the MAC (maximal
allowable concentration) value of $0.05 mg/m^3$. Nevertheless, it is important to
minimize the exposure of nursing staff to HN_2 by appropriate shielding (49). Patients
mixing and applying the medication at home are exposed to the same risks.

Results

Complete responses lasting from 4–14 years have been reported in 20% of patients
with patch or plaque phase mycosis fungoides (stage IA or IB) treated with topical
mechlorethamine (HN_2). Relapses are seen in 17% of these patients, occurring within
8 years of discontinuing maintenance topical chemotherapy. The main complications
from topical HN_2 chemotherapy include contact hypersensitivity reactions in about
40% of patients, xerosis, hyperpigmentation and an increased risk for the development of squamous cell carcinoma (50,51).

Combination with Other Modalities

When PUVA is used in combination with HN_2 (52,53), it may reduce the rate of sensitization. Further, HN_2 also has been used in combination with TSEB therapy (38).

Comments

Topical HN_2 is the first choice for many treatment centers in the United States but is
rarely used in Europe except Scandinavian countries (49). It is a very effective form
of treatment for patients with early patch/plaque stage disease.

Carmustine (BCNU)

Introduction

Carmustine is a nitrosourea agent that serves as an alternative cytostatic drug for the
local therapy of patch/thin plaque type CTCL. It was introduced into the therapeu-

tic armamentarium for CTCL by Zackheim (54–56). Like HN_2, BCNU preparations can be applied topically to the entire skin surface.

Mode of Action

The BCNU is an alkylating agent exhibiting cytostatic effects.

Indications

Whereas PUVA and topical HN_2 are the most frequent treatment modalities for the management of patch/thin plaque stage of lymphoproliferative disorders, BCNU has its major indication when these techniques cannot be used for either geographical reasons (PUVA not available within a reasonable distance) or in cases of allergic hypersensitivity against HN_2.

Practical Application

The stock solution is prepared by dissolving 100 mg BCNU powder (Bristol Laboratories) in 50 ml of 95% or absolute alcohol, yielding a concentration of 2 mg/mL. This stock solution is stable at a temperature of 2–8°C in the refrigerator for at least 3 months. In order to prepare the solution for the treatment of lesions, 5 mL of the stock solution (corresponding to 10 mg of BCNU) is added to 60 mL of cool tap water (57). The resulting aqueous solution is unstable and should be used immediately. The solution is applied once daily (58) for 8–10 weeks to the general body surface with exception of the head, genitals, body folds, palms and soles unless they are involved. If large areas are clearly uninvolved, they need not be treated. Total dose applied should not exceed 200–600 mg BCNU, even though cumulative doses of 6700 mg have been reached in occasional patients (59).

For spot therapy an ointment preparation (4 mg/gm BCNU in white petrolatum) is easier to use and causes fewer cutaneous reactions than the solution. Because of increased absorption, it may pose a greater hazard of myelosuppression (46).

Results

In a large series of patients with long term follow up (up to 15 years) treated with topical carmustine (BCNU), a complete response was obtained in 86% of those with limited extent (less than 10%) plaques (T1 stage), in 48% of those with extensive (greater than or equal to 10%) plaques (T2 stage), and in 21% of those with erythroderma. The median time to achieve complete response was 11.5 weeks (59).

Adverse effects include cutaneous irritation in most patients, telangiectases, hyperpigmentation and the potential for carcinogenesis. Mild hematopoietic depression may occur (less than 10% of patients (59)) and can be avoided by limiting the total dose of topical BCNU to less than 600 mg per course.

Combination with Other Modalities

Even though not explicitly reported, there should not be any contraindications against using topical glucocorticosteroids or systemic nonaggressive agents such as retinoids or interferons in combination with BCNU. There is no proven evidence for a synergistic beneficial effect of such combinations.

Comments

Carmustine is an alternative cytostatic drug for local therapy to HN_2 with efficacy comparable to that of mechlorethamine hydrochloride or PUVA (56). The advantages are similar to HN_2, except that a remission is generally achieved earlier than with HN_2. Moreover carmustine can be used in patients allergic to mechlorethamine.

REFERENCES

1. Schreus HT. (Karl Linser's discovery of heliotherapy of mycosis fungoides). Dermatol Wochenschr 1965; 151:1069–1074.
2. Bloch H. Solartheology, heliotherapy, phototherapy, and biologic effects: a historical overview. J Natl Med Assoc 1990; 82:517–521.
3. Arlett CF, Lowe JE, Harcourt SA, Waugh AP, Cole J, Roza L, Diffey BL, Mori T, Nikaido O, Green MH. Hypersensitivity of human lymphocytes to UV-B and solar irradiation. Cancer Res 1993; 53:609–614.
4. Kasibhatla S, Brunner T, Genestier L, Echeverri F, Mahboubi A, Green DR. DNA damaging agents induce expression of Fas ligand and subsequent apoptosis in T lymphocytes via the activation of NF-kappa B and AP-1. Mol Cell 1998; 1:543–551.
5. Tomimori Y, Ikawa Y, Oyaizu N. Ultraviolet-irradiated apoptotic lymphocytes produce interleukin-10 by themselves. Immunol Lett 2000; 71:49–54.
6. Vink AA, Moodycliffe AM, Shreedhar V, Ullrich SE, Roza L, Yarosh DB, Kripke ML. The inhibition of antigen-presenting activity of dendritic cells resulting from UV irradiation of murine skin is restored by in vitro photorepair of cyclobutane pyrimidine dimers. Proc Natl Acad Sci U S A 1997; 94:5255–5260.
7. Ullrich SE. Mechanism involved in the systemic suppression of antigen-presenting cell function by UV irradiation. Keratinocyte-derived IL-10 modulates antigen-presenting cell function of splenic adherent cells. J Immunol 1994; 152:3410–3416.
8. Alora MB, Fitzpatrick TB, Taylor CR. Total body heliotherapy. Photodermatol Photoimmunol Photomed 1997; 13:178–180.
9. Kim TY, Kripke ML, Ullrich SE. Immunosuppression by factors released from UV-irradiated epidermal cells: selective effects on the generation of contact and delayed hypersensitivity after exposure to UVA or UVB radiation. J Invest Dermatol 1990; 94:26–32.
10. El-Ghorr AA, Pierik F, Norval M. Comparative potency of different UV sources in reducing the density and antigen-presenting capacity of Langerhans cells in C3H mice. Photochem Photobiol 1994; 60:256–261.
11. Avalos-Diaz E, Alvarado-Flores E, Herrera-Esparza R. UV-A irradiation induces transcription of IL-6 and TNF alpha genes in human keratinocytes and dermal fibroblasts. Rev Rhum Engl Ed 1999; 66:13–19.
12. Tokura Y, Seo N, Yagi H, Takigawa M. Photoactivational cytokine-modulatory action of 8-methoxypsoralen plus ultraviolet A in lymphocytes, monocytes, and cutaneous T cell lymphoma cells. Ann N Y Acad Sci 2001; 941:185–193.
13. Ramsay DL, Lish KM, Yalowitz CB, Soter NA. Ultraviolet-B phototherapy for early-stage cutaneous T-cell lymphoma. Arch Dermatol 1992; 128:931–933.
14. Hofer A, Cerroni L, Kerl H, Wolf P. Narrowband (311 nm) UV-B therapy for small plaque parapsoriasis and early-stage mycosis fungoides. Arch Dermatol 1999; 135:1377–1380.
15. Clark C, Dawe RS, Evans AT, Lowe G, Ferguson J. Narrowband TL-01 phototherapy for patch-stage mycosis fungoides. Arch Dermatol 2000; 136:748–752.
16. Gilchrest BA, Parrish JA, Tanenbaum L, Haynes HA, Fitzpatrick TB. Oral methoxsalen photochemotherapy of mycosis fungoides. Cancer 1976; 38:683–689.
17. Honigsmann H, Brenner W, Rauschmeier W, Konrad K, Wolff K. Photochemotherapy for cutaneous T cell lymphoma. A follow-up study. J Am Acad Dermatol 1984; 10:238–245.

18. Roenigk H, Kuzel TM, Skoutelis AP, Springer E, Yu G, Caro W, Gilyon K, Variakojis D, Kaul K, Bunn PJ et al. Photochemotherapy alone or combined with interferon alpha-2a in the treatment of cutaneous T-cell lymphoma. J Invest Dermatol 1990; 95: 198S–205S.

19. Spittle MF. Mycosis fungoides: electron beam therapy in England. Cancer Treat Rep 1979; 63:639–641.

20. Stadler R, Otte HG, Luger T, Henz BM, Kuhl P, Zwingers T, Sterry W. Prospective randomized multicenter clinical trial on the use of interferon-2a plus acitretin vs. interferon-2a plus PUVA in patients with cutaneous T-cell lymphoma stages I and II. Blood 1998; 92:3578–3581.

21. Godar DE. UVA1 radiation triggers two different final apoptotic pathways. J Invest Dermatol 1999; 112:3–12.

22. von Kobyletzki G, Heine O, Stephan H, Pieck C, Stucker M, Hoffmann K, Altmeyer P, Mannherz HG. UVA1 irradiation induces deoxyribonuclease dependent apoptosis in cutaneous T-cell lymphoma in vivo. Photodermatol Photoimmunol Photomed 2000; 16:271–277.

23. Morita A, Werfel T, Stege H, Ahrens C, Karmann K, Grewe M, Grether-Beck S, Ruzicka T, Kapp A, Klotz LO, Sies H, Krutmann J. Evidence that singlet oxygen-induced human T helper cell apoptosis is the basic mechanism of ultraviolet-A radiation phototherapy. J Exp Med 1997; 186:1763–1768.

24. Plettenberg H, Stege H, Megahed M, Ruzicka T, Hosokawa Y, Tsuji T, Morita A, Krutmann J. Ultraviolet A1 (340–400 nm) phototherapy for cutaneous T-cell lymphoma. J Am Acad Dermatol 1999; 41:47–50.

25. Zane C, Leali C, Airo P, De Panfilis G, Pinton PC. "High-dose" UVA1 therapy of widespread plaque-type nodular erythrodermic mycosis fungoides. J Am Acad Dermatol 2001; 44:629–633.

26. Migita K, Eguchi K, Kawabe Y, Nakamura T, Shirabe S, Tsukada T, Ichinose Y, Nakamura H, Nagataki S. Apoptosis induction in human peripheral blood T lymphocytes by high-dose steroid therapy. Transplantation 1997; 63:583–587.

27. Perrin-Wolff M, Mishal Z, Bertoglio J, Pallardy M. Position 16 of the steroid nucleus modulates glucocorticoid-induced apoptosis at the transcriptional level in murine T-lymphocytes. Biochem Pharmacol 1996; 52:1469–1476.

28. Bucks DA, McMaster JR, Maibach HI, Guy RH. Bioavailability of topically administered steroids: a "mass balance" technique. J Invest Dermatol 1988; 91:29–33.

29. Zackheim HS, Kashani-Sabet M, Amin S. Topical corticosteroids for mycosis fungoides. Experience in 79 patients (see comments). Arch Dermatol 1998; 134:949–954.

30. Scholtz W. Über den Einfluss der Röntgenstrahlen auf die Haut in gesundem und krankem Zustand. Arch Derm Syphil 1902; 59:421–449.

31. Goldschmidt H. Radiation therapy of other cutaneous tumors. In: Goldschmidt H., Panizzon R. (eds). Modern Dermatologic Radiation Therapy. Springer, New York, Berlin, Heiddberg 1991: 123–132.

32. Schirren C. Roentgen irradiation at a distance using soft radiation from beryllium- window tubes. J Invest Dermatol 1955; 24:463–467.

33. Goldschmidt H, Lukacs S, Schoefinius HH. Teleroentgen therapy for mycosis fungoides. J Dermatol Surg Oncol 1978; 4:600–605.

34. Wiskemann A, Buck C. Radiotherapy of mycosis fungoides: twenty years of experience with teleroentgen and low-voltage X-ray therapy. J Dermatol Surg Oncol 1978; 4: 606–610.

35. Jones GW, Hoppe RT, Glatstein E. Electron beam treatment for cutaneous T-cell lymphoma. Hematol Oncol Clin North Am 1995; 9:1057–1076.

36. Jones GW, Rosenthal D, Wilson LD. Total skin electron radiation for patients with erythrodermic cutaneous T-cell lymphoma (mycosis fungoides and the Sezary syndrome). Cancer 1999; 85:1985–1995.

37. Quiros PA, Jones GW, Kacinski BM, Braverman IM, Heald PW, Edelson RL, Wilson LD. Total skin electron beam therapy followed by adjuvant psoralen/ultraviolet-A light in the management of patients with T1 and T2 cutaneous T-cell lymphoma (mycosis fungoides). Int J Radiat Oncol Biol Phys 1997; 38:1027–1035.

38. Chinn DM, Chow S, Kim YH, Hoppe RT. Total skin electron beam therapy with or without adjuvant topical nitrogen mustard or nitrogen mustard alone as initial treatment of T2 and T3 mycosis fungoides. Int J Radiat Oncol Biol Phys 1999; 43:951–958.

39. Hallahan DE, Griem ML, Griem SF, Medenica M, Soltani K, Lorincz AL, Baron JM. Combined modality therapy for tumor stage mycosis fungoides: results of a 10-year follow-up. J Clin Oncol 1988; 6:1177–1183.

40. Jones G, McLean J, Rosenthal D, Roberts J, Sauder DN. Combined treatment with oral etretinate and electron beam therapy in patients with cutaneous T-cell lymphoma (mycosis fungoides and Sezary syndrome). J Am Acad Dermatol 1992; 26:960–967.

41. Kaye FJ, Bunn PJ, Steinberg SM, Stocker JL, Ihde DC, Fischmann AB, Glatstein EJ, Schechter GP, Phelps RM, Foss FM, Parlette H, Anderson M, Sausville E. A randomized trial comparing combination electron-beam radiation and chemotherapy with topical therapy in the initial treatment of mycosis fungoides. N Engl J Med 1989; 321:1784–1790.

42. Sipos K. Painting treatment of nitrogen mustard in mycosis fungoides. Dermatologica 1965; 130:3–11.

43. Van Scott E, Kalmanson JD. Complete remissions of mycosis fungoides lymphoma induced by topical nitrogen mustard (HN_2). Control of delayed hypersensitivity to HN_2 by desensitization and by induction of specific immunologic tolerance. Cancer 1973; 32:18–30.

44. Smith KJ, Smith WJ, Hamilton T, Skelton HG, Graham JS, Okerberg C, Moeller R, Hackley, BE Jr. Histopathologic and immunohistochemical features in human skin after exposure to nitrogen and sulfur mustard. Am J Dermatopathol 1998; 20:22–28.

45. Zackheim HS, Amin S, Kashani-Sabet M, McMillan A. Prognosis in cutaneous T-cell lymphoma by skin stage: long-term survival in 489 patients. J Am Acad Dermatol 1999; 40:418–425.

46. Ramsay DL, Meller JA, Zackheim HS. Topical treatment of early cutaneous T-cell lymphoma. Hematol Oncol Clin North Am 1995; 9:1031–1056.

47. Price NM, Deneau DG, Hoppe RT. The treatment of mycosis fungoides with ointment-based mechlorethamine. Arch Dermatol 1982; 118:234–237.

48. Van Vloten W, Cooijmans AC, Poel J, Meulenbelt J. Concentrations of nitrogen mustard in the air during topical treatment of patients with mycosis fungoides. Br J Dermatol 1993; 128:404–406.

49. Volden G, Larsen TE. Remissions of mycosis fungoides induced by nitrogen mustard (HN_2). Topical treatment and hydration of tumours and plaques with HN_2. Topical desensitization to HN2. A clinical and histopathological controlled study. Dermatologica 1978; 156:129–141.

50. Vonderheid EC, Van SE, Wallner PE, Johnson WC. A 10-year experience with topical mechlorethamine for mycosis fungoides: comparison with patients treated by total-skin electron-beam radiation therapy. Cancer Treat Rep 1979; 63:681–689.

51. Vonderheid EC, Tan ET, Kantor AF, Shrager L, Micaily B, Van Scott EJ. Long-term efficacy, curative potential, and carcinogenicity of topical mechlorethamine chemotherapy in cutaneous T cell lymphoma. J Am Acad Dermatol 1989; 20:416–428.

52. Monk BE, Vollum DI, du VA. Combination topical nitrogen mustard and photochemotherapy for mycosis fungoides. Clin Exp Dermatol 1984; 9:243–247.

53. du Vivier A, Vollum DI. Photochemotherapy and topical nitrogen mustard in the treatment of mycosis fungoides. Br J Dermatol 1980; 102:319–322.

54. Zackheim HS. Treatment of mycosis fungoides with topical nitrosourea compounds. Arch Dermatol 1972; 106:177–182.

55. Zackheim HS, Epstein EJ. Treatment of mycosis fungoides with topical nitrosourea compounds: Further studies. Arch Dermatol 1975; 111:1564–1570.
56. Zackheim HS. Topical carmustine (BCNU) for patch/plaque mycosis fungoides. Semin Dermatol 1994; 13:202–206.
57. Zackheim H. Topical mechlorethamine and carmustine for cutaneous T-cell lymphoma. Semin Dermatol 1983; 2:307–318.
58. Zackheim HS. Cutaneous T cell lymphoma: update of treatment. Dermatology 1999; 199:102–105.
59. Zackheim, Epstein EJ, Crain WR. Topical carmustine (BCNU) for cutaneous T cell lymphoma: a 15-year experience in 143 patients. J Am Acad Dermatol 1990; 22:802–810.

Systemic Therapies

Günter Burg, Reinhard Dummer, Werner Kempf, Sonja Michaelis, Philippa Golling, and Frank O. Nestle
Department of Dermatology, University Hospital, Zürich, Switzerland

NONAGGRESSIVE SYSTEMIC THERAPIES

Nonaggressive treatment modalities are intended to control the disease and usually do not cause severe side effects exceeding WHO class 1 (mild) after long term (more than 3 months) use.

Low Dose Chemotherapy with Chlorambucil

Introduction

Early reports demonstrated the beneficial effect of chlorambucil in CTCL (1).

Indication

The main indications are erythrodermic CTCL and Sézary Syndrome(SS) with intractable pruritus. This regimen also is an important and relatively nontoxic chemotherapeutic option for palliation of advanced SS (2).

Results

Low dose chlorambucil (4 mg/day) as single agent chemotherapy in combination with prednisone (20 mg/day) in patients with CTCL produced good results at the Mayo Clinic (3,4). In a series of 40 patients with SS on this regimen, median survival (6.2 years) was longer than with other regimens (3.05 years). The addition of x-ray or additional chemotherapy did not produce significant long-term benefits (5). Patients with erythroderma, circulating Sézary cell levels less than 1000 cells/mm^3, and a chronic course were diagnosed as having preSS. Most of these patients achieved partial or complete remission on low dose chlorambucil and prednisone therapy (5).

497

Combination with Other Modalities

Combination with topical application of nitrogen mustard has been reported (6).

Comments

Prednimustine, a chlorambucil ester of prednisolone, was not found particularly advantageous for the treatment of MF in advanced stage of the disease (7).

Low Dose Chemotherapy with Methotrexate
Mode of Action

Methotrexate (MTX) is an inhibitor of the enzyme dihydrofolate reductase.

Indication

Low dose MTX is considered to be a valuable first-line treatment for the majority of patients with early to intermediate-stage erythrodermic CTCL (8). In addition, MTX is very effective in controlling lymphomatoid papulosis (9,10) and other primary cutaneous CD30–positive lymphoproliferative disorders (11).

Practical Application

As a low dose chemotherapeutic agent MTX is given in a dosage of 15–25 mg once per week.

Results

Low dose MTX was given to patients with SS for periods of up to 5 years with overall low toxicity. A complete response was achieved in 41%, and 35% achieved a partial response with an estimated 5-year survival rate of 71%. Toxicity was minor and self-limited, occurring in only one patient (12).

Combination with Other Modalities

Combination chemotherapy programs consisting of methotrexate and bleomycin, doxorubicin, etoposide or prednimustine and topical nitrogen mustard daily have been used in patients with advanced stage MF (13,14).

Comments

Even the mild immunosuppression that occurs with MTX therapy of rheumatoid arthritis may place patients at added risk for developing lymphoproliferative diseases (15–17) and also cutaneous pseudolymphoma (18,19).

Extracorporeal Photopheresis (ECP)
Introduction

The ECP is based on extracorporeal irradiation of circulating pathogenic T cells (e.g., malignant or autoimmune cells) with UV-A light in the presence of photosensitizing psoralens. It was developed in the late 1970s and early 1980s by Edelson and colleagues at the National Institutes of Health and later Yale University with the primary goal to treat patients with a leukemic form of cutaneous T-cell lymphoma i.e., SS. One rationale for targeting phototherapy to blood cells circulating in SS patients was the fact that PUVA therapy was shown to be successful in the treatment of MF.

To reach the systemically circulating neoplastic cells in SS patients, a device was developed to irradiate blood derived mononuclear cells with UV-A light in the presence of 8-methoxypsoralen (8-MOP) in an extracorporeal photopheresis chamber.

Mode of Action

The complete mode of action of ECP is not fully understood. There were early suggestions about a vaccine effect against pathogenic circulating T lymphocytes since only 10% of the circulating lymphocytes are irradiated. A simple destruction of malignant lymphocytes would therefore not explain the effects of ECP. Recent data support the notion that antigen presenting dendritic cells are activated in the photopheresis chamber, take up pathogenic T cells such as malignant CTCL cells and present them to the immune system after re-infusion (20). The ECP might be therefore considered as some sort of dendritic cell vaccination (21). Further evidence support the notion that ECP induces TNF alpha which has a wide range of antitumorigenic actions as well as apoptosis in malignant T-cell clones (22).

Indication

The main indication of ECP is Sézary Syndrome(SS). In a 1994 consensus conference ECP was proposed to be the first line treatment of this disease (23). Another excellent indication is "Red Man" syndrome (24). Available data on MF are less convincing. Apart from CTCL, other major indications include solid organ transplantation, graft vs. host reaction and atopic dermatitis.

Practical Application

The current treatment protocol is still based on the originally described procedure (25). Access is obtained via an antecubital vein. During six treatment cycles, red blood cells are separated from white blood cells in a centrifuge. Red blood cells are immediately returned to the patient, while the white blood cells (buffy coat) are collected and circulate extracorporally through the photopheresis chamber. One of the major recent developments is the injection of photosensitizing methoxypsoralens directly in the photopheresis chamber instead of giving it to the patient before treatment. After a total dose of 2 Joule/cm^2 UV-A irradiation, cells are returned to the patient. Therapy is performed on two consecutive days, every 2–4 weeks depending on the treatment protocol.

Results

The first published study on ECP treatment in CTCL patients showed that approximately two-thirds of patients respond to therapy (25). The same was true for those with nodal involvement. In a follow-up study, an increase in survival time compared to historical controls was shown (26). However, a randomized study has not yet been performed.

Combination with Other Modalities

The modality most often combined with ECP is IFN-alpha 1.5–5 million units, three times per week, increase the effectiveness of ECP (27). Case reports have shown beneficial effects of adding acitretin 25–50 mg per day.

Comments

The ECP is a very well tolerated therapy with high patient compliance for the treatment of SS and other indications such as solid organ transplantation. The therapy generally achieves treatment success in about two-thirds of SS patients and should be tried as first line therapy in this otherwise difficult to treat disease.

Interferon-alpha

Introduction

Interferon-alpha (IFN-α) is a cytokine produced by many cell types during viral infection or inflammation. It has been successfully used for more than two decades. Today, recombinant IFN-α is used mainly in low nontoxic dosages of $3–9 \times 10^6$ U three times weekly. In general, it is combined with retinoids or PUVA (28).

Mode of Action

IFN-α can have antiproliferative effects on various tumor cell types. However, interferon-resistant tumor cells in cutaneous lymphomas have been reported (29). Besides direct effects on tumor cells, IFN-α stimulates innate and specific immune responses.

Indication

IFN-α is effective in MF and SS, preferentially combined with other treatment modalities. In addition, it works in CD30+ lymphoproliferative disorders and cutaneous B-cell lymphomas. In the latter tumors, intralesional application is preferred (30).

Practical Application

IFN-α is injected subcutaneously three times per week. Also direct intralesional injection is feasible.

Results

The maximally tolerated dose was $50 \, MU/m^2$ three times a week for at least three months and resulted in a partial response in 45% of the CTCL patients (Fig. 1). There are several studies regarding interferon-alpha treatment in CTCL. The literature suggests that lower doses [$3–9 \, MU/m^2$] are as effective, but are less toxic.

The side effects from IFN-α during initial exposure to the drug are fever, chills, myalgias, and malaise which could be easily controlled with antipyretics. Dose related side effects are gastrointestinal complaints, metallic taste, anorexia, leucopoenia, decrease in platelet count, elevation of liver function tests as well as stupor, psychosis and peripheral neuropathy.

Combination with Other Modalities

IFN-α is typically combined with other treatment modalities. Several studies report the combination of retinoids with interferon. However, a prospective randomized trial has shown that the combination of PUVA plus interferon is more efficient than the combination of retinoids plus interferon alpha, at least in early stages of cutaneous T-cell lymphomas (28).

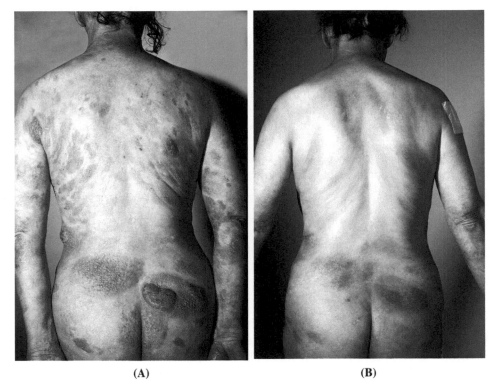

(A)   (B)

Figure 1 Mycosis fungoides before (left) and after (right) treatment with acitretin and interferon-alpha. The tumor has been removed by additional local orthovolt radiotherapy.

Comments

IFN-α has been extensively studied in cutaneous lymphomas. It is well tolerated in most situations and is suitable for combination therapy. Today, it is one of the most important systemic agent for the treatment of cutaneous lymphomas (31).

Retinoid
Introduction

Retinoids are analogs of vitamin A. Vitamin A acid (tretinoin) was discovered in 1946 and came into clinical use in 1969 (32). The first generation of synthetic vitamin A analogues (retinoids) were tretinoin (all-trans-retinoic acid) and isotretinoin (13-cis-tretinoin) (33,34), followed by etretinate and acitretin. Bexarotene represents the third and novel generation of retinoids, the first rexinoid or arotinoid that is selective for the retinoid X receptors (RXRs).

Mode of Action

Retinoids belong to the group of biologic response modifiers. They have antiproliferative, antiangiogenic, immunomodulating effects and modulate cellular differentiation (35,36). Retinoids exhibit their effect through binding to the retinoid A receptor (RAR) or the retinoid X receptor (RXR) in the nuclei of cells either directly or indirectly via nuclear transcription factors (NTFs), regulating the expression of a wide range of target genes. Depending on their action, panagonists binding to both receptors can be distinguished from selective RAR or RXR agonists. They modulate cell growth and differentiation in a variety of human tumor cell types. Retinoids inhibit cell growth by arresting cells in the G1-phase or inducing apoptosis, in particularly in T-cell and Hodgkin lymphoma cell lines (37–39). In addition, retinoids exhibit immunomodulatory effects. They enhance IFN-α production, which is partially mediated via IL-12 induction and is synergistic with interleukin 2 (40,41). This produces an up-regulation of MHC complexes and a shift from T-helper 2 (TH2) cells, which are increased in CTCL (42), to TH1 cells. In addition, RA enhances cytotoxic activity of natural killer (NK) cells mimicking some of the biologic effects of IFN (43).

Indication

Retinoids alone or in combination with other agents play an important role in the treatment of cutaneous T-cell lymphomas, especially MF and SS. There are only a few reports on the use of retinoids in CL other than MF.

Practical Application

Most retinoids of the first and second generation were usually used orally with dosages of 1–2 mg/kg/day. The most commonly reported side effects of these agents are dryness of the skin and mucous membranes, pruritus, increased levels of liver enzymes, hypertriglyceridemia, hypercholesterolemia, axial osteoarthropathy with bone pain, arthralgias, myalgias, and hair loss. Most of these side effects are reversible except for axial osteoarthropathy resulting in stiffness of spine and decreased axial mobility.

Isotretinoin and etretinate have subsequently been replaced by acitretin and the third generation of retinoids, bexarotene, for the treatment of CTCL. An optimal dose of bexarotene of $300 \, mg/m^2/day$ is recommended. Although higher doses $(500–600 \, mg/m^2/day)$ may be more effective, dose-limiting hypertriglyceridemia with pancreatitis is more common. The most significant side effects of bexarotene are hypertriglyceridemia, hypercholesterolemia, leukopenia, central hypothyroidism, and headache. Hypertriglyceridemia occurs in 82% of the patients and requires additional treatment with lipid-lowering agents such as fenofibrate, HMG-CoA reductase inhibitors or statins. Gemfibrozil is not recommended since it increases bexarotene-induced hypertriglyceridemia (44).

Topical retinoid treatment of MF is usually well tolerated although local irritation occurs in up to 80% of the patients independent of the type of topically applied retinoid (44). This irritation can usually easily be managed by dose reduction or by adding topical steroids.

Results

First studies using isotretinoin as single agent in CTCL were reported 20 years ago (45). Isotretinoin showed an overall response rate (ORR) between 43% and up to 100%. Symptomatic relief of pruritus and fading of skin lesions occurred within few weeks and lasted for several months in most of the studied patients (46). Combined therapy with isotretinoin (1 mg/kg/day) and low dose IFN-α 2b (2 Mio U three times per week subcutaneously.) was shown to be effective with responses maintained for up to 15 months under maintenance therapy (47). Etretinate was one of the most widely used retinoids in CTCL and showed response rates similar to isotretinoin, but it is no longer available. More than 70 patients with MF and SS have been followed in studies using a combined therapy with etretinate and IFN-α (48–52) with ORR of at least 50% (50). Combined therapy with etretinate and IFN-2α was able to induce remission in patients with MF, especially in early stages. The combination of retinoids (etretinate, acitretin) with chemotherapy was effective in patients with advanced stage of MF (53–55).

In a large prospective randomized multicenter trial of 98 patients with MF stage I and II, Stadler et al. (28) compared the use of IFN-α plus acitretin vs. IFN-α plus PUVA. Also, IFN-α was administered at 9 MU three times weekly, subcutaneously. Acitretin was used at an initial dosage of 25 mg per day during first week, and 50 mg from weeks 2 to 48. The complete remission rate (CRR) in the group treated with IFN-α plus PUVA was 70% compared to 38.1% in the group with IFN-α and acitretin (28). In addition, time to response in the IFN-α plus PUVA group was significantly shorter than in the other group at 18.6 vs. 21.8 weeks, respectively. Side effects did not differ in the two groups. Based on these data, the authors concluded that a combined treatment of MF stage I and II with IFN-α plus PUVA is more effective than with IFN-α and acitretin.

Oral bexarotene, a RXR-selective retinoid, was approved by the FDA in 1999 for the cutaneous manifestations of CTCL in both early and advanced stages to other therapies (56,57). The efficacy of bexarotene has been well documented in early-stage MF as well as advanced stages of CTCL (58,59). The median duration of response was 10 months (299 days). The recurrence rate after response was 36%. Remarkably, bexarotene was effective also in cases of transformation of MF and erythrodermic MF as well as in patients with SS. A rapid improvement of erythroderma and pruritus occurred within 2 weeks in all four patients with erythrodermic CTCL (60).

Topical retinoids have also been employed in the treatment of early stages of CTCL (stage I and II). Bexarotene (Targretin®) as a topical gel achieved an Overall response rate (ORR) of 58% of the treated lesions (44). Lesions with no previous treatment responded at a higher rate (75% vs. 67%) than lesions that had received previous topical therapy (61). The topical therapy with bexarotene gel could be continued for more than 12 months in one-third of the patients. After long-term use, higher response rates (86% ORR and 28% CRR) were observed than after short-term use (60). A 30% response rate to topical alitretinoin gel 0.1% (Panretin®), the only topical retinoid possessing both RAR and RXR activity, was seen in the phase I study conducted in MF patients with stage IA disease.

Combination with Other Modalities

Retinoids can be combined with photochemotherapy (so called Re-PUVA), IFN-α, and chemotherapy. Bexarotene may be combined with topical steroids, phototherapy or with DAB 8389/IL-2 (denileukin diftitox, Ontak®) (62).

Comments

Clinical response after retinoid therapy does not necessarily imply histological clearing of skin lesions.(46). The persisting lymphoid infiltrates are most probably the source of recurrences. Nevertheless, retinoids as monotherapy or in combination with other nonaggressive treatment modalities represent a low-risk treatment alternative that is especially suitable for controlling early stages of MF and other CTCL. Combined modality therapies may be more effective in controlling CTCL as it was shown for combination of IFN-α together with retinoids and recently with bexarotene and other modalities.

AGGRESSIVE SYSTEMIC THERAPIES

High Dose Mono-Chemotherapy

Introduction

High dose mono-chemotherapy implies an intravenous systemic application of a cytotoxic drug candidates for this type of therapy are methotrexate (63) and liposomal doxorubicin (64).

Mode of Action

Methotrexate is an inhibitor of the enzyme dihydrofolate reductase. Liposomal doxorubicin is a new formulation of adriamycin. Both have significant antitumor activity.

Practical Application

Due to the beneficial side-effect profile, we today recommend only liposomal doxorubicin as a mono-chemotherapy for cutaneous lymphoma. It can be given in a dosage of $20 \, \mathrm{mg/m^2}$ body surface every two or four weeks.

Indication

We recommend liposomal doxorubicin for tumor stage MF but also for other multi-lesional lymphomas that are resistant to other milder approaches such as low dose methotrexate and cannot be irradiated.

Results

Liposomal doxorubicin can induce partial and complete remissions in more than 70% of the cases (64) (Fig. 2).

Combination with Other Modalities

There are few reports on the simultaneous application of liposomal doxorubicin and IFN-α. It is not known whether this improves the results.

Comments

Since there is no treatment modality for advanced stages of cutaneous lymphoma whose effectiveness has been shown in evidence/based fashion, we recommend administering this type of treatment only in the context of controlled clinical trials, preferentially organized by a large organization such as the international society of cutaneous lymphoma or the European Organization for Research and Treatment of Cancer (EORTC).

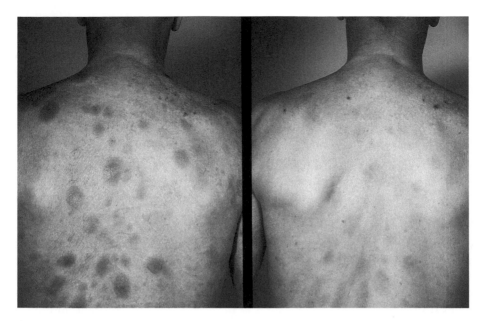

Figure 2 Mycosis fungoides before (left) and after (right) treatment with liposomal doxorubicin.

High Dose Poly-Chemotherapy

Introduction

Poly-chemotherapy is applied for all types of nonHodgkin lymphomas and thus for cutaneous lymphomas. Until now, there is no evidence that this toxic approach has any beneficial impact on survival. Therefore, it should not be routinely used (65).

Mode of Action

Depending on the drugs used, there are different possibilities to block cell proliferation. The chemotherapy most commonly used is the CHOP therapy. It contains cyclophosphamide, vincristine (oncovin) and adriamycin combined with prednisone. Cyclophosphamide is an alkylating agent requiring metabolism by the liver. Vincristine binds to the protein tubulin resulting in an arrest of cells in metaphase with subsequent lysis. Doxorubicin (adriamycin) belongs to the group of anthracyclines, antitumor antibiotics.

Indication

Aggressive types of cutaneous lymphomas, especially advanced cases with systemic involvement, can be targeted by this approach.

Practical Application

The patient should be protected from emesis by a serotonin antagonist. The cytotoxic drugs are given by an experienced treatment team intravenously. The patient's blood counts and cardiac function have to be monitored regularly.

Results

Depending on the subtypes of lymphoma, remissions which are usually shortly last-ing can be expected in approximately 50–70% of the cases (66). There is no proven impact on survival (65,67). The immunosuppressive effects of poly-chemotherapy result in infectious complications such as reactivation of herpes or fungal infections in many patients.

Combination with Other Modalities

Although it is theoretically possible to combine with biological response modifiers or retinoids, these combinations should be avoided due to additional toxicities.

Comments

Poly-chemotherapy may rarely be helpful in advanced stages of cutaneous lymphoma in very critical clinical situations. We recommend that these treatment approaches be administered by experienced centers. Due to the limited information available, we urgently recommend treating this patient population in the context of clinical trials.

Bone Marrow Transplantation

In an initial limited pilot study, six patients received autologous bone marrow trans-plantation (ABMT) (68). They had no life-threatening infections. Only two patients were alive without disease one year after transplantation. There also have been more favorable reports in high grade malignant lymphoma with primary skin involvement going into complete remission lasting for 2–4+ years after high dose chemotherapy, total body irradiation and autologous bone marrow transplantation (69–71). Patients with poor prognosis of CTCL can undergo ABMT without developing life-threatening infections and even achieve prolonged complete recovery.

Allo-bone marrow transplantation also has been reported as highly effective treatment for advanced poor-prognosis lymphoid malignancies with acceptable toxicity (72).

REFERENCES

1. Mante C, Brodkin RH, Cohen F. Chlorambucil in mycosis fungoides. Report of a case of successful treatment. Acta Derm Venereol Stockh 1968; 48:60–63.
2. Harland CC, Balsitis M, Millard LG. Sezary-type cutaneous T-cell leukaemia. Response to Winkelmann regimen. Acta Derm Venereol 1990; 70:251–253.
3. Winkelmann R, P-H Muller SA, Schroeter AL, Jordon RE, Rogers RS. Treatment of Sezary syndrome. Mayo Clin Proc 1974; 49:590–592.
4. Winkelmann R. Nontoxic low dose chemotherapy. Cutis 1977; 19:309–313.
5. Winkelmann RK, Diaz PJ, Buechner SA. The treatment of Sezary syndrome. J Am Acad Dermatol 1984; 10:1000–1004.
6. Hamminga L, Hartgrink GC van VW. Sezary's syndrome: a clinical evaluation of eight patients. Br J Dermatol 1979; 100:291–296.
7. Molin L, Thomsen K, Volden G, Bergqvist KA, Hellbe L. Prednimustine in mycosis fun-goides: a report from the Scandinavian mycosis fungoides study group. Acta Derm Venereol Stockh 1979; 59:87–88.

8. Zackheim HS, Kashani SM, Hwang ST. Low-dose methotrexate to treat erythrodermic cutaneous T-cell lymphoma: results in twenty-nine patients. J Am Acad Dermatol 1996; 34:626–631.

9. Lynch PJ, Saied NK. Methotrexate treatment of pityriasis lichenoides and lymphomatoid papulosis. Cutis 1979; 23:634–636.

10. Lange WG, Thomsen K. Methotrexate in lymphomatoid papulosis. Br J Dermatol 1984; 111:93–95.

11. Vonderheid EC, Sajjadian A, Kadin ME. Methotrexate is effective therapy for lymphomatoid papulosis and other primary cutaneous CD30–positive lymphoproliferative disorders. J Am Acad Dermatol 1996; 34:470–481.

12. Zackheim HS, Epstein EJ. Low-dose methotrexate for the Sezary syndrome. J Am Acad Dermatol 1989; 21:757–762.

13. Zakem MH, Davis BR, Adelstein DJ, Hines JD. Treatment of advanced stage mycosis fungoides with bleomycin, doxorubicin, and methotrexate with topical nitrogen mustard (BAM-M). Cancer 1986; 58:2611–2616.

14. Doberauer C, Ohl S. Advanced mycosis fungoides: chemotherapy with etoposide, methotrexate, bleomycin, and prednimustine. Acta Derm Venereol 1989; 69:538–540.

15. Ellman MH, Hurwitz H, Thomas C, Kozloff M. Lymphoma developing in a patient with rheumatoid arthritis taking low dose weekly methotrexate (see comments). J Rheumatol 1991; 18:1741–1743.

16. Kingsmore SF, Hall BD, Allen NB, Rice JR, Caldwell DS. Association of methotrexate, rheumatoid arthritis and lymphoma: report of 2 cases and literature review. J Rheumatol 1992; 19:1462–1465.

17. Taillan B, Garnier G, Castanet J, Ferrari E, Pesce A, Dujardin P. Lymphoma developing in a patient with rheumatoid arthritis taking methotrexate. Clin Rheumatol 1993; 12:93–94.

18. Delaporte E, Catteau B, Cardon T, Flipo RM, Lecomte HM, Piette F, Delcambre B, Bergoend H. Cutaneous pseudolymphoma during treatment of rheumatoid polyarthritis with low-dose methotrexate. Ann Dermatol Venereol 1995; 122:521–525.

19. Viraben R, Brousse P, Lamant L. Reversible cutaneous lymphoma occurring during methotrexate therapy. Br J Dermatol 1996; 135:116–118.

20. Berger CL, Longley J, Hanlon D, Girardi M, Edelson R. The clonotypic T cell receptor is a source of tumor-associated antigens in cutaneous T cell lymphoma. Ann N Y Acad Sci 2001; 941:106–122.

21. Edelson RL. Cutaneous T cell lymphoma: the helping hand of dendritic cells. Ann N Y Acad Sci 2001; 941:1–11.

22. Vowels BR, Cassin M, Boufal MH, Walsh LJ, Rook AH. Extracorporal photochemotherapy induces the production of tumor necrotis factor-alpha by monocytes: implications for the treatment of cutaneous T-cell lymphoma and systemic siderosis. J Invest Dermatol 1992; 98:686–692.

23. Demierre MF, Foss FM, Koh HK. Proceedings of the international consensus conference on cutaneous t-cell lymphoma (CTCL) Treatment recommendations. Boston, MA, Oct 1–2, 1994. J Am Acad Dermatol 1997; 36:460–466.

24. Zachariae H, Bjerring P, Brodthagen U, Sogaard H. Photopheresis in the red man or pre-Sezary syndrome (see comments). Dermatology 1995; 190:132–135.

25. Edelson R, Berger C, Gasparro F, Jegasothy B, Heald P, Wintroub B, Vonderheid E, Knobler R, Wolff K, Plewigal G et al. Treatment of cutaneous T-cell lymphoma by extracorporeal photochemotherapy. Preliminary results. N Engl J Med 1987; 316:297–303.

26. Heald P, Rook A, Perez M, Wintroub B, Knobler R, Jegasothy B, Gasparro F, Berger C, Edelson R. Treatment of erythrodermic cutaneous T-cell lymphoma with extracorporeal photochemotherapy. J Am Acad Dermatol 1992; 27:427–433.

27. Vonderheid EC, Bigler RD, Greenberg AS, Neukum SJ, Micaily B. Extracorporeal photopheresis and recombinant interferon alfa 2b in Sezary syndrome. Use of dual marker labeling to monitor therapeutic response. Am J Clin Oncol 1994; 17:255–263.

28. Stadler R, Otte HG, Luger T, Henz BM, Kuhl P, Zwingers T, Sterry W. Prospective randomized multicenter clinical trial on the use of interferon-2a plus acitretin vs. interferon-2a plus PUVA in patients with cutaneous T-cell lymphoma stages I and II. Blood 1998; 92:3578–3581.

29. Dummer R, Döbbeling U, Geertsen R, Willers J, Burg G, Pavlovic J. Interferon resistance of cutaneous T-cell lymphoma-derived clonal T-helper 2 cells allows selective viral replication. Blood 2001; 97:523–527.

30. Kutting B, Bonsmann G, Metze D, Luger TA, Cerroni L. Borrelia burgdorferi-associated primary cutaneous B cell lymphoma: complete clearing of skin lesions after antibiotic pulse therapy or intralesional injection of interferon alfa-2a. J Am Acad Dermatol 1997; 36:311–314.

31. Kalinke D-U, Dummer R, Burg G. Mangement of cutaneous T-cell lymphoma. Curr Opinion Dermatol 1996; 3:71–76.

32. Kligman AM, Fulton JE Jr, Plewig G. Topical vitamin A acid in acne vulgaris. Arch Dermatol 1969; 99:469–476.

33. Peck R, Bollag W. Potentiation of retinoid-induced differentiation of HL-60 and U937 cell lines by cytokines. Eur J Cancer 1991; 27:53–57.

34. Bollag W. Retinoids and interferon: a new promising combination? Br J Haematol 1991; 87:87–91.

35. Frey JR, Peck R, Bollag W. Antiproliferative activity of retinoids, interferon alpha and their combination in five human transformed cell lines. Cancer Lett 1991; 57:223–227.

36. Orfanos CE, Zouboulis CC, Almond-Roesler B, Geilen CC. Current use and future potential role of retinoids in dermatology. Drugs 1997; 53:358–388.

37. Cheng AL, Chuang SE, Su IJ. Factors associated with the therapeutic efficacy of retinoic acids on malignant lymphomas. J Formos Med Assoc 1997; 96: 525–534.

38. Fujimura S, Suzumiya J, Anzai K, Ohkubo K, Hata T, Yamada Y, Kamihira S, Kikuchi M, J Ono. Retinoic acids induce growth inhibition and apoptosis in adult T-cell leukemia (ATL) cell lines. Leuk Res 1998; 22:611–618.

39. Collins SJ. The role of retinoids and retinoic acid receptors in normal hematopoiesis. Leukemia 2002; 16:1896–1905.

40. Rook AH, Kubin M, Fox FE, Niu Z, Cassin M, Vowels BR, Gottleib SL, Vonderheid EC, Lessin SR, Trinchieri G. The potential therpaeutic role of interleukin-12 in cutaneous T-cell lymphoma Ann NY Acad Scu 1996; 735:310–318.

41. Fox FE, Kubin M, Cassin M, Niu Z, Trinchieri G, Cooper KD, Rook AH. Retinoids synergize with interleukin-2 to augment IFN-gamma and interleukin-12 production by human peripheral blood mononuclear cells. J Interferon Cytokine Res 1999; 19:407–415.

42. Dummer R, Kohl O, Gillessen J, Kagi M, Burg G. Peripheral blood mononuclear cells in patients with nonleukemic cutaneous T-cell lymphoma. Reduced proliferation and preferential secretion of a T helper-2-like cytokine pattern on stimulation. Arch Dermatol 1993; 129:433–436.

43. Pigatto PD, Bersani L, Colotta F, Morelli M, Altomare GF, Polenghi MM. Effect of retinoids on natural killer cell activity. Arch Dermatol Res 1986; 278:507–509.

44. Apisarnthanarax N, Talpur R, Duvic M. Treatment of cutaneous T cell lymphoma: current status and future directions. Am J Clin Dermatol 2002; 3:193–215.

45. Kessler JF, Meyskens FJ, Levine N, Lynch PJ, Jones SE. Treatment of cutaneous T-cell lymphoma (mycosis fungoides) with 13-cis-retinoic acid. Lancet 1983; 1:1345–1347.

46. Kessler JF, Jones SE, Levine N, Lynch PJ, Booth AR, Meyskens FJ. Isotretinoin and cutaneous helper T-cell lymphoma (mycosis fungoides). Arch Dermatol 1987; 123: 201–204.

47. Knobler RM, Trautinger F, Radaszkiewicz T, Kokoschka EM, Micksche M. Treatment of cutaneous T cell lymphoma with a combination of low-dose interferon alfa-2b and retinoids. J Am Acad Dermatol 1991; 24:247–252.

48. Thestrup-Pedersen K, Halkier SL, Sogaard H, Zachariae H. The red man syndrome. Exfoliative dermatitis of unknown etiology: a description and follow-up of 38 patients. J Am Acad Dermatol 1988; 18:1307–1312.

49. Altomare GF, Capella GL, Pigatto PD, Finzi AF. Intramuscular low dose alpha-2B interferon and etretinate for treatment of mycosis fungoides. Int J Dermatol 1993; 32:138–141.

50. Dreno B. Roferon-A (interferon alpha 2a) combined with Tigason (etretinate) for treatment of cutaneous T cell lymphomas. Stem Cells (Dayton, Ohio) 1993; 11:269–275.

51. Dreno B, Celerier P, Litoux P. Roferon-A in combination with Tigason in cutaneous T-cell lymphomas. Acta Haematol 1993; 1:28–32.

52. Aviles A, Guzman R, Garcia EL, Diaz-Maqueo JC. Biological modifiers (etretinate (changed from etetrinate) and alfa 2a) in the treatment of refractory cutaneous T-cell lymphoma. Cancer Biother Radiopharm 1996; 11:21–24.

53. Ippolito F, Giacalone B. (A case of mycosis fungoides with tumoral manifestations treated with RO 10–9359 (Tigason)). Ann Dermatol Venereol 1982; 109:65–72.

54. Zachariae H, Grunnet E, Thestrup PK, Molin L, Schmidt H, Starfelt, Thomsen FK. Oral retinoid in combination with bleomycin, cyclophosphamide, prednisone and transfer factor in mycosis fungoides. Acta Derm Venereol Stockh 1982; 62:162–164.

55. Molin L, Thomsen K, Volden G, Aronsson A, Hammar H, Hellbe L, Wantzin GL, Roupe G. Oral retinoids in mycosis fungoides and Sezary syndrome: a comparison of isotretinoin and etretinate. A study from the Scandinavian mycosis fungoides group. Acta Derm Venereol Stockh 1987; 67:232–236.

56. Hurst RE. Bexarotene ligand pharmaceuticals. Curr Opin Investig Drugs 2000; 1:514–523.

57. Lowe MN, Plosker GL. Bexarotene. Am J Clin Dermatol 2000; 1:245–250; discussion 251–242.

58. Duvic M, Hymes K, Heald P, Breneman D, Martin AG, Myskowski P, Crowley C, Yocum RC. Bexarotene is effective and safe for treatment of refractory advanced-stage cutaneous T-cell lymphoma: multinational phase II–III trial results. J Clin Oncol 2001; 19:2456–2471.

59. Duvic M, Martin AG, Kim Y, Olsen E, Wood GS, Crowley CA, Yocum RC. Phase 2 and 3 clinical trial of oral bexarotene (targretin capsules) for the treatment of refractory or persistent early-stage cutaneous T-cell lymphoma. Arch Dermatol 2001; 137:581–593.

60. Heald P. The treatment of cutaneous T-cell lymphoma with a novel retinoid. Clin Lymphoma 2000; 1(suppl 1):S45–S49.

61. Breneman D, Duvic M, Kuzel T, Yocum R, Truglia J, Stevens VJ. Phase 1 and 2 trial of bexarotene gel for skin-directed treatment of patients with cutaneous T-cell lymphoma. Arch Dermatol 2002; 138:325–332.

62. Duvic M. Treatment of cutaneous T-cell lymphoma from a dermatologist's perspective. Clin Lymphoma 2000; 1(suppl 1):S15–S20.

63. Schappell DL, Alper JC, McDonald CJ. Treatment of advanced mycosis fungoides and Sezary syndrome with continuous infusions of methotrexate followed by fluorouracil and leucovorin rescue. Arch Dermatol 1995; 131:307–313.

64. Wollina U, Graefe T, Kaatz M. Pegylated doxorubicin for primary cutaneous T cell lymphoma: a report on ten patients with follow-up. Ann N Y Acad Sci 2001; 941:214–216.

65. Kaye FJ, Bunn PJ, Steinberg SM, Stocker JL, Ihde DC, Fischmann AB, Glatstein EJ, Schechter GP, Phelps RM, Foss FM, Parlette, Anderson M, Sausville E. A randomized trial comparing combination electron-beam radiation and chemotherapy with topical therapy in the initial treatment of mycosis fungoides. N Engl J Med 1989; 321:1784–1790.

66. Fierro MT, Quaglino P, Savoia P, Verrone A, Bernengo MG. Systemic polychemotherapy in the treatment of primary cutaneous lymphomas: a clinical follow-up study of 81 patients treated with COP or CHOP. Leuk Lymphoma 1998; 31:583–588.

67. Dummer R, Häffner AC, Hess M, Burg G. A rational approach to the therapy of cutaneous T-cell lymphomas (CTCL). Onkologie 1996; 19:226–230.

68. Bigler RD, Crilley P, Micaily B, Brady LW, Topolsky D, Bulova S, VonderheidI Brodsky EC. Autologous bone marrow transplantation for advanced stage mycosis fungoides. Bone Marrow Transplant 1991; 7:133–137.

69. Moreau P, LeTortorec S, Mahe MA, Mahe B, Moreau A, Bourdin S, Bulabois CE, Bureau B, Harousseau JL, Milpied N. Autologous bone marrow transplantation using TBI and CBV for disseminated high/intermediate grade cutaneous non-epidermotropic non-Hodgkin's lymphoma. Bone Marrow Transplant 1994; 14:775–778.

70. Zeitoun C, Baccard M, Marolleau JP, Rybojad M, Baruchel A, Morel P, Brice P. Bone marrow autograft in the treatment of cutaneous lymphoma. Ann Dermatol Venereol 1996; 123:79–84.

71. Molina A, Nademanee A, Arber DA, Forman SJ. Remission of refractory Sezary syndrome after bone marrow transplantation from a matched unrelated donor. Biol Blood Marrow Transplant 1999; 5:400–404.

72. Bernard M, Dauriac C, Drenou B, Leberre C, Branger B, Fauchet R, Le Prise PY, Lamy T. Long-term follow-up of allogeneic bone marrow transplantation in patients with poor prognosis non-Hodgkin's lymphoma. Bone Marrow Transplant 1999; 23:329–333.

Experimental Therapies

Günter Burg, Reinhard Dummer, Werner Kempf, and Frank O. Nestle
Department of Dermatology, University Hospital, Zürich, Switzerland

TOPICAL EXPERIMENTAL THERAPIES

Imiquimod

Introduction

Imiquimod is a novel immune-response modifier for nonaggressive topical therapy. Imiquimod cream 5% recently became available for the treatment of genital and perianal warts. The topical mechanism of action of imiquimod is not fully understood. Imiquimod is a potent antiviral and antitumor agent in animal models.

Mode of Action

Imiquimod is known to bind toll-like receptor (TLR) 7 (1,2). The TLRs belong to the group of pattern-recognition receptors, namely receptors that are present on innate immune cells which are capable of directly recognizing highly conserved pathogen-associated molecular patterns, mounting a rapid defensive response (3). Imiquimod is capable of inducing a variety of cytokines, including interferon (IFN) -α and tumor necrosis factor-α as well as interleukins 1, 6, 8, and 12. In animal models, imiquimod has demonstrated antiviral, antitumor, and adjuvant activity.

Indications

Patches and thin plaques of CTCL are the major indications for treatment with imiquimod.

Practical Application

Imiquimod 5% cream is applied twice daily for 8–10 days until a strong local inflammatory reaction occurs; treatment should be interrupted at that time and restarted when the skin is once again normal.

511

Results

Treatment of stage IA CTCL with topical application of the immune response modifier imiquimod has been reported recently (4,5). Personal experience has shown beneficial effects in patch and thin plaque type lesions of CTCL.

Combination with Other Modalities

Even though the issue has not been specifically studied, there are probably no contraindications to combining other systemic treatments with imiquimod.

Comments

This modality seems to be very promising for the early stages of CTCL. There is no information on its long-term use for widespread skin lesions or on possible late side effects with respect to carcinogenicity or delayed type hypersensitivity. Moreover, costs still are prohibitive for treatment of larger skin areas.

Phosphocholine

Introduction

Miltefosine (6% hexadecylphosphocholine) solution is well established as a nonaggressive topical effective palliative treatment option for cutaneous metastases from breast cancer (6). The topical application of this phospholipid also has been tested in patients with cutaneous lymphoma (7).

Mode of Action

The phospholipid analog hexadecylphosphocholine inhibits proliferation and phosphatidylcholine biosynthesis of human epidermal keratinocytes in vitro (8). It exerts its cytotoxicity by acting on cell membrane phospholipids and can be administered topically. In addition, it may have immunoregulatory properties (9).

Indication and Practical Application

Miltefosine solution has been used topically for the treatment of CTCL, CBCL, and lymphomatoid papulosis.

Practical Application

Six percent miltefosine solution (Miltex[®]; Asta Medica, Frankfurt, Germany) is applied topically twice a day on the lesions for 8 weeks.

Results

Complete remission, partial remissions, and stable disease have been seen. Histological monitoring demonstrated only a partial clearing of infiltrating lymphocytes in lesions that showed a partial or complete response clinically. Two patients with lymphomatoid papulosis experienced transient complete remission, which might have been due to the spontaneous course of the disease. An objective response rate (partial and complete response) of 56% (10/18) was achieved in the patients with cutaneous lymphoma (7).

Combination with Other Modalities
There is no information on this topic.

Comments
Hexadecylphosphocholine is the prototype of a new class of antitumor agents suitable for local application. Its role in cutaneous neoplasms still remains to be defined by larger studies.

Photodynamic Therapy

Introduction
Photodynamic therapy (PDT) in its topical form using porphyrin compounds has become a promising therapeutic modality for various superficial tumors, especially epithelial neoplasms (10). Although PDT was introduced in 1903, only a small number of clinical studies on topical PDT for the treatment of CL have been reported. The data on PDT demonstrate its efficacy in patients with localized patch and plaque stage disease.

Mode of Action
Photodynamic therapy is based on the photo-oxidative effects (i.e., generation of oxygen radicals) creating by illuminating porphyrins and their derivates that have accumulated in tumor cells after topical application. The tumor-selective effect of PDT is due to the preferential uptake of aminolevulinic acid (ALA) into tumor cells. The ratio of uptake of ALA between tumor and normal skin in CTCL is 5:1 (11). The most widely used photosensitizer for topical PDT is delta-ALA. Its uptake results in accumulation of protoporphyrin IX (PpIX) that exerts in vitro toxic effects on both, T- and B-lymphocytes during PDT (12). Photodynamic therapy is capable of inhibiting proliferation of transformed T-cells, in a manner similar to PUVA (13).

Apart from its cytotoxic effects, PDT exhibits immunomodulatory properties. Antigen-presenting cells such as Langerhans' cells and T-cells are activated by PDT with low light dosages that lead to changes in the cytokine milieu (14). It has still to be clarified which biologic effects of PDT are responsible for its therapeutic efficacy observed in CL.

Indication
Photodynamic therapy is an alternative therapeutic approach for limited disease (stage 1) MF with few lesions or lesions at difficult locations which are not easily accessible to other therapeutic modalities. Due to the limited tissue penetration of light, topical PDT is only efficient in superficial tumors such as patch or plaque stage MF.

Practical Application
The photosensitizer, usually ALA 10% or 20% cream, is applied for 3–5 hr on the lesion prior to illumination with red light at wavelength of 600–700 nm and 20–180 J/cm^2. Aminolevulinic acid 10% seems to be less efficient than ALA 20% cream (15). Illumination of larger lesional areas (more than 5 cm) is accompanied by pain and requires local anesthesia in most cases.

Results

Single treatments of MF patch lesions with topical PDT and 20% ALA cream can induce clinical clearance of lesions (16). Repeated (up to five) sessions with 20% ALA cream resulted in clearance of even plaque stage MF lesions with maintained remission in one patient at 14 months after intervention (17). In another study, seven of nine plaque stage MF lesions cleared clinically and histologically, using 20% ALA cream and illumination at 88–180 J/cm^2. Repeated sessions may be necessary to induce clearance of plaque MF lesions (18). Controversial data have been reported on the efficacy of PDT on tumor MF lesions. While in one study, complete clearance of a tumor lesion was observed (19), none of the two tumor lesions responded to topical PDT under similar conditions in another trial. Prolonged application time of ALA in combination with illumination by laser light may be more effective, as shown by complete response in stage 1 CTCL of two patients (20). Apart from MF, PDT has been successfully employed in a patient with a medium to large cell pleomorphic CD8+ CD30– primary cutaneous T-cell lymphoma with involvement of the ear (21).

Comments

Similar to other therapeutic interventions in CTCL, clinical response of lesions does not necessarily imply histological clearance (22). In contrast to treating epithelial tumors, several sessions seem to be necessary to induce remission of CTCL lesions by PDT. Although efficacy of topical PDT in CTCL, especially patch and plaque stage MF, has been demonstrated, larger studies are needed to assess its role. Moreover, parameters such as concentration and application time of the photosensitizer, light dosimetry, and number of sessions have to be standardized to enable comparison of studies.

SYSTEMIC EXPERIMENTAL THERAPIES

Rituximab (anti-CD20 antibody)

Introduction

Rituximab is a chimeric monoclonal antibody directed against the CD20 antigen expressed by B-lymphocytes. This protein is produced by recombination biotechnology.

Mode of Action

The monoclonal antibody binds to all C20+ B-lymphocytes. After binding, the cells can be killed by activation of the complement cascade or by antibody-dependent cellular cytotoxicity. In addition, the antibody may induce apoptosis directly (23).

Indication

Rituximab can be used in primary cutaneous B-cell lymphomas, which do not respond to usual measures or recur. Because of the high cost, its use should be restricted to difficult situations. We recommend performing immunohistochemistry for CD20 before the treatment is initiated since those cutaneous B-cell lymphomas which fail to express CD20 are less responsive.

Practical Application

According to the recommendations of the manufacturer, the antibody should be given intravenously by slow infusion in a dosage of 375 mg/m^2 body surface every 4 weeks (24). This protocol clears CD20+ B-cells from the circulation for several months. Because of the great expense of high dose systemic use, topical approaches have been explored. Intralesional injection is reported to be well-tolerated in a dosage of 30 mg 3 times weekly (25).

Results

Remission can be induced in more than 70% of the patients, either by systemic use or by local injections with acceptable side effects (24). Nonaggressive primary cutaneous B-cell lymphomas respond excellently. The efficacy of this drug in the more aggressive diffuse large cell B-cell lymphomas still remains to be determined (24–27).

Combination with Other Modalities

Theoretically, this antibody can be combined with chemotherapy, IFN-α or even other biological response modifiers such as interleukin (IL) -2. Since experience is so limited, combinations are not yet recommended for treating cutaneous lymphomas.

Comments

This antibody is a powerful but expensive treatment tool for primary cutaneous B-cell lymphoma which should be explored in large multicenter trials.

Fusion Proteins

Introduction

Development of a number of receptor-targeted fusion toxins has been based on a detailed understanding of the structure–function relationships of both diphtheria toxin and pseudomonas exotoxin A, and availability of the nucleic acid sequences of each structural gene. The IL-2 receptor is an attractive target for T-cell-directed therapy. Agents including monoclonal antibodies, single-chain antibody immunoconjugates, radioimmunoconjugates, and, most recently, ligand fusion toxins have demonstrated activity in vitro and in clinical trials in both hematological malignancies and diseases characterized by proliferation of activated T-cells, such as graft vs. host disease (28). DAB389IL-2 and its predecessor DAB486IL-2 are ligand fusion toxins consisting of the full-length sequence of the IL-2 gene genetically fused to the enzymatically active and translocating domains of diphtheria toxin.

Mode of Action

These fusion toxins preferentially damage cells expressing the high-affinity IL-2 receptor in vitro and are active in a variety of animal model systems (29) DAB389IL-2 is able to bind selectively to the high-affinity IL-2R in a concentration-dependent manner, and once bound is internalized via receptor-mediated endocytosis. The ADP-ribosyltransferase activity of diphtheria toxin is cleaved in the endosome and is translocated into the cytosol where it inhibits protein synthesis, leading to apoptosis (30).

Interleukin-7 induces cell growth in hematological malignancies such as acute lymphoblastic leukemia, chronic lymphocytic leukemia, acute myelogenous leukemia, and Sézary syndrome (31). The recombinant fusion protein, DAB389IL-7, composed of the catalytic and transmembrane domains of diphtheria toxin (DT), fused to IL-7 may possess potential as a therapeutic agent against IL-7 receptor-bearing hematological malignancies (32).

Indications

The use of fusion protein therapeutics is indicated in all hematopoietic disorders, provided the tumor cells bear the respective receptor for which the fusion toxin is specifically constructed.

Practical Application

Treatment consists of DAB389IL-2 at 9 or 18 μg/kg as a 15 min intravenous infusion daily for 5 days every 3 weeks for eight cycles. Side effects such as myalgias, acute infusion-related hypersensitivity reactions (in 70% of patients), and vascular leak syndrome (VLS) with transient edema, hypoalbuminemia, and weight gain (in 27%) may be more common during the first cycle (28,33). Steroid premedication significantly improves the tolerability of DAB(389)IL-2 without compromising the clinical response (28).

Results

DAB(389)IL-2 and DAB(486)IL-2 were the first fusion toxins to be evaluated in CTCL patients who had already failed multiple approaches (34,35).

In a series of 35 patients with cutaneous T-cell lymphomas, objective response was achieved in 37% and complete response in 14% of the patients even in those with extensive erythroderma and tumor stage MF (36).

In a large multicenter study, the median time to response was 2 months and the duration of response was 2–39+ months. Approximately, half of the patients had significant titers of antibody to diphtheria toxin or to DAB389IL-2 at the time of enrollment, as compared with 92% with titers at the end of treatment. The presence of antibody did not preclude clinical response (37).

Combination with Other Modalities

The decreased efficiency of uptake by neoplastic cells which do not express the high-affinity IL-2R represents a potential limitation. Interleukin-1 alpha can increase the cytotoxicity of an IL-2-diphtheria toxin fusion protein against neoplastic lymphocytes by inducing high-affinity IL-2R expression (38).

Comments

The IL-2 fusion protein Ontak® is registered for the use in IL-2 receptor positive CTCL. These cases typically are advanced cases. We recommend this drug for patients in therapy-resistant stage IIb to IVb disease.

Acyclovir

Introduction

The use of the antiviral acyclovir in the treatment of cutaneous lymphoma was first reported by Resnick et al.(39). The positive therapeutic effect was confirmed by some authors (40), but not by others (41).

Mode of Action

Since herpes simplex virus, cytomegalovirus, Epstein–Barr virus and varicella-zoster do not play an etiologic role in CL and since HTLV-I virus, due to its lack of thymidine kinase, cannot activate ACV, the drug does not act in its usual antiviral role. Instead, the following mechanisms may explain its possible effectiveness in lymphoproliferative diseases: a direct cytopathic effect; activation of ACV by the thymidine kinase of viruses not yet detected in cutaneous lymphoproliferative disorders; or ACV activation by cellular thymidine kinase, which has been found to be elevated in lymphoproliferative disorders (40).

Indications

This treatment is a relatively risk-free alternative especially in rapidly proliferating lymphoproliferative disorders like lymphomatoid papulosis. There is little evidence for its effectiveness.

Practical Application

Acyclovir is given intravenously.

Results

We are aware of 23 patients (10 of our own, 13 reported in personal communications and in the literature) suffering from lymphoproliferative diseases who were treated with ACV. In 5 patients (3 of 18 with cutaneous T-cell lymphomas, 2 of 5 with lymphomatoid papulosis) , partial remission was achieved (40). Intravenous acyclovir for treatment of disseminated herpes zoster resulted in almost complete disappearance of generalized erythroderma and pruritus in a patient with Sézary syndrome (42).

Post-transplantation cutaneous B-cell lymphomas with (43) or without (44) monoclonal Epstein–Barr virus infection have responded to acyclovir along with a reduction in immunosuppression.

Combination with Other Modalities

There are no limitations for combining acyclovir with other modalities of therapy in cutaneous lymphomas.

Interleukin-2

Introduction

Interleukin-2 is a recombinant cytokine that is used for the treatment of melanomas and renal cell carcinomas. Although it was originally described as T-cell growth factor, it does not promote the growth of tumor cells derived from cutaneous T-cell lymphomas (45).

Mode of Action

Interleukin-2 stimulates the activity of T-lymphocytes and natural killer cells. These effectors are able to kill tumor cell populations not only in cutaneous T-cell lymphomas but also cutaneous B-cell lymphomas.

Indications

Theoretically, IL-2 could be employed in cutaneous B-cell lymphomas or in cutaneous T-cell lymphomas that are characterized by a T-helper 2 cytokine profile (46). Since recombinant IL-2 was not further developed, there is very limited information on other modes of application such as subcutaneous or intralesional injection.

Practical Application

We have used IL-2 in a combined intravenous/subcutaneous application modus (47) or in intralesional therapy. Daily dosage was between 0.5 and 2 mg.

Results

Interleukin-2 was administered by continuous infusion at relatively high doses for several days during a phase II multicenter study for various types of lymphoma. During this study, several cases of MF were treated and 5 out of 7 patients responded (48).

Combination with Other Modalities

Fritz et al.(47) reported the combined use of extracorporeal photopheresis, IFN-α, and IL-2 for Sézary syndrome.

Comments

Recombinant IL-2 still remains an experimental treatment for cutaneous T-cell lymphomas. Additional clinical studies are necessary to determine its value for these diseases.

Interleukin-12

Introduction

Interleukin-12 is a heterodimeric cytokine, supporting the development of T-helper 1 lymphocytes and cytotoxic lymphocytes.

Mode of Action

Several extensive investigations have shown that the tumor cell populations are characterized by the secretion of T-helper 2 associated cytokines such as IL-10 or IL-5 and cytokines inhibiting IFN-γ activities such as IK-protein (49). Therefore, the application of cytokines restoring the reduced T-helper 1 activity appears beneficial. Recombinant IL-12 was reported to restore the IFN-γ production of CTCL derived T-cells in vitro (50).

Indications

Recombinant IL-12 can be used in various stages of cutaneous T-cell lymphomas.

Practical Application

Dose levels ranged from 15 to 300 ng/kg per injection. Two injections per week were performed subcutaneously. Intralesional injection was also done. Treatment duration was up to 6 months.

Results

Overall response rate was reported to be approximately 50% in 32 patients (51).

Combination with Other Modalities

There is little information on combination therapies. Therefore, combinations should only be applied in the context of clinical trials.

Comments

Interleukin-12 holds promise for the treatment of cutaneous T-cell lymphomas based on the immune biology of these diseases (52). Its clinical role is not yet defined.

VACCINATION THERAPY

Introduction

Vaccination for the treatment of CTCL has the aim to achieve a tumor antigen-specific immune response against malignant T-cells. The specific targeting of tumor cells with activated cytolytic effector cells should ideally destroy tumor cells in the absence of significant side effects. Dendritic cell vaccination is a powerful vaccination approach which has been mainly used in melanoma (53). Recent evidence supports the notion that this approach might also be applicable to CTCL (54). Extracorporeal photopheresis, a well-established therapeutic approach in CTCL, has recently been proposed to be a form of DC vaccination (55).

Mode of Action

Evidence for an involvement of the immune system in disease pathogenesis stems from several lines of evidence. Early ultramorphological studies have demonstrated the close apposition of dendritic antigen presenting cells and CTCL cells. Pautrier microabscesses, a histological hallmark of CTCL, represent a collection of epidermal dendritic cells (Langerhans' cells) and intact/apoptotic/necrotic CTCL cells as well as keratinocytes. Migration of LCs from the epidermis is facilitated by the inflammatory environment of the typical MF lesions with lesional production of chemokines critical for DC migration. Inflamed CTCL lesions provide a constant migratory flow of tumor antigen-loaded DC towards draining lymph nodes and presentation of CTCL tumor antigens to the specific adaptive T-cell mediated immune system and to the generation of CTCL tumor antigen-specific effector cells. It is tempting to speculate that CTCL tumor antigen-specific immune response keeps the development of the disease in check and contributes to the well known slow development of the disease. The often-made observation that chemotherapy leads to short-term response with relapse of a more aggressive transformed tumor might be due to the fact that this type of treatment does not only destroy neoplastic helper T-cells but also tumor immunosurveillance mechanisms operative at the site of the lesion. It has been further demonstrated that CTCL skin lesions contain tumor-infiltrating lymphocytes (TIL) that express an activated phenotype (56). Presence of TILs in lesions of CTCL patients was positively correlated with long-term survival. MHC class I restricted cytotoxic CD4 as well as CD8+ T-cells have been isolated form CTCL lesions and shown to kill CTCL cells in a granzyme/perforin dependent pathway (57). Taken together, there is accumulating evidence about an ongoing immunosurveillance which keeps CTCL lesions in check, at the same time, immune escape mechanisms present in CTCL lesions might overcome the immunosurveillance system.

There is evidence for immune escape mechanisms operative at the tumor site. Production of the inhibitory cytokine TGF beta by CTCL cells might lead to inhibition of the antitumor response through suppressive effects on the proliferation, differentiation, and activation of CTL responses, specifically through inhibition of IL-12 and its signaling. Recent in vitro data suggest that expression of natural killer cell inhibitory receptors leads to the inhibition of CTCL specific T-cell responses (58). As TGF beta has been shown to increase the expression of NK inhibitory receptors on T-lymphocytes, these mechanisms could act synergistically to decrease the antitumor specific T-cell response in CTCL patients.

Indication

There are few available data regarding DC vaccination for CTCL. Early pilot data suggest that DC vaccination induces immune responses as well as clinical responses in selected CTCL patients (54). Patients with lower tumor burden seem to respond better.

Practical Application

Dendritic cells are generated ex vivo from monocyte precursors in the presence of cytokines such as IL-4, GM-CSF, and further maturation stimuli. Dendritic cells are incubated with autologous tumor lysate, washed extensively, and injected into uninvolved inguinal lymph nodes. Injections are preformed every two weeks; both immune and clinical response is evaluated after eight injections (54).

Comments

Proof of principle studies in CTCL patients suggests that vaccination approaches might be successful in this disease. CTCL generally takes a slow course and can be followed with molecular markers (e.g., TCR gene rearrangement analysis). Furthermore, correlation of vaccine administration with the clinical course is easily established. CTCL might be especially suited for pilot trials in future vaccine approaches.

Adenoviral Vector Encoding for Human Interferon-γ (TG1042)

Introduction

TG1042 is an adenoviral vector of the 3rd generation encoding the gene for IFN-γ under the control of a cytomegalovirus promoter.

Mode of Action

The vector is injected into lesions of cutaneous lymphomas and induces the local production of IFN-γ. For T-cell lymphoma, we know that IFN-γ is counteracting the local cytokine milieu since the tumor cells express IL-10 (59) and the interferon inhibiting cytokine IK (49). In cutaneous B-cell lymphomas, it interferes with the cytokine milieu of the follicular center cell reaction.

Indications

Early reports indicate that it can be used for MF, CD30+ lymphoproliferative disorders, follicular B-cell lymphomas and marginal zone lymphomas.

Practical Application

TG1042 is weekly injected into the cutaneous tumor.

Results

In a pilot study with 9 patients with cutaneous lymphomas, we have observed regressions in MF, CD30+ lymphoproliferative disorders, and cutaneous B-cell lymphomas.

Combination with Other Modalities

TG1042 has only been used as monotherapy.

Comments

This adenoviral vector has been demonstrated to be effective in several types of cutaneous lymphomas. Additional studies are required.

REFERENCES

1. Hemmi H, Kaisho T, Takeuchi O, Sato S, Sanjo H, Hoshino K, Horiuchi T, Tomizawa H, Takeda K, Akira S. Small anti-viral compounds activate immune cells via the TLR7 MyD88-dependent signaling pathway. Nat Immunol 2002; 3:196–200.
2. Jurk M, Heil F, Vollmer J, Schetter C, Krieg AM, Wagner H, Lipford G, Bauer S. Human TLR7 or TLR8 independently confer responsiveness to the antiviral compound R-848. Nat Immunol 2002; 3:499.
3. Armant MA, Fenton MJ. Toll-like receptors: a family of pattern-recognition receptors in mammals. Genome Biol Rev 2002; 3:3011.
4. Suchin KR, Junkins-Hopkins JM, Rook AH. Treatment of stage IA cutaneous T-cell lymphoma with topical application of the immune response modifier imiquimod. Arch Dermatol 2002; 138:1137–1139.
5. Dummer R, Urosevic M, Kempf W, Kazakov D, Burg G. Imiquimod induces complete clearance of a PUVA resistant plaque in mycosis fungoides. Dermatology 2003; 207: 116–118 .
6. Leonard R, Hardy J, van Tienhoven G, Houston S, Simmonds P, David M, Mansi J. Randomized, double-blind, placebo-controlled, multicenter trial of 6% miltefosine solution, a topical chemotherapy in cutaneous metastases from breast cancer. J Clin Oncol 2001; 19:4150–4159.

7. Dummer R, Krasovec M, Roger J, Sindermann H, Burg G. Topical administration of hexadecylphosphocholine in patients with cutaneous lymphomas: results of a phase I/II study. J Am Acad Dermatol 1993; 29:963–970.
8. Detmar M, Geilen CC, Wieder T, Orfanos CE, Reutter W. Phospholipid analogue hexadecylphosphocholine inhibits proliferation and phosphatidylcholine biosynthesis of human epidermal keratinocytes in vitro. J Invest Dermatol 1994; 102:490–494.
9. Smorenburg CH, Seynaeve C, Bontenbal M, Planting AS, Sindermann H, Verweij J. Phase II study of miltefosine 6% solution as topical treatment of skin metastases in breast cancer patients. Anticancer Drugs 2000; 11:825–828.
10. Ibbotson SH, Morton CA, Brown SB, Collins S, Ibbotson S, Jenkinson H, Kurwa H, Langmack K, McKenna K, Moseley H, Pearse AD, Stringer M, Taylor DK, Wong G, Rhodes LE. Topical 5-aminolaevulinic acid photodynamic therapy for the treatment of skin conditions other than non-melanoma skin cancer. Guidelines for topical photodynamic therapy: report of a workshop of the British Photodermatology Group. Br J Dermatol 2002; 146:178–188.
11. Svanberg K, Andersson T, Killander D, Wang I, Stenram U, Andersson Engels S, Berg R, Johansson J, Svanberg S. Photodynamic therapy of non-melanoma malignant tumours of the skin using topical delta-amino levulinic acid sensitization and laser irradiation. Br J Dermatol 1994; 130:743–751.
12. Grebenova D, Cajthamlova H, Bartosova J, Marinov J, Klamova H, Fuchs O, Hrkal Z, Holada K, Jirsa M. Selective destruction of leukaemic cells by photo-activation of 5-aminolaevulinic acid-induced protoporphyrin-IX. Photodynamic effects of meso-tetra (4-sulfonatophenyl) porphine on human leukemia cells HEL and HL60, human lymphocytes and bone marrow progenitor cells. J Photochem Photobiol B 1998; 47:74–81.
13. Boehncke WH, Konig K, Ruck A, Kaufmann R, Sterry W. In vitro and in vivo effects of photodynamic therapy in cutaneous T cell lymphoma. Acta Derm Venereol 1994; 74:201–205.
14. Kalka K, Merk H, Mukhtar H. Photodynamic therapy in dermatology. J Am Acad Dermatol 2000; 42:389–413.
15. Shandler SD, Wan W, Whitaker JE. Photodynamic therapy with topical delta-aminolevulinic acid for the treatment of cutaneous carcinomas and cutaneous T-cell lymphoma. J Invest Dermatol 1993; 100(602):680A.
16. Ammann R, Hunziker T. Photodynamic therapy for mycosis fungoides after topical photosensitization with 5-aminolevulinic acid. J Am Acad Dermatol 1995; 33:541.
17. Wolf P, Fink Puches R, Reimann Weber A, Kerl H. Development of malignant melanoma after repeated topical photodynamic therapy with 5-aminolevulinic acid at the exposed site. Dermatology 1997; 194:53–54.
18. Leman JA, Dick DC, Morton CA. Topical 5-ALA photodynamic therapy for the treatment of cutaneous T-cell lymphoma. Clin Exp Dermatol 2002; 27:516–518.
19. Markham T, Sheahan K, Collins P. Topical 5-aminolaevulinic acid photodynamic therapy for tumour-stage mycosis fungoides. Br J Dermatol 2001; 144:1262–1263.
20. Orenstein A, Haik J, Tamir J, Winkler E, Trau H, Malik Z, Kostenich G. Photodynamic therapy of cutaneous lymphoma using 5-aminolevulinic acid topical application. Dermatol Surg 2000; 26:765–769.
21. Eich D, Eich HT, Otte HG, Ghilescu V, Stadler R. Photodynamische Therapie kutaner T-zell-lymphome in besonderer lokalisation. Hautarzt 1999; 50:109–114.
22. Edstrom DW, Ros AM, Porwit A. Topical 5-aminolevulinic acid based photodynamic therapy for mycosis fungoides: a study of cell proliferation and apoptosis before and after therapy. J Dermatol Sci 1998; 16:229.
23. Shan D, Ledbetter JA, Press OW. Apoptosis of malignant human B cells by ligation of CD20 with monoclonal antibodies. Blood 1998; 91:1644–1652.
24. Heinzerling L, Dummer R, Kempf W, Hess-Schmid M, Burg G. Intralesional therapy with anti-CD20-antibody in primary cutaneous B-cell Lymphoma. Arch Derm 2000; 136:374–378.

25. Paul T, Radny P, Krober SM, Paul A, Blaheta HJ, Garbe C. Intralesional rituximab for cutaneous B-cell lymphoma. Br J Dermatol 2001; 144:1239–1243.

26. Heinzerling ML, Urbanek M, Funk JO, Peker S, Bleck O, Neuber K, Burg G, von den Driesch P, Dummer R. Reduction of tumor burden and stablization of disease by systemic therapy with anti-CD20 antibody (rituximab) in patients with primary cutaneous B-cell lymphomas. Cancer 2000; 89:1835–1844.

27. Gellrich S, Muche JM, Pelzer K, Audring H, Sterry W. Der anti-CD20-antikorper bei primar kutanen B-zell-lymphomen. Erste erfahrungen in der dermatologischen anwendung [Anti-CD20 antibodies in primary cutaneous B-cell lymphoma. Initial results in dermatologic patients]. Hautarzt 2001; 52:205–210.

28. Foss FM, Bacha P, Osann KE, Demierre MF, Bell T, Kuzel T. Biological correlates of acute hypersensitivity events with DAB(389)IL-2 (denileukin diftitox, ONTAK) in cutaneous T-cell lymphoma: decreased frequency and severity with steroid premedication. Clin Lymphoma 2001; 1:298–302.

29. Woodworth TG, Nichols JC. Recombinant fusion toxins—a new class of targeted biologic therapeutics. Cancer Treat Res 1993; 68:145–160.

30. Foss FM. DAB(389)IL-2 (ONTAK): a novel fusion toxin therapy for lymphoma. Clin Lymphoma 2000; 1:110–116, discussion 117.

31. Dalloul A, Laroche L, Bagot M, Mossalayi MD, Fourcade C, Thacker DJ, Hogge DE, Merle BH, Debre P, Schmitt C. Interleukin-7 is a growth factor for Sezary lymphoma cells. J Clin Invest 1992; 90:1054–1060.

32. Sweeney EB, Foss FM, Murphy JR, van der Spek JC. Interleukin 7 (IL-7) receptor-specific cell killing by DAB389 IL-7: a novel agent for the elimination of IL-7 receptor positive cells. Bioconjug Chem 1998; 9:201–207.

33. Duvic M, Cather J, Maize J, Frankel AE. DAB389IL2 diphtheria fusion toxin produces clinical responses in tumor stage cutaneous T cell lymphoma. Am J Hematol 1998; 58:87–90.

34. Hesketh P, Caguioa P, Koh H, Dewey H, Facada A, McCaffrey R, Parker K, Nylen P, Woodworth T. Clinical activity of a cytotoxic fusion protein in the treatment of cutaneous T-cell lymphoma. J Clin Oncol 1993; 11:1682–1690.

35. Kuzel TM, Rosen ST, Gordon LI, Winter J, Samuelson E, Kaul K, Roenigk HH, Nylen P, Woodworth T. Phase I trial of the diphtheria toxin/interleukin-2 fusion protein DAB486IL-2: efficacy in mycosis fungoides and other non-Hodgkin's lymphomas. Leuk Lymphoma 1993; 11:369–377.

36. Saleh MN, LeMaistre CF, Kuzel TM, Foss F, Platanias LC, Schwartz G, Ratain M, Rook A, Freytes CO, Craig F, Reuben J, Sams MW, Nichols JC. Antitumor activity of DAB389IL-2 fusion toxin in mycosis fungoides. J Am Acad Dermatol 1998; 39:63–73.

37. LeMaistre CF, Saleh MN, Kuzel TM, Foss F, Platanias LC, Schwartz G, Ratain M, Rook A, Freytes CO, Craig F, Reuben J, Nichols JC. Phase I trial of a ligand fusion-protein (DAB389IL-2) in lymphomas expressing the receptor for interleukin-2. Blood 1998; 91:399–405.

38. Salard D, Kuzel TM, Samuelson E, Rosen S, Bakouche O. Interleukin-1 alpha increases the preferential cytotoxicity of an interleukin-2-diphtheria toxin fusion protein against neoplastic lymphocytes from patients with the Sezary syndrome compared to normal lymphocytes. J Clin Immunol 1998; 18:223–234.

39. Resnick L, Schleider KN, Horwitz SN, Frost P. Remission of tumor-stage mycosis fungoides following intravenously administered acyclovir. JAMA 1984; 251:1571–1573.

40. Burg G, Klepzig K, Kaudewitz P, Wolff H, Braun-Falco O. Acyclovir in mycosis fungoides and lymphomatoid papulosis. Hautarzt 1986; 37:533–536.

41. Mahrle G, Thiele B, Steigleder GK. Treatment of mycosis fungoides with Zovirax (acyclovir). Study of 2 patients. Z Hautkr 1985; 60:602–607.

42. Scheman AJ, Steinberg I, Taddeini L. Abatement of Sezary syndrome lesions following treatment with acyclovir. Am J Med 1986; 80:1199–1202.

43. Mozzanica N, Cattaneo A, Fracchiolla N, Boneschi V, Berti E, Gronda E, Mangiavacchi M, Finzi AF, Neri A. Posttransplantation cutaneous B-cell lymphoma with monoclonal Epstein–Barr virus infection, responding to acyclovir and reduction in immunosuppression. J Heart Lung Transplant 1997; 16:964–968.

44. Wong R, Harrison P. Non EBV-related B-cell lymphoma in a renal transplant patient responding to acyclovir and reduction in immunosuppression. Postgrad Med 1992; J 1992 145–146.

45. Dobbeling U, Dummer R, Laine E, Potoczna N, Qin JZ, Burg G. Interleukin-15 is an autocrine/paracrine viability factor for cutaneous T-cell lymphoma cells. Blood 1998; 92:252–258.

46. Dummer R, Heald PW, Nestle FO, Ludwig E, Laine E, Hemmi S, Burg G. Sézary syndrome's T-cell clones display T helper 2 cytokines and express the accessory factor-1 (interferon gamma receptor beta chain). Blood 1996; 88:1383–1389.

47. Fritz T, Kleinhans M, Nestle F, Burg G, Dummer R. Combination treatment with extracorporeal photopheresis, Interferon alfa and interleukin-2 in a patient with the Sézary syndrome. Br J Dermatol 1999; 140:1144–1147.

48. Gisselbrecht C, Maraninchi D, Pico JL, Milpied N, Coiffier B, Divine M, Tiberghien P, Bosly A, Tilly H, Boulat O, et al. Interleukin-2 treatment in lymphoma: a phase II multicenter study. Blood 1994; 83:2081–2085.

49. Willers J, Haeffner A, Zepter K, Storz M, Urosevic M, Burg G, Dummer R. The interferon inhibiting cytokine IK is overexpressed in cutaneous T cell lymphoma derived tumor cells that fail to upregulate major histocompatibility complex class II upon interferon-gamma stimulation. J Invest Dermatol 2001; 116:874–879.

50. Rook AH, Kubin M, Cassin M, Vonderheid EC, Vowels BR, Wolfe JT, Wolf SF, Singh A, Trinchieri G, Lessin SR. IL-12 reverses cytokine and immune abnormalities in Sezary syndrome. J Immunol 1995; 154:1491–1498.

51. Rook AH, Zaki MH, Wysocka M, Wood GS, Duvic M, Showe LC, Foss F, Shapiro M, Kuzel TM, Olsen EA, Vonderheid EC, Laliberte R, Sherman ML. The role for interleukin-12 therapy of cutaneous T cell lymphoma. Ann N Y Acad Sci 2001; 941:177–184.

52. Dummer R, Willers J, Kamarashev J, Urosevic M, Döbbeling U, Burg G. Pathogenesis of cutaneous lymphomas. Semin Cutan Med Surg 2000; 19:78–86.

53. Nestle FO, Banchereau J, Hart D. Dendritic cells: On the move from bench to bedside. Nat Med 2001; 7:761–765.

54. Maier T, Tun-Kyi A, Tassis A, Jungius KP, Burg G, Dummer R, Nestle FO. Vaccination of cutaneous T-cell lymphoma patients using intranodal injection of autologous tumor lysate pulsed dendritic cells. Blood 2003;102:2338–2344.

55. Edelson RL. Cutaneous T cell lymphoma: the helping hand of dendritic cells. Ann N Y Acad Sci 2001; 941:1–11.

56. Wood GS. Lymphocyte activation in cutaneous T-cell lymphoma. J Invest Dermatol 1995; 105:105S–109S.

57. Echchakir H, Bagot M, Dorothee G, Martinvalet D, Le Gouvello S, Boumsell L, Chouaib S, Bensussan A, Mami-Chouaib F. Cutaneous T cell lymphoma reactive CD4+ cytotoxic T lymphocyte clones display a Th1 cytokine profile and use a fas-independent pathway for specific tumor cell lysis. J Invest Dermatol 2000; 115:74–80.

58. Bagot M, Martinvalet D, Echchakir H, Chabanette-Schirm F, Boumsell L, Bensussan A, Martinvallet D. Functional inhibitory receptors expressed by a cutaneous T cell lymphoma-specific cytolytic clonal T cell population. J Invest Dermatol 2000; 115:994–999.

59. Dummer R, Häffner AC, Hess M, Burg G. A rational approach to the therapy of cutaneous T-cell lymphomas. Onkologie 1996; 19:226–230.

Stage-Adjusted Treatment of Cutaneous Lymphomas: The Practical Approach

Günter Burg, Reinhard Dummer, Werner Kempf, Sonja Michaelis, Philippa Golling, and Frank O. Nestle
Department of Dermatology, University Hospital, Zürich, Switzerland

CUTANEOUS T-CELL LYMPHOMAS (CTCL)

CTCL is a heterogeneous group of rare diseases. Large randomized therapeutic trials with sufficient yet statistically significant stratification of subgroups are almost completely lacking (1). In addition, the early diagnosis in eczematous lesions is difficult, even if immunohistochemistry and molecular biology techniques are applied. In general, dermatopathologists in the United States use different criteria to establish the diagnosis of MF (2) and tend to avoid diagnoses such as small plaque parapsoriasis or large plaque parapsoriasis (an obligate precursor of MF). This fact has to be kept in mind when comparing American studies with European ones.

Thus, the utility of therapeutic guidelines for CTCL could be questioned. We believe that the following recommendations are at least useful for small cell CTCL such as MF, SS, and some cases of pleomorphic CTCL, which account for some 80% of the cases. In large cell primary CTCL with a solitary nodular skin lesion without extracutaneous disease (CD30+), aggressive local treatment such as surgery or radiotherapy may be sufficient. If multiple lesions are present, the treatment options discussed below have to be considered.

Since early aggressive treatment of CTCL does not improve the long-term disease-free period (3), stage-adapted therapy is currently recommended. The treatment approach depends on the extent and the aggressiveness of the CTCL, age of the patient, the presence of concurrent disease, the availability of various treatments, and the patient's compliance. The treatment suggestions summarized in Table 1 are based on published data (4).

Table 1 Recommendations for a Stage-Adapted Therapy for CTCL

Stage	Definition	Therapy
IA	Eczematous lesions and thin plaques, <10% of body surface	Nonaggressive, topical
IB	Eczematous lesions and thin plaques, >10% of body surface	Nonaggressive, topical, PUVA, HN2
IIA	Skin involvement with dermatopathic lymphadenopathy (N1)	1. PUVA + IFN-α 2. PUVA + retinoids 3. IFN-α + retinoids
IIB	Tumors with or without dermatopathic lymphadenopathy (N1)	Aggressive topical therapy: surgery, soft X-rays, total skin electron beam (TSEB) In case of progression or blastic transformation: systemic polychemotherapy
III	Erythroderma ($\pm$N1)	1. Extracorporeal photopheresis $\pm$ IFN-α/retinoics 2. PUVA + IFN-α 3. MTX, Chlorambucil + prednisone, electron beam, HN2
IVA/IVB	Specific involvement of lymph nodes (IVA) and dissemination with involvement of organs (IVB)	Systemic chemotherapy with or without radiotherapy
Lymph. Pap.		MTX, low dose

Source: From Ref. 4.

Stage Ia, Ib, and IIa

1. Heliotherapy, topical glucocorticosteroids, psoralens with UVA (PUVA) or retinoids with PUVA (Re-PUVA) (Europe).
2. Generalized topical nitrogen mustard (HN2, mechlorethamine) or topical carmustine (BCNU) (USA mainly).

If disease progression occurs: PUVA with IFN-α or retinoids with IFN-α, total skin electron beam therapy (TSEB), low dose chlorambucil, or methotrexate.

Stage IIb

1. PUVA with IFN-α or retinoids with IFN-α combined with soft X-ray radiation (6–8×200 cGy, 50 kV, twice/week).
2. TSEB with boost radiation to tumors with optional follow-up topical therapies to maintain response.

If disease progression occurs: systemic chemotherapy including mechlorethamine, CHOP (cyclophosphamide, vincristine, adriamycin, and prednisone) and high dose chlorambucil plus prednisone.

Stage III

1. Photopheresis. If no remission: add methotrexate or IFN-α in combination with retinoids.
2. IFN-α or PUVA with IFN-α low dose chlorambucil.

If disease progression occurs: palliative PUVA, topical HN2, teleroentgen or TSEB, IFN-α, retinoids, and systemic chemotherapy.

Stage IVa, IVb

Palliative treatment using systemic chemotherapy, interferons, retinoids, and photopheresis (if leukemic) or experimental protocols.

CUTANEOUS B-CELL LYMPHOMAS

The better prognosis of CBCL as compared to CTCL should be taken into consideration, when therapeutic strategies for CBCL are planned. Once again, the stage is the most important prognostic factor and appropriate treatment of CBCL depends on the results of the staging procedures. Besides systemic or intralesional steroids, combination with systemic antibiotic therapy (5) may be effective in some cases. PUVA therapy is another possible approach for superficial CBCL. For solitary lesions without extracutaneous involvement, radiotherapy or surgical excision are the preferred first line treatment modalities (6–8).

In advanced stages, chemotherapy may be indicated. Most polychemotherapy regimens including CHOP (cyclophosphamide, doxorubicin, vincristine, and prednisone with or without bleomycin), CVP (cyclophosphamide, vincristine, and prednisone) or ACVD (doxorubicin, cyclophosphamide, vindesine, bleomycin, and prednisone) are able to induce complete remissions in CBCL patients (9). When discussing treatment options, one has to keep in mind that aggressive treatment has not been shown to improve survival of these patients.

REFERENCES

1. Vonderheid EC, Micaily B. Treatment of cutaneous T-cell lymphoma. Dermatol Clin 1985; 3:673–687.
2. King ID, Ackerman AB. Guttate parapsoriasis/digitate dermatosis (small plaque parapsoriasis) is mycosis fungoides [see comments]. Am J Dermatopathol 1992; 14:518–530.
3. Kaye FJ, Bunn PJ, Steinberg SM, Stocker JL, Ihde DC, Fischmann AB, Glatstein EJ, Schechter GP, Phelps RM, Foss FM, Parlette H, Anderson M, Sausville E. A randomized trial comparing combination electron-beam radiation and chemotherapy with topical therapy in the initial treatment of mycosis fungoides. N Engl J Med 1989; 321:1784–1790.
4. Dummer R, Häffner AC, Hess M, Burg G. A rational approach to the therapy of cutaneous T-cell lymphomas (CTCL). Onkologie 1996; 19:226–230.
5. Cerroni L, Signoretti S, Hofler G, Annessi G, Putz B, Lackinger E, Metze D, Giannetti A, Kerl H. Primary cutaneous marginal zone B-cell lymphoma: a recently described entity of low-grade malignant cutaneous B-cell lymphoma. Am J Surg Pathol 1997; 21:1307–1315.
6. Santucci M, Pimpinelli N, Arganini L. Primary cutaneous B-cell lymphoma: a unique type of low-grade lymphoma. Clinicopathologic and immunologic study of 83 cases. Cancer 1991; 67:2311–2326.
7. Watsky KL, Longley BJ, Dvoretzky I. Primary cutaneous B-cell lymphoma. Diagnosis, treatment, and prognosis. J Dermatol Surg Oncol 1992; 18:951–954.
8. Zemtsov A, Camisa C. Treatment of primary cutaneous B cell lymphoma with local radiotherapy. Cutis 1990; 45:435–438.
9. Joly P, Thomine E, Lauret P. Cutaneous lymphomas other than mycosis fungoides. Semin Dermatol 1994; 13:172–179.

48

Prognosis

48.1. Prognostic Parameters in Cutaneous Lymphomas

Günter Burg, Werner Kempf, and Monika Hess Schmid
Department of Dermatology, University Hospital, Zürich, Switzerland

The course and prognosis of cutaneous lymphomas (CL) differs significantly from that of their nodal lymphomas with similar histological and cytological features. Moreover, there is a broad variety in biologic behavior among the various types of CL. To assess prognosis in an individual patient is of importance for the choice of an adequate therapeutic strategy. The prognostic parameters that have been identified over the last few years are described. In addition, a prognostic index is presented which may serve as a method to assess prognosis in individual patients.

PROGNOSTIC PARAMETERS IN CUTANEOUS T-CELL LYMPHOMAS

Various prognostic parameters have been identified in CTCL, which are summarized in Table 1 and described in more detail. The clinical stage at the time of diagnosis, determined by either the TNM staging system or the tumor burden index (TBI) (see Chapter 11), represents the most relevant prognostic factor. In addition to clinical stage of the disease, there are many additional parameters, including histological features, immunophenotype of the tumor cells, presence of tumor cells in the peripheral blood, and serological findings.

Clinical Parameters

The most important clinical parameter is the stage of the disease, as discussed in Chapter 11 (1,2). TNM stages 1 and 2 do much better than stages with erythroderma or extracutaneous involvement stages 3 and 4.

Other prognostic parameters are ulceration of tumors (3), bone marrow involvement (4), size of atypical circulating cells ($<11\,nm$, $>11\,nm$) (5), and percentage of T cells in the peripheral blood (more or less than 55%) (6). Detection of a peripheral blood T-cell clone seems to be an independent prognostic marker in mycosis fungoides (7).

Table 1 Prognostic Parameters in Cutaneous T-cell Lymphomas

	Favorable prognosis	Poor prognosis
Demographic factors		
Race	White	Black
Age	Young	Advanced
Sex	Identical	Identical
Occupation in manufacturing industry	No	Yes
Clinical parameters		
T-stages	1,2	3,4
Percentage of skin involvement	<25	>25
Ulceration of skin lesions	No	Yes
Involvement of lymph nodes and visceral organs	No	Yes
Bone marrow involvement	No	Yes
Peripheral blood involvement	No	Yes
Size of atypical circulating cells (nm)	<11	>11
Percentage of T cells in the peripheral blood	>55	<55
Oral manifestation	No	Yes
Histopathology		
Cytomorphology	Pleomorphic,small-cell	Immunoblastic/anaplastic
Nuclear volume (nm^3)	<104	>104
Large cell lymphoma (LCL)	Solitary	Multiple
Cytological transformation	No	Yes
Tumor thickness	Thin	Thick
Granulomatous features	Identical	Identical
Hemophagocytosis	No	Yes
DNA cytophotometry	Diploid	Ana-/tetraploid
Immunophenotype		
HML-1	Positive	Negative
CD	4+, 8−	4−, 8+

	Primary	Secondary
Ki-1 positivity		
CD8+	2+, 7−	2−, 7+
Epidermal Langerhans cells (LC)	>90 cells/mm² [188 LC/1000 lyc]	<90 cells/m³ [34 LC/1000 lyc]
Transferrin receptor expression (%)	25–75	100
Loss of antigens	No	Yes
LCL CD30+	Yes	No
Percentage of PCNA positive cells	Low	High
CD 28 (Leu 6) positive cells	Few	Many
Apoptosis (bcl-2−, FAS+)	−	+
Peripheral blood		
Atypical lymphocytes (per mm³)	<1000	>1000
CD4/CD8 ratio	<10	>10
Size of atypical circulating cells (nm)	<11	>11
Percentage of T cells	>55	<55
Aberrant loss of expression of pan T-cell markers	−	+
Serologic factors		
EBV antibodies	No	
Serum IL-2, IL-1	Low	High
LDH	Low	High

Histological Parameters
Infiltration

The thickness of the clinically thickest lesion (measured from the granular layer to the lower limit of the infiltrate, as in malignant melanoma) (8) has been reported to be significantly correlated with prognosis in CTCL, which is not surprising since the histologically measurable infiltrate correlates with the clinical stage of the disease: patchy eczematous lesions histologically show a patchy infiltrate in the papillary dermis; in the plaque stage, there is a dense subepidermal infiltrate, filling the papillary dermis, whereas in the tumor stage there is a dense, diffuse infiltrate reaching into or filling the reticular dermis and even the subcutaneous fat. The presence of granulomatous features in CTCL does not have prognostic implications, as cases with aggressive, but also with a prolonged, course have been described (9,10).

Nuclear Atypia

The nuclear contour index (NCI) taken alone has very poor diagnostic value (11). The combination of the NCI and the nuclear surface area has a highly significant prognostic value. The best electron microscopic discrimination between benign and mycosis fungoides groups occurred when the proportion of cells with an NCI of 7 or more and the proportion of cells with a nuclear profile area greater than $30 \, \mu m^2$ were used together (12). In one study, nuclear volume (more or less than $104 \, nm^3$) appeared to be a good prognostic indicator in plaque and tumor stage of mycosis fungoides (13).

Transformation

Histological and cytological transformation is thought to be associated with worsening of the prognosis (14–16). Transformation may be found even before progression of the disease (17). The prognosis of lymphoma complicated by hemophagocytosis is reported to be very poor (18–20).

DNA Cytometry

The prognostic significance of DNA cytometry in cutaneous malignant lymphomas (21) is of limited value today, as better markers for cytological characterization are available.

Immunophenotypic Markers
T-cell Markers

Aberrant loss or expression of pan-T-cell markers (loss of one or more of T-cell markers CD7, CD5, CD8, and rarely CD3) by flow cytometry in the peripheral blood is a poor prognostic marker in cutaneous T-cell lymphomas (14,22). Loss of antigenicity and prognosis do not necessarily correlate (23). Simultaneously occurring plaques and tumors in patients with mycosis fungoides and Sézary syndrome can show phenotypic deviation or loss of antigens on tumor cells between plaques and tumors, indicating that different immunophenotypes can occur simultaneously in an individual patient (24). TCRdelta1 expression in cutaneous lymphomas is an independent prognostic factor associated with decreased survival (25).

CD30

CD30 expression is an important prognostic parameter (26). A large study including more than 200 patients confirmed the favorable prognosis of primary cutaneous CD30(+) lymphoproliferative disorders and the close relationship between lymphomatoid papulosis and primary cutaneous CD30(+) lymphomas (27–32). The anaplastic morphology does not change the favorable biologic behavior.

Cytotoxic Phenotype

The expression of aberrant or suppressor T-cell phenotypes in CTCL is not of independent prognostic significance. Stage and histology are more important (33). Granzyme B (GrB) and T-cell-restricted intracellular antigen (TIA-1) are cytotoxic proteins that are specifically expressed by cytotoxic CD4 or CD8+ T cells and natural killer cells. Recent studies demonstrated frequent expression of GrB and TIA-1 by neoplastic cells in primary cutaneous CD30(+) large T-cell lymphomas and lymphomatoid papulosis, which both have a favorable prognosis, but not in CD30(–) large T-cell lymphomas, which have a poor prognosis (34). Correlation between GrB/TIA-1 expression biopsies taken sequentially from patches or plaques of patients with early stage mycosis fungoides did not give any evidence of these proteins being of prognostic significance (35).

Proliferation and Apoptosis

The apoptosis and proliferation indexes assessed using terminal deoxyuridine triphosphate (dUTP) -biotin nick end labeling (TUNEL) (36) or percentage of PCNA positive cells (37) may be useful markers in the determination of the prognosis for patients with lymphoproliferative disorders of the skin. A decrease in the number of bcl-2+ (antiapoptotic) cells and an increase in Fas+ cells were associated with disease progression (38). High proportions of CD8+ cytotoxic tumor infiltrating T cells in CTCL correlated with a better prognosis, suggesting that these cells could play an important role in the antitumor response (39). It has been speculated that Fas ligand expression by neoplastic T lymphocytes mediates elimination of CD8+ cytotoxic T lymphocytes in mycosis fungoides and provides a potential mechanism of tumor immune escape (40). A higher number of epidermal Langerhans cells assessed by staining with CD1a have been shown to correlate with better prognosis (24,41–43).

Chemokines and Their Receptors

Expression of the lymphocyte homing receptor CD44 and its splice variants has been linked to tumor dissemination and poor prognosis in non-Hodgkin lymphoma, while CD44v6 expression was associated with aggressive behavior of cutaneous lymphomas (44). These findings were not confirmed in other studies (45). The T-cell chemokine receptor CXCR3 is highly expressed in low-grade mycosis fungoides (46). Large cell transformation may be accompanied by loss of CXCR3 expression. In contrast, CLA expression levels in mycosis fungoides do not differ among low-grade and transformed cases (46). When progression from mycosis fungoides to Sézary syndrome occurs, a significant decrease in the number of IFN-producing T cells has been reported (47,48).

Serological Factors

Epstein–Barr Virus Antibodies

Epstein–Barr virus (EBV)-associated recurrent necrotic papulovesicle, simulating classic hydroa vacciniformia, are a distinct lymphoproliferative clinicopathologic entity with systemic involvement, development of lymphoma, and poor prognosis in most cases (49). Latent EBV infection has been reported to be frequently detected in subcutaneous lymphoma associated with hemophagocytosis (50–53).

Soluble Interleukin-2 Receptor

The degree of elevation of soluble interleukin-2 receptor (sIL-2R) levels was correlated with advanced clinical stage of disease and with increased numbers of PCNA positive cells (37). Although sIL-2R is not a specific parameter for cutaneous T-cell lymphoma, a value above 1000 units/mL is correlated with clinical disease activity and is a parameter indicating a serious prognosis (54). Elevated sIL-2R levels may account for diminished NK activity by neutralizing interleukin-2 in CTCL patients (55).

Selenium

Serum selenium concentrations were found to correlate with disease severity in cutaneous lymphoma. Before treatment, it was higher in CTCL with good response to treatment (89 ± 36) than in those without response (62 ± 30) ($p < 0.01$) (56).

Lactate Dehydrogenase

In an evaluation of prognostic parameters, serum LDH levels were significantly associated with survival (57).

PROGNOSTIC PARAMETERS IN CUTANEOUS B-CELL LYMPHOMAS

There is still no widely used system for staging classification of CBCL. Attempts have been made according to TNM (58,59), taking into account number of lesions and spread of the disease. In contrast to CTCL, type and spread of tumor do not correlate well with prognosis in CBCL. Various prognostic parameters have been identified, as summarized in Table 2 and described in greater detail.

Clinical Parameters

Primary B-cell lymphomas of the skin differ significantly from nodal lymphomas (60). Almost 50% of cutaneous B-cell lymphoproliferative infiltrates are MALT-type lymphomas or are derived from follicle center cells (FCCs). Among these, about 25% show a rapidly progressive course, whereas about 75% account for flattening of the survival curve after about 7 years. The FCC-derived lymphomas of the skin most frequently occur in the head and neck area and have an excellent prognosis (61). When on the back, FCC-derived lymphomas—originally referred to as "reticulohistiocytosis dorsi" by Crosti (62,63)—also have a favorable prognosis (64). Primary cutaneous large B-cell lymphoma of the legs in elderly women has been considered a distinct type of cutaneous B-cell lymphoma with an intermediate or poor prognosis

Table 2 Prognostic Parameters in Cutaneous B-cell Lymphomas

	Favorable prognosis	Poor prognosis
Clinical parameters		
Localization	Head and neck	Lower leg
Distribution	Solitary or regional	Disseminated
Histopathology		
Growth pattern	Follicular	Diffuse
Cytomorphology	Large	Small
Admixture of plasma cells	+	−
Intravascular proliferation	−	+
Phenotype and cytogenetics		
bcl-2	−	+
t(14;18)	−	+
CD21	Present; regular networks	Absent or irregular networks

by some (65,66) and with the same prognosis as seen with the same cytological large cell type in any other localization by others (67).

Multicentricity of skin lesions rather than solitary lesions or lesions confined to one area of the body is significantly related to death (66,68,69). Others claim that the number, type, and localization of the lesions are not associated with variations in either survival or recurrence-free survival (70).

Histological Parameters

Growth Pattern

Follicular growth pattern has a more favorable prognosis than diffuse growth pattern composed of centroblasts and/or immunoblasts (large round cells) (71).

Intravascular proliferation of large neoplastic B cells within blood vessels has a poor prognosis (72–75).

Cytomorphology

The morphologic spectrum of large B-cell lymphoma is broad. Several unusual variants have been described, such as lymphoma with myxoid stroma, sclerosing B-cell lymphoma, signet ring-cell lymphoma, multilobated B-cell lymphoma, and epidermotropic B-cell lymphoma (76,77). The prognostic significance of these features has not been sufficiently studied. In a minor proportion of CBCL, the infiltrate is composed of small cleaved follicle center cells, as seen in nodal mantle cell lymphoma. The few reports available suggest a rather poor prognosis for cutaneous lymphomas with this morphology (78–80). Primary T-cell-rich B-cell lymphoma of the skin, in contrast to its nodal counterpart, shares a favorable diagnosis with most other types of CBCL (81).

Tumor-Infiltrating Lymphocytes

The presence and percentage of CD8+ tumor-infiltrating T cells have been shown to correlate with differentiation and prognosis in various neoplasms. The number of cytotoxic CD8+ cells in large B-cell lymphoma was significantly lower than in B-cell

Table 3 Prognostic Index for Cutaneous T-cell Lymphomas

Score class	1	2	3
Criterium			
Tumor Burden Index (TBI)	1	>1-3	>3
Stage (TNM)	Ia, Ib	IIa, IIb	III, IVa, IVb
Cytomorphology	Small	Medium	Large
Age at diagnosis (years)	<45	46–65	>65
Time prior to diagnosis (years)	<5	6–12	>12
Gender	–	F	M

pseudolymphomas, follicular lymphomas, and MALT-type lymphomas of the skin (82). The prognostic significance of these findings, however, is unclear.

Immunophenotypic Markers
Bcl-2

Expression of bcl-2 protein and t(14;18) translocation is found in most cases of nodal FCC lymphomas. Bcl-2 reactivity, however, is absent in FCC-derived B-cell lymphomas of the skin in the head, neck, and trunk areas, whereas it is frequently found in B-cell lymphomas of the leg (83), indicating a worse prognosis or a secondary manifestation of primary nodal lymphoma. Even though t(14;18) translocation and bcl-2 expression have been found to be present in a subset of primary cutaneous follicular lymphoma without site-specific differences (67,84), they are absent in most FCC-derived cases of the skin (85–87), indicating that the detection of a t(14;18) translocation in cutaneous B-cell lymphoma should suggest the presence of systemic disease (88,89).

Comparison between the bcl-2 and/or t(14;18)(q32;q21) -positive and t(14;18)(q32;q21) -negative cases revealed no significant difference in age, site, clinical course, or outcome (90).

Adhesion Molecules

A relation between the expression of adhesion molecules and the differences in clinical behavior between different groups of primary and secondary cutaneous follicle center cell lymphomas has been suggested (91). The expression of adhesion molecules ICAM-1 and LFA-1 was studied in prognostically different groups of cutaneous

Table 4 Groups Within the Prognostic Index (PI[a]; 1–3), Prognosis, and Survival Time in Cutaneous T-cell Lymphoma

PI range	Prognosis	Survival
1–1.3	Favorable	> 14 years
> 1.3–1.8	Good	9–14 years
> 1.8–2.4	Moderate	3–8 years
> 2.4–3.0	Poor	< 2 years

[a]PI(1–3): sum of score values divided by total number of prognostic criteria.

B-cell lymphomas. Absence of both ICAM-1 and LFA-1 on the neoplastic B cells was correlated with a poor prognosis (91).

Serological Factors

The occurrence of monoclonal gammopathy and paraproteinemia may be a hint for a plasmacytoma that is secreting immunoglobulins.

THE PROGNOSTIC INDEX

So far, no widely accepted scheme for the assessment of the prognosis of CL is available. We propose a prognostic index (PI), which can be calculated for each individual patient by dividing the sum of score classes by the number of criteria examined (Table 3).

The calculation of PI results in a value between 1 and 3, reflecting favorable (PI 1–1.3; survival > 14 years), good (PI 1.3–1.8; survival 9–14 years), moderate (PI 1.8–2.4; survival 3–8 years), and poor (PI 2.4–3.0; survival < 2 years) prognosis, as shown in Table 4.

In the patients studied so far (unpublished results), this ranking (1–3) system significantly correlates with survival time.

REFERENCES

1. Lamberg SI, Bunn PJ. Proceedings of the Workshop on Cutaneous T-Cell Lymphomas (Mycosis Fungoides and Sézary Syndrome). Introduction. Cancer Treat Rep 1979; 63:561–564.
2. Hoppe RT, Wood GS, Abel EA. Mycosis fungoides and the Sézary syndrome: pathology, staging, and treatment. Curr Probl Cancer 1990; 14:293–371.
3. Helm KF, Su WP, Muller SA, Kurtin PJ. Malignant lymphoma and leukemia with prominent ulceration: clinicopathologic correlation of 33 cases. J Am Acad Dermatol 1992; 27:553–559.
4. Graham SJ, Sharpe RW, Steinberg SM, Cotelingam JD, Sausville EA, Foss FM. Prognostic implications of a bone marrow histopathologic classification system in mycosis fungoides and the Sézary syndrome. Cancer 1993; 72:726–734.
5. Schechter GP, Sausville EA, Fischmann AB, Soehnlen F, Eddy J, Matthews M, Gazdar A, Guccion J, Munson D, Makuchal R. Evaluation of circulating malignant cells provides prognostic information in cutaneous T cell lymphoma. Blood 1987; 69:841–849.
6. van der Loo E, Meijer CJ, Scheffer E, van Vloten WA. The prognostic value of membrane markers and morphometric characteristics of lymphoid cells in blood and lymph nodes from patients with mycosis fungoides. Cancer 1981; 48:738–744.
7. Fraser-Andrews EA, Woolford AJ, Russell-Jones R, Seed PT, Whittaker SJ. Detection of a peripheral blood T cell clone is an independent prognostic marker in mycosis fungoides. J Invest Dermatol 2000; 114:117–121.
8. Marti RM, Estrach T, Reverter JC, Mascaro JM. Prognostic clinicopathologic factors in cutaneous T-cell lymphoma. Arch Dermatol 1991; 127:1511–1516.
9. Fischer M, Wohlrab J, Audring TH, Sterry W, Marsch WC. Granulomatous mycosis fungoides. Report of two cases and review of the literature. J Eur Acad Dermatol Venereol 2000; 14:196–202.
10. Dabski K, Stoll HL Jr. Granulomatous reactions in mycosis fungoides. J Surg Oncol 1987; 34:217–229.
11. Simon GT. The value of morphometry in the ultrastructural diagnosis of mycosis fungoides. Ultrastruct Pathol 1987; 11:687–691.

12. McNutt NS, Heilbron DC, Crain WR. Mycosis fungoides: diagnostic criteria based on quantitative electron microscopy. Lab Invest 1981; 44:466–474.

13. Brooks B, Sorensen FB, Thestrup-Pedersen K. Estimates of nuclear volume in plaque and tumor-stage mycosis fungoides. A new prognostic indicator. Am J Dermatopathol 1994; 16:599–606.

14. Salhany KE, Cousar JB, Greer JP, Casey TT, Fields JP, Collins RD. Transformation of cutaneous T cell lymphoma to large cell lymphoma. A clinicopathologic and immunologic study. Am J Pathol 1988; 132:265–277.

15. Dmitrovsky E, Matthews MJ, Bunn PA, Schechter GP, Makuch RW, Winkler CF, Eddy J, Sausville EA, Ihde DC. Cytologic transformation in cutaneous T cell lymphoma: a clinicopathologic entity associated with poor prognosis. J Clin Oncol 1987; 5:208–215.

16. Cerroni L, Rieger E, Hodl S, Kerl H. Clinicopathologic and immunologic features associated with transformation of mycosis fungoides to large-cell lymphoma. Am J Surg Pathol 1992; 16:543–552.

17. Vergier B, de Muret A, Beylot-Barry M, Vaillant L, Ekouevi D, Chene G, Carlotti A, Franck N, Dechelotte P, Souteyrand P, Courville P, Joly P, Delaunay M, Bagot M, Grange F, Fraitag S, Bosq J, Petrella T, Durlach A, De Mascarel A, Merlio JP, Wechsler J. Transformation of mycosis fungoides: clinicopathological and prognostic features of 45 cases. French Study Group of Cutaneous Lymphomas. Blood 2000; 95:2212–2218.

18. Chan YF, Lee KC, Llewellyn H. Subcutaneous T-cell lymphoma presenting as panniculitis in children: report of two cases. Pediatr Pathol 1994; 14:595–608.

19. Romero LS, Goltz RW, Nagi C, Shin SS, Ho AD. Subcutaneous T-cell lymphoma with associated hemophagocytic syndrome and terminal leukemic transformation. J Am Acad Dermatol 1996; 34:904–910.

20. Nakajima A, Abe T, Takagi T, Satoh N, Sakuragi S, Miura I, Wakui H, Oshima A, Horiuchi T, Ono S, Miura AB. Two cases of malignant lymphoma complicated by hemophagocytosis resembling orbital cellulitis. Jpn J Ophthalmol 1997; 41:186–191.

21. Vogt T, Stolz W, Braun-Falco O, Kaudewitz P, Eckert F, Abmayr W, Dummer R, Burg G. Prognostic significance of DNA cytometry in cutaneous malignant lymphomas. Cancer 1991; 68:1095–1100.

22. Vonderheid EC, Bernengo MG, Burg G, Duvic M, Heald P, Laroche L, Olsen E, Pittelkow M, Russell-Jones R, Takigawa M, Willemze R. Update on erythrodermic cutaneous T-cell lymphoma: report of the International Society for Cutaneous Lymphomas. J Am Acad Dermatol 2002; 46:95–106.

23. Mukai HY, Hasegawa Y, Kojima H, Okoshi Y, Takei N, Yamashita Y, Nagasawa T, Mori N. Nodal CD8 positive cytotoxic T-cell lymphoma: a distinct clinicopathological entity. Mod Pathol 2002; 15:1131–1139.

24. Preesman AH, Toonstra J, van der Putte SC, van Vloten WA. Immunophenotyping on simultaneously occurring plaques and tumours in mycosis fungoides and Sézary syndrome. Br J Dermatol 1993; 129:660–666.

25. Toro JR, Liewehr DJ, Pabby N, Sorbara L, Raffeld M, Steinberg SM, Jaffe ES. Gamma delta ({gamma}{delta}) T-cell phenotype is associated with significantly decreased survival in cutaneous T-cell lymphoma. Blood 2003; 101:3407–3412.

26. Beljaards RC, Meijer CJ, Scheffer E, Toonstra J, van Vloten WA, van der Putte SC, Geerts ML, Willemze R. Prognostic significance of CD30 (Ki-1/Ber-H2) expression in primary cutaneous large-cell lymphomas of T-cell origin. A clinicopathologic and immunohistochemical study in 20 patients. Am J Pathol 1989; 135:1169–1178.

27. Kaudewitz P, Kind P, Sander CA. CD30+ anaplastic large cell lymphomas. Semin Dermatol 1994; 13:180–186.

28. Romaguera JE, Manning JT Jr, Tornos CS, Rodriguez J, Brooks TE, Pugh WC, Ordonez NG, Goodacre AM, Cabanillas F. Long-term prognostic importance of primary Ki-1 (CD30) antigen expression and anaplastic morphology in adult patients with diffuse large-cell lymphoma. Ann Oncol 1994; 5:317–322.

29. Beljaards RC, Meijer CJ, van der Putte SC, Hollema H, Geerts ML, Bezemer PD, Willemze R. Primary cutaneous T-cell lymphoma: clinicopathological features and prognostic parameters of 35 cases other than mycosis fungoides and CD30-positive large cell lymphoma. J Pathol 1994; 172:53–60.

30. Romaguera JE, Garcia-Foncillas J, Cabanillas F. 16-Year experience at M. D. Anderson Cancer Center with primary Ki-1 (CD30) antigen expression and anaplastic morphology in adult patients with diffuse large cell lymphoma. Leuk Lymphoma 1995; 20:97–102.

31. Paulli M, Berti E, Rosso R, Boveri E, Kindl S, Klersy C, Lazzarino M, Borroni G, Menestrina F, Santucci M. CD30/Ki-1-positive lymphoproliferative disorders of the skin—clinicopathologic correlation and statistical analysis of 86 cases: a multicentric study from the European Organization for Research and Treatment of Cancer Cutaneous Lymphoma Project Group. J Clin Oncol 1995; 13:1343–1354.

32. Bekkenk MW, Geelen FA, van Voorst Vader PC, Heule F, Geerts ML, van Vloten WA, Meijer CJ, Willemze R. Primary and secondary cutaneous CD30(+) lymphoproliferative disorders: a report from the Dutch Cutaneous Lymphoma Group on the long-term follow-up data of 219 patients and guidelines for diagnosis and treatment. Blood 2000; 95:3653–3661.

33. Ralfkiaer E, Wollf-Sneedorff A, Thomsen K, Vejlsgaard GL. Immunophenotypic studies in cutaneous T-cell lymphomas: clinical implications. Br J Dermatol 1993; 129:655–659.

34. Kummer JA, Vermeer MH, Dukers D, Meijer CJ, Willemze R. Most primary cutaneous CD30-positive lymphoproliferative disorders have a CD4-positive cytotoxic T-cell phenotype. J Invest Dermatol 1997; 109:636–640.

35. Vermeer MH, Geelen FA, Kummer JA, Meijer CJ, Willemze R. Expression of cytotoxic proteins by neoplastic T cells in mycosis fungoides increases with progression from plaque stage to tumor stage disease. Am J Pathol 1999; 154:1203–1210.

36. Kikuchi A, Nishikawa T. Apoptotic and proliferating cells in cutaneous lymphoproliferative diseases. Arch Dermatol 1997; 133:829–833.

37. Neish C, Charlry M, Jegasothy B, Tharp M, Deng JS. Proliferation cell nuclear antigen and soluble interleukin 2 receptor levels in cutaneous T cell lymphoma: correlation with advanced clinical diseases. J Dermatol Sci 1994; 8:11–17.

38. Nevala H, Karenko L, Vakeva L, Ranki A. Proapoptotic and antiapoptotic markers in cutaneous T-cell lymphoma skin infiltrates and lymphomatoid papulosis. Br J Dermatol 2001; 145:928–937.

39. Vermeer MH, van Doorn R, Dukers D, Bekkenk MW, Meijer CJ, Willemze R. CD8+ T cells in cutaneous T-cell lymphoma: expression of cytotoxic proteins, Fas ligand, and killing inhibitory receptors and their relationship with clinical behavior. J Clin Oncol 2001; 19:4322–4329.

40. Ni X, Hazarika P, Zhang C, Talpur R, Duvic M. Fas ligand expression by neoplastic T lymphocytes mediates elimination of CD8+ cytotoxic T lymphocytes in mycosis in mycosis fungoides: a potential mechanism of tumor immune escape? Clin Cancer Res 2001; 7:2685–2692.

41. Igisu K, Watanabe S, Shimosato Y, Kukita A. Langerhans cells and their precursors with S100 protein in mycosis fungoides. Jpn J Clin Oncol 1983; 13:693–702.

42. Meissner K, Michaelis K, Rehpenning W, Loning T. Epidermal Langerhans' cell densities influence survival in mycosis fungoides and Sézary syndrome. Cancer 1990; 65: 2069–2073.

43. Meissner K, Loning T, Rehpenning W. Epidermal Langerhans cells and prognosis of patients with mycosis fungoides and Sézary syndrome. In Vivo 1993; 7:277–280.

44. Dommann SN, Ziegler T, Dommann SC, Meyer J, Panizzon R, Burg G. CD44v6 is a marker for systemic spread in cutaneous T-cell lymphomas. A comparative study between nodal and cutaneous lymphomas. J Cutan Pathol 1995; 22:407–412.

45. Orteu CH, Li W, Allen MH, Smith NP, Barker JN, Whittaker SJ. CD44 variant expression in cutaneous T-cell lymphoma. J Cutan Pathol 1997; 24:342–349.

46. Lu D, Duvic M, Medeiros LJ, Luthra R, Dorfman DM, Jones D. The T-cell chemokine receptor CXCR3 is expressed highly in low-grade mycosis fungoides. Am J Clin Pathol 2001; 115:413–421.

47. Lee BN, Duvic M, Tang CK, Bueso-Ramos C, Estrov Z, Reuben JM. Dysregulated synthesis of intracellular type 1 and type 2 cytokines by T cells of patients with cutaneous T-cell lymphoma. Clin Diagn Lab Immunol 1999; 6:79–84.

48. Dummer R, Dobbeling U, Geertsen R, Willers J, Burg G, Pavlovic J. Interferon resistance of cutaneous T-cell lymphoma-derived clonal T-helper 2 cells allows selective viral replication. Blood 2001; 97:523–527.

49. Yoon TY, Yang TH, Hahn YS, Huh JR, Soo Y. Epstein–Barr virus-associated recurrent necrotic papulovesicles with repeated bacterial infections ending in sepsis and death: consideration of the relationship between Epstein–Barr virus infection and immune defect. J Dermatol 2001; 28:442–447.

50. Iwatsuki K, Harada H, Ohtsuka M, Han G, Kaneko F. Latent Epstein–Barr virus infection is frequently detected in subcutaneous lymphoma associated with hemophagocytosis but not in nonfatal cytophagic histiocytic panniculitis. Arch Dermatol 1997; 133:787–788.

51. Magana M, Sangueza P, Gil-Beristain J, Sanchez-Sosa S, Salgado A, Ramon G, Sangueza OP. Angiocentric cutaneous T-cell lymphoma of childhood (hydroa-like lymphoma): a distinctive type of cutaneous T-cell lymphoma. J Am Acad Dermatol 1998; 38:574–579.

52. Iwatsuki K, Xu Z, Takata M, Iguchi M, Ohtsuka M, Akiba H, Mitsuhashi Y, Takenoshita H, Sugiuchi R, Tagami H, Kaneko F. The association of latent Epstein–Barr virus infection with hydroa vacciniforme. Br J Dermatol 1999; 140:715–721.

53. Iwatsuki K, Xu Z, Ohtsuka M, Kaneko F. Cutaneous lymphoproliferative disorders associated with Epstein–Barr virus infection: a clinical overview. J Dermatol Sci 2000; 22:181–195.

54. Zachariae C, Larsen CS, Kaltoft K, Deleuran B, Larsen CG, Thestrup PK. Soluble IL2 receptor serum levels and epidermal cytokines in mycosis fungoides and related disorders. Acta Derm Venereol 1991; 71:465–470.

55. Dummer R, Posseckert G, Nestle F, Witzgall R, Burger M, Becker JC, Schafer E, Wiede J, Sebald W, Burg G. Soluble interleukin-2 receptor inhibit interleukin 2-dependent proliferation and cytotoxicity: explanation for diminished natural killer cell activity in cutaneous T-cell lymphomas in vivo? J Invest Dermatol 1992; 98:50–54.

56. Deffuant C, Celerier P, Boiteau HL, Litoux P, Dreno B. Serum selenium in melanoma and epidermotropic cutaneous T-cell lymphoma. Acta Derm Venereol 1994; 74:90–92.

57. Grange F, Hedelin G, Joly P, Beylot-Barry M, D'Incan M, Delaunay M, Vaillant L, Avril MF, Bosq J, Wechsler J, Dalac S, Grosieux C, Franck N, Esteve E, Michel C, Bodemer C, Vergier B, Laroche L, Bagot M. Prognostic factors in primary cutaneous lymphomas other than mycosis fungoides and the Sézary syndrome. The French Study Group on Cutaneous Lymphomas. Blood 1999; 93:3637–3642.

58. Burg G, Braun-Falco O. . Cutaneous Lymphomas, Pseudolymphomas, and Related Disorders. Berlin: Springer, 1983.

59. Burg G, Kerl H, Przybilla B, Braun-Falco O. Some statistical data, diagnosis, and staging of cutaneous B-cell lymphomas. J Dermatol Surg Oncol 1984; 10:256–262.

60. Kerl H, Cerroni L. Primary B-cell lymphomas of the skin. Ann Oncol 1997; 2(suppl 8):29–32.

61. Pimpinelli N, Santucci M, Bosi A, Moretti S, Vallecchi C, Messori A, Giannotti B. Primary cutaneous follicular centre-cell lymphoma—a lymphoproliferative disease with favourable prognosis. Clin Exp Dermatol 1989; 14:12–19.

62. Crosti A. Micosi fungoid e reticulo-istiocitomi cutanei maligni. Minerva Dermatol 1951; 26:3–11.

63. Cerutti P, Santoianni P. A relatively benign reticulosis: Crosti's "reticulohistiocytoma of the back". Int J Dermatol 1973; 12:35–40.

64. Berti E, Alessi E, Caputo R. Reticulohistiocytoma of the dorsum (Crosti's disease) and other B-cell lymphomas. Semin Diagn Pathol 1991; 8:82–90.

65. Vermeer MH, Geelen FA, van Haselen CW, van Voorst Vader PC, Geerts ML, van Vloten WA, Willemze R. Primary cutaneous large B-cell lymphomas of the legs. A distinct type of cutaneous B-cell lymphoma with an intermediate prognosis. Dutch Cutaneous Lymphoma Working Group. Arch Dermatol 1996; 132:1304–1308.

66. Grange F, Bekkenk MW, Wechsler J, Meijer CJ, Cerroni L, Bernengo M, Bosq J, Hedelin G, Fink Puches R, van Vloten WA, Joly P, Bagot M, Willemze R. Prognostic factors in primary cutaneous large B-cell lymphomas: a European multicenter study. J Clin Oncol 2001; 19:3602–3610.

67. Paulli M, Viglio A, Vivenza D, Capello D, Rossi D, Riboni R, Lucioni M, Incardona P, Boveri E, Bellosta M, Orlandi E, Borroni G, Lazzarino M, Berti E, Alessi E, Magrini U, Gaidano G. Primary cutaneous large B-cell lymphoma of the leg: histogenetic analysis of a controversial clinicopathologic entity. Hum Pathol 2002; 33:937–943.

68. Watsky KL, Longley BJ, Dvoretzky I. Primary cutaneous B-cell lymphoma. Diagnosis, treatment, and prognosis. J Dermatol Surg Oncol 1992; 18:951–954.

69. Kurtin PJ, DiCaudo DJ, Habermann TM, Chen MG, Su WP. Primary cutaneous large cell lymphomas. Morphologic, immunophenotypic, and clinical features of 20 cases. Am J Surg Pathol 1994; 18:1183–1191.

70. Fernandez-Vazquez A, Rodriguez-Peralto JL, Martinez MA, Platon EM, Algara P, Camacho FI, Lopez-Rios F, Zarco C, Sanchez-Yus E, Fresno MF, Barthe L, Aliaga A, Fraga M, Forteza J, Oliva H, Piris MA. Primary cutaneous large B-cell lymphoma: the relation between morphology, clinical presentation, immunohistochemical markers, and survival. Am J Surg Pathol 2001; 25:307–315.

71. Wechsler J, Bagot M. Primary cutaneous large B-cell lymphomas. Semin Cutan Med Surg 2000; 19:130–132.

72. Sheibani K, Battifora H, Winberg CD, Burke JS, Ben-Ezra J, Ellinger GM, Quigley NJ, Fernandez BB, Morrow D, Rappaport H. Further evidence that "malignant angioendotheliomatosis" is an angiotropic large-cell lymphoma. N Engl J Med 1986; 314:943–948.

73. Petroff N, Koger OW, Fleming MG, Fishelder A, Bergfeld WF, Tuthill R, Tubbs R. Malignant angioendotheliomatosis: an angiotropic lymphoma. J Am Acad Dermatol 1989; 21:727–733.

74. Perniciaro C, Winkelmann RK, Daoud MS, Su WP. Malignant angioendotheliomatosis is an angiotropic intravascular lymphoma. Immunohistochemical, ultrastructural, and molecular genetics studies. Am J Dermatopathol 1995; 17:242–248.

75. Asagoe K, Fujimoto W, Yoshino T, Mannami T, Liu Y, Kanzaki H, Arata J. Intravascular lymphomatosis of the skin as a manifestation of recurrent B-cell lymphoma. J Am Acad Dermatol 2003; 48:S1–S4.

76. Chui CT, Hoppe RT, Kohler S, Kim YH. Epidermotropic cutaneous B-cell lymphoma mimicking mycosis fungoides. J Am Acad Dermatol 1999; 41:271–274.

77. Cerroni L, El-Shabrawi-Caelen L, Fink-Puches R, LeBoit PE, Kerl H. Cutaneous spindle-cell B-cell lymphoma: a morphologic variant of cutaneous large B-cell lymphoma. Am J Dermatopathol 2000; 22:299–304.

78. Geerts ML, Burg G, Schmoeckel C, Braun-Falco O. Alkaline phosphatase activity in non-Hodgkin's lymphomas and pseudolymphomas of the skin. J Dermatol Surg Oncol 1984; 10:306–312.

79. Bertero M, Novelli M, Fierro MT, Bernengo MG. Mantle zone lymphoma: an immunohistologic study of skin lesions. J Am Acad Dermatol 1994; 30:23–30.

80. Geerts ML, Busschots AM. Mantle-cell lymphomas of the skin. Dermatol Clin 1994; 12:409–417.

81. Dommann S, Dommann-Scherer C, Müller B, Hassam S, Burg G. Cutaneous T-cell rich B-cell lymphoma. Verh Dtsch Ges Path 1994; 78:334.

82. Kamarashev J, Schaerer L, Burg G, Schmid MH, Müller B, Kempf W. Tumor-infiltrating T cells in primary cutaneous B-cell lympho-proliferative disorders. J Cutan Pathol 2001; 28:448–452.

83. Geelen FA, Vermeer MH, Meijer CJ, van der Putte SC, Kerkhof E, Kluin PM, Willemze R. Bcl-2 protein expression in primary cutaneous large B-cell lymphoma is site-related. J Clin Oncol 1998; 16:2080–2085.

84. Lawnicki LC, Weisenburger DD, Aoun P, Chan WC, Wickert RS, Greiner TC. The t[14;18] and bcl-2 expression are present in a subset of primary cutaneous follicular lymphoma: association with lower grade. Am J Clin Pathol 2002; 118:765–772.

85. Cerroni L, Arzberger E, Putz B, Hofler G, Metze D, Sander CA, Rose C, Wolf P, Rutten A, McNiff JM, Kerl H. Primary cutaneous follicle center cell lymphoma with follicular growth pattern. Blood 2000; 95:3922–3928.

86. Cerroni L, Kerl H. Primary cutaneous follicle center cell lymphoma. Leuk Lymphoma 2001; 42:891–900.

87. Goodlad JR, Krajewski AS, Batstone PJ, McKay P, White JM, Benton EC, Kavanagh GM, Lucraft HH. Primary cutaneous follicular lymphoma: a clinicopathologic and molecular study of 16 cases in support of a distinct entity. Am J Surg Pathol 2002; 26:733–741.

88. Marzano AV, Berti E, Alessi E. Primary cutaneous B-cell lymphoma with a dermatomal distribution. J Am Acad Dermatol 1999; 41:884–886.

89. Child FJ, Russell-Jones R, Woolford AJ, Calonje E, Photiou A, Orchard G, Whittaker SJ. Absence of the t[14;18] chromosomal translocation in primary cutaneous B-cell lymphoma. Br J Dermatol 2001; 144:735–744.

90. Mirza I, Macpherson N, Paproski S, Gascoyne RD, Yang B, Finn WG, Hsi ED. Primary cutaneous follicular lymphoma: an assessment of clinical, histopathologic, immunophenotypic, and molecular features. J Clin Oncol 2002; 20:647–655.

91. RC Beljaards. Van Beek P, Willemze R. Relation between expression of adhesion molecules and clinical behavior in cutaneous follicle center cell lymphomas. J Am Acad Dermatol 1997; 37:34–40.

48.2. Survival Rates in Cutaneous Lymphomas

Günter Burg and Werner Kempf

Department of Dermatology, University Hospital, Zürich, Switzerland

The type of therapy employed—early aggressive vs. nonaggressive treatment modalities—does not have significant impact on disease-free or overall survival (1). In 650 cases from nine population-based cancer registries in the United States, the median survival time was 7.8 yr (2).

In a study of the EORTC group, survival times were evaluated retrospectively in 772 patients with cutaneous lymphoma (582 CTCL, 190 CBCL). Actuarial survival was 0.63 for both B- and T-cell lymphomas after 7 yr and 0.52 for CTCL and 0.57 for CBCL after 10 yr (3).

Many differences in the survival rates of cutaneous lymphomas result from varying diagnostic concepts. In CTCL, the biggest variable is whether or not parapsoriasis, red man syndrome, or pre-Sézary-syndrome are included. In CBCL, the discrepancies concern the often difficult discrimination between pseudolymphoma (lymphoid hyperplasia) and malignant B-cell lymphoma, in particular of MALT type.

The following tables reflect some data from the literature (Table 1) and from the EORTC classification (Table 2), which is preferentially based on the material of the Dutch Lymphoma Group.

Table 3 gives some epidemiological data on cutaneous lymphoma, based on the EORTC-Registry 1982–1992 (12), classified according to the Kiel classification at that time (13).

These examples, even though informative, show the difficulties which result from frequent changes in classification concepts, especially if in addition different "organ-specific" classifications contribute to the Babylonian confusion.

Table 1 Survival Data of Cutaneous Lymphoma Patients

Cutaneous lymphoma	Study	Survival
Mycosis fungoides Sézary syndrome	Historical study of 144 cases by the NCI between 1954 and 1969 (5)	Observed SR at 5 yr: <30% Specific SR at 5 yr: 45% Median observed survival and relative SR: 3 and 4 yr, respectively
	Prospective study in the United States comparing two therapeutic methods (1)	Median observed survival: 7.8 yr
	US study of nine registries; approximately 10% of the US population (6)	Relative SR at 5 and 10 yr: 77% and 69%, respectively
	Dutch retrospective study of 309 MF cases (7)	Observed and specific SR at 5 yr: 80% and 89%, respectively Observed and specific SR at 10 yr: 57% and 75%, respectively
Lymphomatoid papulosis	Long term follow-up of 118 cases by the Dutch Cutaneous Lymphoma Group (8)	Observed and specific SR at 5 yr: 98% and 100%, respectively
Large cell CTCL, CD30+	Study of 30 cases from the Groupe Francaise d'Etudes des Lymphomes Cutanés (9)	Relative SR at 5 yr: 88%
	Long term follow-up of 79 cases by the Dutch Cutaneous Lymphoma Group (8)	Observed and specific SR at 5 yr: 83% and 96%, respectively
Large cell CTCL, CD30-	Study of 36 Dutch cases (10)	Specific SR at 5 yr: 15%
	Study of 16 cases from the Groupe Francaise d'Etudes des Lymphomes Cutanés (9)	Relative SR at 5 yr: 21%
Pleomorphic CTCL with small and medium cells	Study of 27 cases from the Groupe Francaise d'Etudes des Lymphomes Cutanés (9)	Relative SR at 5 yr: 82%
Immunocytomas and marginal-zone B-cell lymphoma	Study of 18 Dutch cases (10) Study of 12 Dutch cases (10)	Specific SR at 5 yr: 62% Specific SR at 5 yr: 100%
Primary cutaneous B cell lymphoma with follicle-center cells	Study of 84 Dutch cases (10)	Specific SR at 5 yr: 97%
Large-cell B lymphomas of the lower limbs	European multicenter study including 48 cases (11)	Specific and relative SR at 5 yr: 52% and 57%, respectively

Source: Adapted from Ref. 4.

Table 2 Relative Frequency and 5-Year Survival of the Main Entities of Primary Cutaneous Lymphoma According to the EORTC-Classification

Diagnosis	Number of patients	Frequency (%)	5-Yr survival (%)
Mycosis fungoides	278	44	87
Pagetoid reticulosis	5	<1	100
CTCL, large cell (CD 30+)	57	9	90
Lymphomatoid papulosis	70	11	100
CTCL, large cell (CD 30–)	36	5	15
Sézary syndrome	12	2	11
CRCL, pleomorphic small/medium	18	3	62
CBCL, follicle center cell	84	13	97
Immunocytoma/MALT-type CBCL	12	2	100
Large B-cell lymphoma (of the leg)	18	3	58
Intravascular BCL	4	<1	50

These data are based on more than 600 patients with a cutaneous malignant lymphoma, registered by the Dutch Cutaneous Lymphoma Working Group between 1986 and 1994 (10).
Source: From Ref. 10.

Table 3 Cutaneous Lymphoma: Epidemiological Data (Based on the EORTC-Registry 1982–1992)

	CTCL		CBCL	
	Mycosis fungoides and Sézary syndrome[a]	Large cell (CD30–)[b]	MALT-type and follicle center cell[a]	Large cell type[b]
Prediagnostic phase (yr)	5.5 ($n = 452$)	2.6 ($n = 20$)	2.4 ($n = 96$)	1.5 ($n = 28$)
Average age of onset (yr)	60 (Sézary: 68)	64	59	72
Survival time (yr)	4.0 ($n = 117$)	1.2 ($n = 6$)	2.3 ($n = 22$)	1.4 ($n = 9$)

Patients: $n = 827$ (male: 478; female: 349) from 27 clinics. Follow-up: 1–23 yr (1956–1992).
[a] Low grade malignancy according to the former Kiel-classification (13).
[b] High grade malignancy according to the former Kiel-classification (13).
Source: From Ref. 12.

REFERENCES

1. Kaye FJ, Bunn PJ, Steinberg SM, Stocker JL, Ihde DC, Fischmann AB, Glatstein EJ, Schechter GP, Phelps RM, Foss FM, Parlette H, Anderson M, Sausville E. A randomized trial comparing combination electron-beam radiation and chemotherapy with topical therapy in the initial treatment of mycosis fungoides. N Engl J Med 1989; 321:1784–1790.
2. Weinstock MA, Horm JW. Population-based estimate of survival and determinants of prognosis in patients with mycosis fungoides. Cancer 1988; 62:1658–1661.
3. Burg G, Schmid MH, Kung E, Dommann S, Dummer R. Semimalignant ("pseudolymphomatous") cutaneous B-cell lymphomas. Dermatol Clin 1994; 12:399–407.

4. Grange F, Bagot M. Prognosis of primary cutaneous lymphomas. Ann Dermatol Venereol 2002; 129:30–40.

5. Epstein EH Jr, Levin DL, Croft JD Jr, Lutzner MA. Mycosis fungoides. Survival, prognostic features, response to therapy, and autopsy findings. Medicine (Baltimore) 1972; 51:61–72.

6. Weinstock MA, Reynes JF. The changing survival of patients with mycosis fungoides: a population-based assessment of trends in the United States. Cancer 1999; 85:208–212.

7. van Doorn R, Van Haselen CW, van Voorst Vader PC, Geerts ML, Heule F, de Rie M, Steijlen PM, Dekker SK, van Vloten WA, Willemze R. Mycosis fungoides: disease evolution and prognosis of 309 Dutch patients. Arch Dermatol 2000; 136:504–510.

8. Bekkenk MW, Geelen FA, van Voorst Vader PC, Heule F, Geerts ML, van Vloten WA, Meijer CJ, Willemze R. Primary and secondary cutaneous CD30(+) lymphoproliferative disorders: a report from the Dutch Cutaneous Lymphoma Group on the long-term follow-up data of 219 patients and guidelines for diagnosis and treatment. Blood 2000; 95:3653–3661.

9. Grange F, Hedelin G, Joly P, Beylot-Barry M, D'Incan M, Delaunay M, Vaillant L, Avril MF, Bosq J, Wechsler J, Dalac S, Grosieux C, Franck N, Esteve E, Michel C, Bodemer C, Vergier B, Laroche L, Bagot M. Prognostic factors in primary cutaneous lymphomas other than mycosis fungoides and the Sézary syndrome. The French Study Group on Cutaneous Lymphomas. Blood 1999; 93:3637–3642.

10. Willemze R, Kerl H, Sterry W, Berti E, Cerroni L, Chimenti S, Diaz Perez JL, Geerts ML, Goos M, Knobler R, Ralfkiaer E, Santucci M, Smith N, Wechsler J, van Vloten WA, Meijer CJ. EORTC classification for primary cutaneous lymphomas: a proposal from the Cutaneous Lymphoma Study Group of the European Organization for Research and Treatment of Cancer. Blood 1997; 90:354–371.

11. Grange F, Bekkenk MW, Wechsler J, Meijer CJ, Cerroni L, Bernengo M, Bosq J, Hedelin G, Fink Puches R, van Vloten WA, Joly P, Bagot M, Willemze R. Prognostic factors in primary cutaneous large B-cell lymphomas: a European multicenter study. J Clin Oncol 2001; 19:3602–3610.

12. Burg G, Kempf W, Heaeffner AC, Nestle FO, Hess Schmid M, Doebbeling U, Mueller B, Dummer R. Cutaneous Lymphomas. Curr Probl Dermatol 1997; 9:137–204.

13. Gérard-Marchant R, Hamlin I, Lennert K, Rilke F, Stansfeld AG, van Unnick JAM. Classification of non-Hodgkin's lymphomas. Lancet 1974; 2:406–408.

49

Concepts, Misconceptions, and Controversies in Cutaneous Lymphomas

Günter Burg
Department of Dermatology, University Hospital, Zürich, Switzerland

Cutaneous lymphoma (CL) in most cases is in the end stage of a stepwise pathogenetic process that originates from a reactive inflammatory chronic stimulation of lymphocytes and dendritic cells. Through the accumulation of mutations in genes that regulate the cell cycle, in oncogenes and in suppressor genes, this inflammatory process transforms into malignant lymphoma.

Research on this complex and vexing disease process has, over the years, resulted in many concepts and misconceptions with regard to various issues: classification and prognostic grading, nomenclature and semantics, diagnostic procedures, pathogenesis and management. Some of these issues will be tackled here.

WHO WAS FIRST?: THERE WILL ALWAYS BE SOMEBODY "BEFORE"

It is a misbelief that Alibert was the first to describe mycosis fungoides (MF). Almost 200 years earlier, Bontius (1) Citing Pesino from Italy described a disease, which today we would classify as cutaneous T-cell lymphoma (CTCL). The erythrodermic and leukemic variant of MF was not described for the first time by Sézary and Bouvrain (2). Twenty years earlier, Leo von Zumbusch at the 9th reunion of the Munich Dermatological Society presented a 71-year-old male patient suffering for 5 months with erythroderma, leukocytosis (21,000/mL) and lymphocytosis (> 70%), with lymphoid skin infiltrates, hair loss, and hyperkeratosis (3). This probably is the first documented description of what we refer to today as Sézary syndrome.

THE INFINITE LOOP OF LYMPHOMA CLASSIFICATION

Classifications have a short half-life. Rappaport, Lukes and Collins, Kiel, REAL, WHO, and EORTC classifications and their updates are a few examples in the infinite loop of attempts to classify lymphoproliferative disorders. Even if there is no International Divine to Everyone Acceptable Lymphoma (IDEAL) classification for lymphomas that can cover the broad spectrum of nodal and extranodal lymphomas, including CL, it is best to adapt the classification of CL to the WHO classification scheme, rather than to create a skin-specific classification system that (almost) nobody understands.

The new WHO classification lists all major nosologic entities of nodal and extranodal lymphomas, so that there is no need for a super-specialized provincial organ-specific, i.e., skin-specific, classification. In order to take into account the requirements of the patient and the physician, categorization of peripheral cutaneous T- and B-cell lymphomas within the WHO classification into grades of different biological and prognostic behavior is recommended, as presented in Chapter 20.

USING THE SAME WORDS DOES NOT MEAN SPEAKING THE SAME LANGUAGE

The misinterpretation of the French word "plaques" is at the root of some conceptual disagreements. "Plaques," in the context of "parapsoriasis en plaques" as described in the French literature, are in fact patches. They are erythematous lesions that are not palpable but only visible. The term "parapsoriasis" is confusing and encompasses a number of different conditions.

Brocq (4) described three major subgroups, one of which is "parapsoriasis en plaques," formally referred to by Brocq as "erythrodermies pityriasiques en plaques disseminés." In the international literature, it has also been referred to as Brocq disease and has been synonymously labeled as digitate dermatosis, which should not be confused with parapsoriasis en gouttes (pityriasis lichenoides chronica of Jadassohn and Juliusberg) which is a completely different disease unrelated to malignant lymphoma. Besides the digitate variant, other forms with large patches ("plaques"), with or without poikiloderma, have been described.

There also is some confusion concerning the term mycosis fungoides (MF). In some countries, this term is used synonymously with cutaneous T-cell lymphoma. However, the term MF should only be used for a well-defined entity, clinically characterized by flat or elevated plaques and/or tumors. These were the types of lesions originally reported by Bontius (1), Alibert (5), Bazin (6), and others.

THE EMPEROR'S NEW CLOTHES: SEEING SOMETHING THAT IS NOT THERE

Early diagnosis is one of the greatest challenges in the management of malignant lymphomas. In skin lymphomas, the anatomical and topographical conditions for early diagnosis are optimal. Nevertheless, a distinct diagnosis must be based on reproducible criteria. Since the diagnosis "MF" can be based on clear-cut, reproducible clinical, histological, phenotypical, and genotypical criteria, those cases in which these criteria are not met should not be referred to as MF.

With respect to parapsoriasis and to early stage MF, i.e., initial nonpalpable macular lesions, one has to confess, that specific diagnostic criteria as found in plaque stage or tumor stage MF are not present. These conditions may be referred to as Brocq disease, parapsoriasis en plaques, prelymphoma or premycosis fungoides but certainly not mycosis fungoides, because this designates a malignant neoplastic disease.

PINK AND BLUE VS. RED AND BROWN

When confronted with lymphoproliferative skin infiltrates, some people tend to perform a plethora of special stains and additional laboratory tests. These techniques in most cases do nothing but create high costs and waste time. They are appropriate only in a minor proportion of cases. Histology is the gold standard for the diagnosis of lymphoproliferative skin infiltrates. However, the microscopic picture should not be over-emphasized and over-interpreted. In cases, in which clear-cut histological and cytological features for a malignant neoplastic process are completely lacking, additional extensive phenotyping and genotyping is also usually inconclusive.

WHAT MAKES THE LYMPHOCYTE ANGRY?

Reactive inflammatory or neoplastic from the very beginning: this is the open question on the pathogenesis of cutaneous lymphomas. Along with modern concepts on tumorigenesis, it is hypothesized that MF arises in a background of chronic inflammation or as a response to chronic stimulation due to various exogenous and/or endogenous pathogenetic factors. Subsequently, a series of mutations results in the stepwise progression from eczematous patches, to plaques, tumors, and eventual hematogeneous dissemination.

WHICH TARGET DO WE REALLY TREAT?

The question if early aggressive or nonaggressive treatment is more beneficial with respect to survival time in CTCL has been decided, favoring disease control by primary nonaggressive treatment modalities (7). Topical glucocorticoids, PUVA and HN2 are effective in clearing patches and thin plaques. The question is how these treatment modalities work. Steroids and UV in the doses applied on top of the epidermis are unable to kill lymphocytes in the dermis. It is much more plausible that through these "soft" approaches, the microenvironment (e.g., pattern of cytokines released by keratinocytes) is changed leading to temporary remission of skin infiltrates without affecting the responsible pathogenetic factors, which continue to attract lymphocytes into the dermis and epidermis.

REFERENCES

1. Bontius J. De medicina Indorum libri IV, Piso, 1642.
2. Sézary A, Bouvrain Y. Erythrodermie avec presence de cellules monstrueuses dans le derme et le sang circulant. Bull Soc Fr Dermatol Syphiligr 1938; 45:254–260.
3. Von Zumbusch H. Fallbericht. Archiv für Dermatologie und Syphilis 1915; 51:119.
4. Brocq L. Les parapsoriasis. Ann Dermatol Syphilol 1902; 3:433–468.
5. Alibert JLM. Tableau du pian fongoide. Description des maladies de la peau, observées à l'Hôpital Saint-Louis et exposition des meilleurs méthodes suivies pour leur traitement Barrois L'Ainé & Fils: Paris, 1806.
6. Bazin A. Leçons sur le traitement des maladies chroniques en général, affections de la peau en particulier, par l'emploi comparé des eaux minérales, de l'hydrothérapie et des moyens pharmaceutiques. Paris: Delahaye, 1806.
7. Kaye FJ, Bunn PAJ, Steinberg SM, Stocker JL, Ihde DC, Fischmann AB, Glatstein EJ, Schechter GP, Phelps RM, Foss FM, Parlette HL, Anderson MJ, Sausville EA. A randomized trial comparing combination electron-beam radiation and chemotherapy with topical therapy in the initial treatment of mycosis fungoides. N Engl J Med 1989; 321: 1784–1790.

Index

T - #1057 - 101024 - C589 - 254/178/27 [29] - CB - 9780824729974 - Gloss Lamination